Nutrition and Cancer

Nutrition and Cancer

Raymond J. Shamberger
The Cleveland Clinic Foundation
Cleveland, Ohio

Plenum Press • New York and London

Library of Congress Cataloging in Publication Data

Shamberger, Raymond J., 1934–
  Nutrition and cancer.

  Includes bibliographies and index.
  1. Cancer — Nutritional aspects. I. Title. [DNLM: 1. Diet — adverse effects.2. Neoplasms — diet therapy. 3. Neoplasms — etiology. QZ 202 S528n]
RC262.S45   1984   616.99′4   84-11774
ISBN 0-306-41553-4

Printed in the United States of America

Preface

The importance of environmental factors in the etiology of the major degenerative diseases, including cancers, is now generally accepted. Evidence obtained from studies with experimental animals and from human populations associates nutritional factors and dietary constituents with the causation of cancers at different sites in the body. Estimates by epidemiologists based on comparisons of various population groups have indicated that as much as 50% of the cancer mortality may be influenced by diet. An important indicator is found in migrants to the United States or to other countries who develop the spectrum of cancers typical for the United States (or other countries) but different from that reported for their native country.

About 20% of all deaths (450,000 per year) in the United States are caused by cancer. In addition, as the population grows the number of cancer cases steadily increases, but the age-adjusted total cancer incidence and mortality rates for sites other than the respiratory tract (cancers primarily attributable to cigarette smoking) have remained stable during the last 30 to 40 years. If one-half of these cancers are associated with dietary practices, an understanding of the process could save about 225,000 lives each year.

The causes of cancer have been an important area of cancer research for many years. Certainly if one understands how the diet or the environment affects cancer, great insights might be gained into the mechanisms of cancer as well.

The objective of this textbook is to summarize the major areas of nutrition and their relationship to cancer. Topics include macronutrients such as lipids, proteins, amino acids, carbohydrates, and fiber; micronutrients such as vitamins and minerals; mutagens and carcinogens in food; food additives and contaminants; unproved cancer diet claims; and cancer cachexia. Reference lists for each chapter were generally reduced to include the most recent sources.

I wish to thank Thelma Brittain, Phyllis Pittman, and Helen Brewster for their excellent typing, as well as my Department Head, Dr. Robert Galen, for his support.

34516

Contents

Nutrition
and Cancer

Scope of the Problem of Nutrition and Cancer

ENVIRONMENTAL CARCINOGENESIS

Diet and Lifestyle

About 70–90% of cancer is thought to be environmentally related, with about 40–60% attributed to lifestyle or dietary practices. About 10–30% is thought to be related to tobacco smoking. It is not possible to give a precise upper limit to the sum of attributable risks, which may be more than 100%, for the total cancer burden in a community. However, in many cases the degree to which a factor might contribute to the total cancer incidence can be estimated in the sense that if the factor is absent, the proportion of all related cancers would not occur. For example, tobacco smoking is responsible for about 85% of the lung cancer in most populations.

Two approaches have been postulated in establishing the proportion of cancers related to environmental factors.[1] One suggested method is to estimate the number of persons exposed in the entire population and then to calculate the number of resulting cancers expected. However, such calculations are not currently possible for any population. The second approach is to examine cancer risk site-by-site for a given population and to determine the proportion of cancers attributable to known or suspected predominant causes and those considered due to lifestyle.

This latter approach is exemplified by analysis that compares local populations. Table 1-1 shows a 10–1000-fold difference when the high-incidence areas are divided by the low-incidence areas. Estimations have been made of the proportion of cancers due to various causes for an English population, (Birmingham and West Midlands) (1968–1972), for an Indian Bombay population (1958–1972), and for a Black Bulawayo, South Africa population (1968–1972) for both males and females. These histograms are shown in Figures 1-1 to 1-3.

The English population resides in a long-established industrial community

1

Table 1-1. Variation in Cancer Incidence[a,b]

Range of rates (high divided by low)	Type of primary cancer	High-incidence areas	Low-incidence areas
1000	Liver (ages 15–44 years)	Lourenço Marques/ Maputo (Mozambique)	Alberta and Saskatchewan (Canada), Norway, Sweden, New York State, Birmingham (Alabama) region
200	Esophagus	Ghurjev district of Kazakhstan (U.S.S.R.)	Alberta and Manitoba (Canada), Netherlands, Ibadan (Nigeria)
100	Penis	Kingston (Jamaica), Uganda	Israel
100	Nasopharynx	Singapore (Chinese)	Uganda, Cali (Colombia), Chile, Finland
50	Lip	Saskatachewan, Alberta, New Brunswick (Canada)	Lourenço Marques/ Maputo, Uganda, Hawaii (Japanese, Hawaiians), Japan, Johannesburg (South Africa) (Africans)
40	Skin	New Brunswick, Saskatchewan, Alberta, Cali (Colombia)	Johannesburg (Africans), Ibadan
40	Bronchus	Liverpool, Birmingham	Uganda, Ibadan
30	Chorion-epithelioma (F) (ages 15–44 years)	Ibadan, Japan	Iceland, Hawaii, Alberta, Manitoba, Newfoundland, Connecticut, Birmingham region, Denmark
30	Pharynx	Puerto Rico	Ibadan, Johannesburg (Africans), Iceland, Japan
20	Mouth	Bombay	Uganda, Hawaii (Hawaiians), Iceland, Denmark, Chile

in which fewer than 2% are employed in agriculture and more than 60% are employed in industry. In the Bombay population more than 50% are industrial workers. Many of these workers are migrants from elsewhere in India. The Bulawayo population would be expected to be predominantly rural.

Mortality data from many sources were used in the preparation of these estimates; they included analytical and correlation studies, sex ratios, changes in population migration, and geographic risk differences.[1] For example, cancer

Table 1-1. (*Continued*)

Range of rates (high divided by low)	Type of primary cancer	High-incidence areas	Low-incidence areas
20	Corpus uteri (F)	Saskatchewan, Hawaii (Caucasians)	Ibadan, Johannesburg (Africans), Lourenço Marques/Maputo, Uganda
20	Cervix uteri (F)	New York (Puerto Ricans), Cali (Colombia), Johannesburg (Africans), Hawaii (Hawaiians)	New York (Jews), Israel, South Metropolitan region (England), Birmingham region
10–15	Rectum	Denmark, New Zealand	Lourenço Marques/Maputo, Johannesburg (Africans), Ibadan
10–15	Thyroid	Cali (Colombia), Hawaii (all groups combined)	Uganda, Johannesburg (Africans), Liverpool, Southwestern England
10	Tongue	Puerto Rico	Lourenço Marques/Maputo, Uganda, Alberta, Japan, Israel
10	Colon	Connecticut, New Zealand	Uganda, Ibadan, Johannesburg (Africans)
10	Testis	Denmark, New Zealand	Ibadan, Uganda, Johannesburg (Africans), Kingston (Jamaica), Japan
10	Kidney	Iceland, Sweden	Ibadan, Uganda, Japan
10	Melanoma	New Zealand, Connecticut, Norway	Hawaii (Japanese, Hawaiians), Japan, Iceland, Ibadan, Johannesburg (Africans)
6	Bladder	Connecticut	Japan

[a]Mean aged 35–64 years, unless specified otherwise.
[b]Schneiderman, M. A., 1978, Eighty percent of cancer is related to the environment. *Laryngoscope* 88:559–574.

incidence for each site in females provides a reference point for evaluation of the impact of these environmental exposures, which mainly affect males, e.g., heavy industry. However, the identical incidence of colon cancer in both sexes in Birmingham suggests common means of exposure. Geographic differences can be evaluated by a similar approach. If assignments were made to a given cause, this would not mean that other factors are not involved; the assignment only means that the factor listed is likely the major dominant cause.

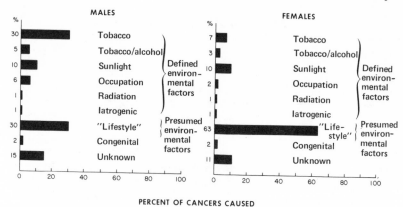

PERCENT OF CANCERS CAUSED

Figure 1-1. Deaths from presumed and defined environmental factors in Birmingham males and females. (By permission of J. Higginson 1980, *J. Prev. Med. 9*:180–188.)

The histograms are clearly approximations, and the proportions ascribed to different causes chosen may depend on the type of population studies; thus in some parts of Africa more than 40% of liver cancers may be attributed to mycotoxins. In these cases hepatitis virus is considered as a promoting, but not necessarily a predominant, factor.

In the three populations of Birmingham, Bombay, and Bulawayo, the lifestyle cancers, which included diet, affected females to a much greater extent than males. In contrast, tobacco or betel nut usage affected males to a much greater extent, who are heavier users of tobacco and betel nut. Higginson[2] has also

BOMBAY (1958-72)

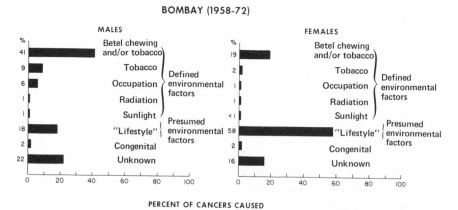

PERCENT OF CANCERS CAUSED

Figure 1-2. Deaths from presumed and defined environmental factors in Bombay males and females:1958–1972. (By permission of J. Higginson 1980, *J. Prev. Med. 9*:180–188.)

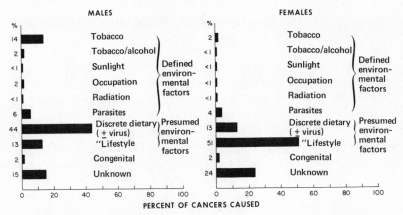

Figure 1-3. Deaths from presumed and defined environmental factors in male and female Black populations, Bulawayo, South Africa: 1968–1972. (By permission of J. Higginson 1980, *J. Prev. Med. 9:* 180–188.)

estimated an overall best estimate for the proportion of cancers attributable to various causes (Fig. 1-4). The relative importance of diet and behavioral or cultural patterns that make up the lifestyle pattern has also been estimated. These estimates, however, are likely only rough estimates.

Most tumors of the gastrointestinal tract and the endocrine-dependent organs have been attributed to lifestyle. Even though some carcinogenic risk factors have been identified, they are insufficient to explain the large geographic and temporal differences in the incidence of cancer between Birmingham and

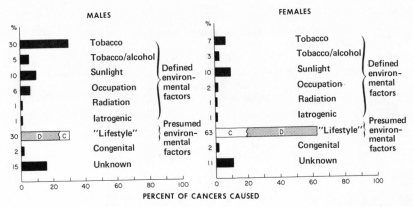

Figure 1-4. John Higginson's best estimates for the proportion of cancers attributable to various causes. The relative importance of diet (D) and behavioral culture pattern (C) in lifestyle are rough estimates. (By permission of J. Higginson 1979, *J. Science 205:*1363–1366. Copyright 1979, American Association for the Advancement of Science.)

Bombay as well as some other parts of the world, e.g., prostate cancer and breast cancer in Japan and stomach cancer in Iceland. However, studies of the Mormons and Seventh-Day Adventists, in whom lower rates are observed for cancers of the breast and gastrointestinal tract as well as for the tobacco- and alcohol-related cancers, suggest that these estimates are reasonable.

Other investigators have also summarized their best estimates of the predominant factors of cancer causation. The estimates of Doll and Peto,[3] Wynder and Gori,[4] and Weisburger et al.[5] are summarized in Table 1-2. Estimates of cancer related to diet ranged from 35 to 56%. The study of Doll and Peto suggests that infection may directly or indirectly cause 10% of cancer.[3] Another study suggests that the cause of 20% of cancer was unknown or congenital.[4] In contrast, one study indicates that some factors such as food additives actually prevent cancers in man and estimate that cancer is actually prevented on an average of 2% in males and females.[5]

Table 1-2. Estimated Causes of Human Cancer in Males and Females[a]

Type	Percentage of total[b]		
	1	2	3
Occupational cancers: various organs	1–5	4	2
Cryptogenic cancers: lymphomas, leukemias, sarcomas, cervix(?) (virus?)	10–15	—	—
Lifestyle-related cancers			
Tobacco-related: lung, pancreas, bladder, kidneys	23	30	18
Diet-related	—	35	48
Nitrate–nitrite, low vitamin C, mycotoxin: stomach, liver	5	—	—
High-fat, low-fiber, broiled, or fried foods: large bowel, pancreas, breast, prostate, ovary, endometrium	44	—	—
Multifactorial			
Tobacco and alcohol: oral cavity, esophagus	5	3	1
Tobacco and asbestos, tobacco mining, tobacco–uranium–radium: lung, respiratory tract	1–5	—	—
Iatrogenic–radiation, drug: various organs	1	1	1
Food additives	—	2	—
Reproductive and sexual behavior	—	7	—
Pollution	—	2	—
Industrial products	—	1	—
Geophysical factors	—	3	—
Infection	—	10?	—
Unknown–congenital	?	?	20
Exogenous hormones	—	—	2

[a]Source: Doll and Peto,[3] Wynder and Gori,[4] and Weisburger et al.[5]
[b]Estimates of (1) Weisburger et al.[5]; (2) Doll and Peto[3]; and (3) Wynder and Gori.[4]

Tobacco

About 10–30% of cancer mortality is thought to be due to smoking or betal nut usage. In most countries 80–85% of lung cancers are also thought to be caused by cigarette smoking. Smoking is also thought to be involved in cancer of the mouth, larynx, pharynx, esophagus, the cardiac end of the stomach, bladder, and possibly the pancreas. There is probably no single measure known that would have as great an impact on cancer mortality as a reduction in the use of tobacco or a change to a less dangerous tobacco substitute. The major impact would be on the incidence of lung cancer, which by late middle age is more than 10 times greater in regular cigarette smokers than in lifelong nonsmokers (see Table 1-3).[3] In addition, a material effect is seen in the incidence of cancers of the mouth, pharynx, larynx, esophagus, bladder, probably the pancreas, and possibly the kidney. The difference in incidence between smokers and nonsmokers is less marked for cancers of the bladder, pancreas, and kidney than for

Table 1-3. Comparison of Numbers of Deaths Observed among a Sample of Male U.S. Cigarette Smokers with the Numbers That Would Have Been Expected If Their Rate of Death Had Been the Same as That of Age-Matched Nonsmokers[a]

Certified cause of death	Deaths by mid-1970 of men who in the 1950s were smokers of cigarettes only			
	No. of deaths observed	No. expected from corresponding nonsmoker experience	Difference between observed and expected	Ratio of observed
Cancer				
Lung	2,609	231	2,378	11.3
Mouth, pharynx, larynx, or esophagus	452	65	387	7.0
Bladder	326	151	175	2.2
Pancreas	459	256	203	1.8
Kidney	175	124	51	1.4
All other cancers	3,660	2,796	864	1.3
Total, all cancers	7,681	3,623	4,058	2.1
Other causes				
Respiratory	2,107	488	1,619	4.3
Cardiovascular disease	21,413	13,572	7,841	1.6
Other certified causes	3,721	2,564	1,157	1.5
Cause not available	1,221	610	611	2.0
Total, all other causes	28,462	17,234	11,228	9.4
Total, all causes	36,143	20,857	15,286	1.7

[a]Source: Doll and Peto.[3]

cancers of the respiratory or upper digestive tracts. The evidence in Table 1-3 suggests that an average consumption of cigarettes about doubles the incidence of cancer of the bladder and probably also of the pancreas, with a more moderate increase in kidney cancer. Although one could predict a direct effect of carcinogens on the respiratory or gastrointestinal tract, the observation that smoking should affect bladder cancer and perhaps kidney cancer is more surprising. It is likely that the mutagens and other chemicals from tobacco smoke are absorbed from the lungs into the bloodstream and circulate through distant organs; they have also been observed in the urine of smokers.

When tobacco is smoked in the form of cigarettes, the ill effects are much greater than from pipes and cigars. It is not likely that the paper or the cigarette additives have any special effect, but the smoke from pipes and cigars is more alkaline than cigarette smoke. The alkaline smoke from pipes and cigars is more irritating than cigarette smoke and therefore is less likely to be taken into the lungs. This phenomenon should decrease the exposure of the lungs to the carcinogens in cigarette smoke. The differences between cigarettes and tobacco from pipes and cigars are greatest in regard to lung, bladder, and pancreatic cancers, but less marked in relationship to cancers of the mouth, pharynx, larynx, and esophagus.

It is possible that the effects of different types of cigarettes may likewise differ. It is likely that the low-tar cigarettes may prove less harmful than the cigarettes of a quarter-century ago. For lung cancer the risk reduction could be as much as 50% or better. These reductions are based on the rapid decreases in male lung cancer now observed in England. However, reliable data, especially on the effects of long-term usage of low-tar cigarettes, are still not available.

Doll and Peto also estimated the percentages of U.S. cancer deaths that might have been avoided if the individuals had not smoked (Table 1-4).[3] The study estimated separately the numbers of deaths in males and females from each type of cancer (e.g., lung, larynx, bladder) caused by smoking.

There were about 95,000 lung cancer deaths in the United States in 1978, of which 80,000–85,000 could be ascribed to tobacco smoking. These statistics were arrived at by comparing the rates for smokers with the rates for another population of nonsmokers. The same method was applied to respiratory, upper digestive, bladder, and pancreatic cancers. These results suggest that there would have been about 40,000 deaths from these four types of cancer in 1978 if Americans had not smoked, instead of the 155,000 actually observed. The difference—115,000—represents an estimate of the number of deaths in the United States from these four types of cancer. It is possible that by changing the basis of these estimates, a slightly different excess mortality might have been calculated.

There is no way to estimate from these statistics the extent to which "passive smoking, i.e., the inhalation of air polluted by other peoples' smoking,

Table 1-4. Cancer Deaths Caused by Tobacco: United States 1978[a]

Certified cause of death	No. of deaths		
	Observed	Estimated, had Americans not smoked	Approximate excess attributed to tobacco
Cancer, males			
Lung	71,006	6,439	64,567
Mouth, pharynx, larynx, or esophagus	14,282	1,792 × 2	10,698
Bladder	6,771	2,960	3,811
Pancreas	11,010	6,585	4,425
Other specified sites	100,799	?	5,000?
Unspecified sites	14,469	8,188	6,281
Total, males	218,337		94,782 (43%)
Cancer, females			
Lung	24,080	5,454	18,626
Mouth, pharynx, larynx, or esophagus	5,100	1,458 × 2	2,184
Bladder	3,078	2,170	908
Pancreas	9,767	7,291	2,476
Other specified sites	127,642	?	1,000?
Unspecified sites	13,951	11,879	2,072
Total, females	183,618		27,266 (15%)
Total, males and females	401,955	—	122,048 (30%)

[a]Source: Doll and Peto.[3]

might affect the incidence of cancer either among smokers or nonsmokers. However, whether or not there were appreciable passive effects on nonsmokers, the effect could become great as the carcinogenity of tobacco smoke depends strongly on the duration of exposure. There is a possibility that lifelong exposure (including childhood) may have as much as four times the effect of exposure limited to adult life. In support of this view, twofold excess risks have already reported among the nonsmoking wives of cigarette smokers.[6,7] The estimate by Doll and Peto[3] of 30% relates to the entire population of the United States and is somewhat higher than the estimate (22%) made by Hammond and Seidman,[8] but slightly lower than 38% estimated from the tables presented by Enstrom.[9]

Lung cancer rates in the United States have been rising. Estimates of the percentage of cancer deaths by smoking will likely increase; Doll and Peto believe they will probably reach a level of about 33% by 1985, assuming no large trends in net mortality from nonrespiratory cancer.[3] How great the increase, or possibly decrease, will depend largely on the effect from current decreases in sales-weighted tar yields and cigarette consumption. Although modest increases over the present 30% can be forecasted, long-term prediction is not possible.

The percentage of cancers due to smoking is somewhat lower in Bombay (Fig. 1-2), where betal quid seems also to have an impact on cancer of the oral cavity, pharynx, and upper esophagus. These cancers are the lowest percentages in the Black Bulawayo population (Fig. 1-3).

Tobacco–Alcohol

Alcohol is considered next, not because it is one of the more important causes of cancer, but because it interacts with smoking. Alcohol has been suspected for more than 60 years to be related to cancer, since it has been shown that cancers of the mouth, pharynx, larynx, and esophagus are more common in men who consume large amounts of alcohol. This initial observation has been confirmed subsequently in several studies of men and women affected by these diseases in Europe. Excessive alcohol consumption is thought to cause cirrhosis of the liver and to increase the incidence of liver cancer. Accurate estimations are difficult, because accurate statistics of alcohol consumption are difficult to obtain. Results are complicated, since total abstainers from alcohol often also avoid the use of tobacco, which may affect the occurrence of cancer associated with alcohol.

Considerable research has been directed at finding out whether the effect of alcohol is due to the alcohol itself or to other chemicals found in spirits, wines, and beers. The carcinogenicity of alcohol may be due to its concentration or to the presence of phenols and benzpyrene, which may be produced through distillation. Nitrosamines have also been found in beer. These carcinogens are also likely produced through heating during production. Some research suggests that the effect is greatest when alcohol is consumed in spirits and that apple-based drinks consumed in Northwest France are especially harmful. Certain areas of Iran have an especially high rate of esophageal cancer, which has also been associated with alcohol-based drinks. However, most evidence suggests that the principal effect is due to the alcohol itself and is unrelated to the form in which it is drunk. This is supported by the observation that the rate of oral cancer is higher among habitual users of strongly alcoholic mouthwashes. Pure alcohol has not been shown in itself to be carcinogenic in animal experiments. Alcohol may exert a carcinogenic effect in humans by facilitating contact between extrinsic carcinogenic chemicals and the contents of the stem cells, which affect the integrity of the lining of the upper digestive tract and larynx.

Nonsmokers who consume large amounts of alcohol have a two to three times increased incidence of cancers of the mouth and pharynx. However, smokers who consume the same amount of alcohol would have a much greater absolute effect (Fig. 1-5). Consumed alcohol seems to multiply the carcinogenic effect of tobacco smoke on the mouth, pharynx, larynx, and esophagus, but has no effect on the lung. It appears that cancers of these sites related to alcohol consumption account for about 7% of all cancer deaths in men and about 3% in women. Doll and Peto estimate that about one-half the cancer deaths now caused by alcohol could have been avoided by the avoidance of smoking, even if alcohol is consumed.[3] Cancer mortality in nonsmoking and nondrinking Mormons and Seventh-Day Adventists in the United States supports these estimates. Estimates of deaths due to alcohol consumption in Bombay (Fig. 1-3) are about 0% as alcohol consumption is relatively rare in that area.

Sunlight

Sunlight is regarded as the major cause of skin cancer. It is difficult, however, to separate exposure from occupational and recreational exposures. Ultraviolet (UV) sunlight is the principal cause of basal cell carcinoma of the face and neck of white-skinned people and also causes a high proportion of the squamous carcinomas. Ultraviolet sunlight also promotes cancer of the lip and melanoma of the skin. Lip cancer is uncommon and is also associated with pipe smoking, which has declined in popularity. If treatment is started soon after the lump appears, death seldom occurs. In contrast, the incidence of melanoma of the skin is increasing rapidly among white-skinned populations and, because it rapidly metastasizes, causes a substantial number of deaths. The incidence of melanoma in different parts of the world correlates fairly closely with the amount

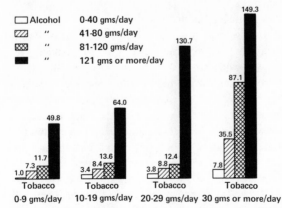

Figure 1-5. Relative risk of developing cancer of the esophagus in relationship to smoking and drinking habits. (By permission of Doll and Peto, 1981, *J. Nat. Cancer Inst. 66*:1192–1308.)

of exposure to UV light. Xeroderma pigmentosum patients who sustain damage from UV light to the DNA of their skin have a markedly elevated risk of melanoma. Because regular exposure to sunlight produces a protective suntan, the dose–response relationship is unusual. It is possible that some of the world-wide increase in melanoma among white-skinned people is due in part to changes in clothing styles and consequent greater exposure of the skin to sunlight than was customary 50 years ago. The relationship is not as clear for basal cell and squamous carcinoma because the distribution of cancer on the body surface does not correspond to this as neatly as melanoma does to the degree of exposure. The appearance of melanomas is not always limited to exposed areas, although it occurs in greater amounts on the exposed areas than elsewhere. Sunlight may affect the incidence of the disease at sites distant from the irradiated area through the hormonal stimulation of melanocytes.

Doll and Peto attribute 90% of lip cancers and 50% or more of melanomas as well as 80% of other skin cancers to UV light.[3] It is apparent, because of the relatively small number of cancers that occur from these causes, that strong sunlight on white skin might account for 1–2% of all cancer deaths. Skin cancer is rare in India and Africa due to darker protective skin pigment. Cancer levels in these countries and in North American Blacks could be used as a reference point in estimating the excess percentage of cancers attributable to sunlight and non-sunlight sources.

Ionizing Radiation

The possible relationship between cancer and ionizing radiation has been a source of much debate. It was previously assumed about 30 years ago that ionizing radiations (whether X-rays, γ-rays, or α- or β-particles) did not produce cancer unless they were intense enough to cause obvious damage to the irradiated tissue. However, it is now known that this is not true, and it is assumed that at low doses and low-dose rates the cancer effect is about proportional to the dose.

Ionizing radiations can also contribute to the production of occupational cancer, cancers due to radioactive pollutants, and those due to the use of ionizing radiation for medical purposes. Estimates have also been made of the effect of cosmic rays and the small amounts of radon and other radionuclides that occur in the air in all natural materials, which accumulate inside houses with restricted air exchange, as well as in the human body.[3] If each individual receives a whole-body dose of about 100 millirems (mrems), the total annual dose received by the total population of the United States would be about 22 million rems. This estimate compares closely with the 20 million rems/year estimated by the Interagency Task Force on the Health Effects of Ionizing Radiation. This exposure might cause about 5500 cancer deaths a year, or 1.4% of the total.

The total number caused by the geophysical factors of sunlight and ionizing radiation accounts for about 3% of all cancer deaths. However, almost none of the 1.4% attributable to background ionizing radiation is avoidable. The proportion of avoidable deaths depends on the way in which melanoma risk depends on the exact hazard from exposure to sunlight, but probably only amounts to about 1–2%.

Occupation

Calculation of the number of occupational cancers in a population is dependent on the measurement of the excess risk for a given site for exposed individuals. The lung and the bladder are the sites most often involved in occupational cancer. Precise determination is difficult, since it requires evaluation of on-the-job exposure, lifestyle factors, and alcohol and tobacco use.

It is important to establish an accurate background cancer measurement to estimate the amount of cancer caused by occupational factors. In the case of lung cancer, the low risk of lung cancer in nonsmoking women and physicians represents a background level that is unassociated with either smoking or occupation. After allowing for smoking and background, Higginson and Muir[1] have attributed the remainder (10%) of all lung cancers to occupation. In addition, all mesotheliomas (0.1% of all male cancers) in Birmingham, England were attributed to occupation, as was 30% of male bladder cancer, and if one can assume that the male–female difference is entirely due to occupation, 30% of leukemia might be attributed to this factor.[1] Because much of the industry in Bombay is artisanal, the proportion of occupational cancer is more difficult to estimate, but a 6% estimate is probably too high. Some employment-associated cancers are attributed to their suspected etiology; for example, esophageal cancer in bartenders may be assigned to alcohol consumption.

The most historic and classical observation of occupational cancer was that of Sir Perceival Pott in 1775, who observed that cancer of the scrotum occurred characteristically in chimney sweeps in whom "the disease . . . seems to derive from a lodgment of soot in the rugae [folds] of the scrotum." After Perceival Pott's initial observation, many other groups of industrial workers were also found to suffer from specific hazards of cancer. Investigations of these cancer hazards have led to the discovery of more substances known to cause cancer in humans than any other method used.

This is not surprising, in view of the widespread use of industrial chemicals. A few simple tests on animals showed them to be toxic, or a brief experience of their use showed them to be carcinogenic. Other chemicals shown to be carcinogenic through epidemiological studies similar to that of Pott are listed in Table 1-5. Several occupational carcinogens were first shown to be carcinogenic in laboratory animals. In addition, certain occupations show a statistical risk of cancer, although the specific substances responsible have not been identified. Usually the hazards that have been recognized markedly increase the relative risk of certain types of cancer. However, there could also be serious occupational hazards that have not been detected because the additional risk is comparatively small. In many cases cancer in humans seldom develops until one or more decades after the initial exposure to a carcinogen. In these cases it is difficult to identify the carcinogenic agent. Other complicating factors are the decrease or increase of certain industrial occupations and the discontinuation or introduction of chemicals, some used on a large scale. Increased plant automation may require less worker exposure during the later stages of manufacture. Exposure time during the primary stages of manufacture will probably not be affected.

Even though it is impossible to make accurate estimates of the proportion of the cancers of today that are attributable to work hazards, one can estimate mortality from cancers that affect organs that might be affected by occupational hazards. Doll and Peto[3] have estimated cancer mortality for these types of cancer on the basis of their interpretation of the literature and clinical impression. These estimates are summarized in Table 1-6. The proportion of cancer deaths from occupational causes was therefore about 17,000 out of 400,000, i.e., about 4% of all United States cancer deaths.

Iatrogenic Causes

Several treatment agents that have been shown to be carcinogenic have been used in the course of medical treatment. These include cyclophosphamide, melphalan, arsenic, busulfan, chlornaphazine, immunosuppressive drugs, ionizing radiation, estrogens, phenactin, polycyclic hydrocarbons, oxymetholone, steroid contraceptives, as well as UV light. It should not be surprising that so many carcinogenic agents have been prescribed medically, because often the treatment requires some modification of the metabolism of human cells. Sometimes these chemicals interfere with the DNA itself. Although there is some risk of death due to the possible development of iatrogenic cancer, this risk is substantially less than if the drug was not used, i.e., busulfan, immunosuppressive drugs, and radiotherapy. This has not always been the case. The medical use of both arsenic and chlornaphazine have been abandoned. In many cases risk versus benefit has yet to be fully assessed, and the agent is used under controlled conditions in the hope that the benefit will outweigh the risks. Agents used in treating other diseases are unlikely to cause more than a few hundred cancers throughout the United States each year.

Table 1-5. Established Occupational Causes of Cancer[a]

Agent	Site of cancer	Occupation
Aromatic amines (4-amino-diphenyl, benzidine, 2-naphthylamine)	Bladder	Dye manufacturers, rubber workers, coal gas manufacturers
Arsenic	Skin, lung	Copper and cobalt smelters, arsenical pesticide manufacturers, some gold miners
Asbestos	Lung, pleura, peritoneum (also probably stomach, large bowel, esophagus)	Asbestos miners, asbestos textile manufacturers, asbestos insulation workers, certain shipyard workers
Benzene	Marrow, especially erythroleukemia	Workers with glues and varnishes
Bischloromethyl ether	Lung	Makers of ion-exchange resins
Cadmium	Prostate	Cadmium workers
Chromium	Lung	Manufacturers of chromates from chrome ore, pigment manufacturers
Ionizing radiation	Lung	Miners of uranium and other ores
Ionizing radiation	Bone	Luminizers
Ionizing radiation	Marrow, all sites	Radiologists, radiographers
Isopropyl oil	Nasal sinuses	Isopropyl alcohol manufacturers
Mustard gas	Larynx, lung	Poison gas manufacturers
Nickel	Nasal sinuses, lung	Nickel refiners
Polycyclic hydrocarbons in soot, tar, oil	Skin, scrotum, lung	Coal gas manufacturers, roofers, asphalters, aluminum refiners; many groups selectively exposed to certan tars and oils
UV light	Skin	Farmers, seaman
Vinyl chloride	Liver (angiosarcoma)	Poly vinyl chloride manufacturers
—	Nasal sinuses	Hardwood furniture manufacturers
—	Nasal sinuses	Leather workers

[a]Source: Doll and Peto.[3]

Table 1-6. Cancers That Definitely Can Be Produced by Occupational Hazards[a]

| | No. of deaths recorded in 1978 | | Cancer deaths ascribed to occupational hazards in 1978 (United States) | | | |
| | | | Male | | Female | |
Type of cancer	Male	Female	N ascribed	% ascribed	N ascribed	% ascribed
Mesentery and peritoneum	652	697	98	15	35	5
Liver and intrahepatic bile ducts	1,812	984	72	4	10	1
Larynx	2,909	550	58	2	6	1
Lung	71,006	24,080	10,651	15	1,204	5
Pleura, nasal, sinuses, and remaining respiratory sites	857	496	214	25	25	5
Bone	997	740	40	4	7	1
Skin other than melanoma	1,061	753	106	10	15	2
Prostate	21,674	—	217	1	—	—
Bladder	6,771	3,078	677	10	154	5
Leukemia	8,683	6,708	868	10	335	5
Other and unspecified cancers	15,445	14,821	1,045	6.8	185	1.2
Subtotal, above sites	131,867	52,907	14,046	—	1,976	—

[a]Source: Doll and Peto.[3]

Ionizing Radiation

Ionizing radiation such as those produced through X-ray often are essential for diagnosis treatment. X-rays probably account for about 85% of the total dose given in the United States, which has been estimated at about 18 million rems/year. The continuation of these present exposure levels would lead to about 4500 fatal cancers per year. In many cases because of severity of illness or advanced age, irradiation is given to people with a life expectation too short for any significant chance of developing radiation-induced cancer. Currently X-ray is used primarily for diagnostic examinations and involve a lower dosage of irradiation than formerly. With the decreased dosage estimate of deaths might decrease to about 2000 per year.[3]

A small percentage (5% or less) of all childhood cancers maybe produced by exposure of the fetus due to radiological examination of the mother's abdomen during pregnancy. In some cases there may be liberal use of X-rays in certain intensive care units for premature babies. The total proportion of cancers due to the medical use of ionizing radiation is probably about 0.5%. It is likely that education in the frequency of use or the dosage of diagnostic irradiation, especially for fetuses (and perhaps children), could prevent several hundred cancer deaths per year.

Estrogens

Estrogens have been given extensively for the relief of postmenopausal symptoms and for the prevention of osteoporosis. There is some debate as to the extent to which their use causes cancer. However, there is a possibility that estrogens have been responsible for the recent increase in the incidence of endometrial cancer.[10] It is difficult to estimate how many cases they are continuing to produce throughout the United States.

Estrogens may have been responsible for one half the cases of endometrial cancer, which is responsible for about 1% of all cancer deaths. However, because endometrial cancer has a relatively good prognosis, and cases associated with the use of estrogen have an especially good prognosis, the percentage of deaths caused by use of the drug is probably only a small fraction of 1%. This conclusion is supported by the continuing steady decline in the rate of death certification attributing to endometrial cancer.

A major uncertainty concerns the role of estrogens in the production of cancer of the breast.[11] Estrogens are probably only responsible for a small proportion of breast cancer, but this disease is so common and has a relatively high fatality rate, with breast cancer accounting for a total of 9% of all cancer deaths, that the causation of even 5% of cases would be important.

Oral Contraceptives

Oral steroid contraceptives, known collectively as "the pill" are taken daily by millions of young women. However, since pregnancy at an early age reduces the risk of cancer of the breast in middle and old age, any effective form of contraception would increase these risks. Components of the pill given in much larger doses to laboratory animals have produced cancers of the breast and liver, and their carcinogenic potential has been well established. There is a possibility that at lower levels the ingredients of the pill might not cause cancer.

One type of pill that has been abandoned has probably caused cancer of the endometrium, but there is no evidence that this pill caused cancer of the breast or cervix uteri. Other types of pills that are still in use have been related to benign tumors of the liver. In some cases, these benign tumors, can cause fatal internal hemorrhage. There is some evidence that the use of the pill may reduce the risk of cancer of the ovary. This reduction may be related to the cyclic activity of the ovary, which the pill suppresses. It is likely that the total number of cancers arising each year from the use of the pill is too small to be accurately determined.

Even though the known iatrogenic hazards may not cause more than 1% of the cancer, this does not imply that there is no greater unknown hazard. Early data from the Boston Collaborative Drug Surveillance Program suggest that the percentage of current cancers caused by long-term drug use, excluding radiation, is at most about 2%, but as more data accumulate, this percentage is likely to decrease.[12]

Congenital, Hereditary, and Unknown Factors

The importance of individual general susceptibility to cancer should not be overlooked. However, no more than 2% of cancers can be related to hereditary or congenital causes alone. There may also be unknown cancers, for which we have no reasonable hypothesis as to etiology. These estimates are large population averages, and the pattern for small groups within these large populations may be quite different.

Infections

Infection has often been suspected of causing cancer, but the statistical evidence establishes beyond doubt that cancer is not, in general, an infectious disease in the sense that medical personnel and others who come in close contact with patients are not at increased risk of developing cancer. There have been reports of unusually large numbers of cases of some rare type of cancer in small communities within a short time at a particular time. However, such "clusters" should be expected to occur periodically by chance in a population as that of the United States. Some weak evidence has shown clustering of acute lymphocytic leukemia and Burkitt's lymphoma.[3]

Although viruses are capable of being transmitted from one person to another and are important in certain types of cancer, it is likely that there are a variety of other factors that determine whether exposure to the virus leads to the development of disease. If cancer is caused by viral infection, it is likely that it does so by becoming integrated with the genetic material of human cells through viral DNA and modifying to become a malignant group of cells.

One virus that seems able to do this is the Epstein-Barr virus, which occurs extensively and is known to cause glandular fever (infectious mononucleosis). Under certain circumstances in tropical Africa and South China the virus may insert itself into the DNA of a reticuloendothelial cell of an epithelial cell in the nasopharynx, resulting in Burkitt's lymphoma or nasopharyngeal carcinoma. These cancer cells are characterized by containing some of the viral DNA in combination with their own cellular DNA. The presence of the viral DNA in the genetic material of the cell has not been shown in any other human cancers, but this may be because the methods of detecting the presence of virus are not sufficiently sensitive. Viral infection may eventually be shown to be an essential factor in the production of various other types of cancer, i.e., cancer of the cervix uteri and of the penis. It has been shown that the wives of men who have cancer of the penis have an abnormally high risk of developing cancer of the cervix uteri, but not of any other type of cancer.[13] Acute lymphatic leukemia in childhood may be virally related because the disease may recur, affecting donated cells from a marrow transplant the patient has received from a healthy relative. Reticulosarcoma may also be affected by virus because it may appear on occasion after a patient has started to receive immunosuppressive drugs for the treatment of some other condition. Apparently the drugs are of sufficient dosage to diminish the body's resistance to viruses.

If all these cancers were depedent on viral infection, the percentage of cancer deaths from infections would have been estimated to be about 4%.[3] However, this percentage might be much greater, as infections, in the same way as diet, may contribute to the production of cancer in a variety of ways.

Bacterial or parasitic infection may contribute to the production of cancer as well. Intestinal bacteria are capable of producing or destroying carcinogenic metabolites in the large bowel. Salivary duct bacteria are capable of converting nitrates into nitrites and can therefore enhance the formation of N-nitroso compounds *in vivo;* bacteria could also contribute directly to the formation of N-nitroso compounds in the stomach and bladder.

Rimington[14] has associated bacterial infection and the subsequent development of chronic bronchitis with an increased risk of lung cancer. Bronchitis may impair the efficiency of the mechanisms for clearing the bronchi, permitting more prolonged contact between inspired carcinogens and the bronchial cells. Infection could also be important in the association between ulcerative colitis and colorectal cancer. Possibly bacteria-related associations exist between bladder cancer and schistosomiasis, a parasitic infection that commonly affects the bladder in parts of Africa, and between cholangiocarcinoma and clonorchiasis, a parasitic infection of the liver that is common in certain parts of China.

The examples cited are unlikely to be the only ways in which infection affects the risk of developing cancer. Doll and Peto[3] have suggested an approximate figure of 10% as an uncertain best estimate of cancer deaths related to infection. About 5% may be attributed to viruses and another 5% for other infectious agents. Infectious agents associated with cancer of the uterine cervix may likely provide a lower limit of at least 1%, but it is difficult to estimate an upper limit.

Reproductive and Sexual Behavior

The most obvious relationship is that between sexual intercourse and cancer of the cervix uteri, which occurs on occasion in virgins, but more commonly in women who have had children. Cervical cancer had been thought to be caused by the trauma of childbirth. Recent evidence indicates that the number of children is not directly related and that the risk is mainly related to the number of sexual partners. Current evidence strongly suggests that one of the primary causes of cervical cancer is an agent passed between partners during intercourse, quite possibly a virus.

Pregnancy and childbirth seem to play an important role in the prevention of cancers of the uterus, ovary, and breast. These are less common in women who have borne children than in women who have had no children. Breast cancer in parous women is less likely as the age of first pregnancy decreases. A pregnancy leading to abortion does not have the same protective value as one that goes to term. It seems that the effect is produced by the first stimulus to lactation, which somehow decreases the risk of development of a cancer. The length of lactation seems to have no material effect. In addition, the risk of cancer of the breast is lessened by a late onset of menstruation, made more likely by undernutrition, and by an early menopause.

Cervical cancer currently accounts for about 1.5% of all cancer deaths in the United States. This number is decreasing, however, because of the widespread use of cervical screening and because of the increasing number of women who have undergone hysterectomy previously and who therefore have no risk of uterine cancer. If one compares the small number of deaths from cancer of the uterine cervix in nuns with deaths in other women, it is apparent that the large majority of cases of cancer of the uterine cervix are due to the presumably infective processes or agents transmitted between sexual partners. Prevention or treatment might reduce total cancer mortality by 1%.[3]

Cancer of the breast, ovary, and endometrium accounts for almost 29% of all female cancer deaths in the United Staes and 13% of all cancer deaths in the United States. These deaths may be preventable when the mechanisms and reproductive factors that influence them are understood. Estimates of the percentage that might be related to the reproductive process range between 0 and 12%. Doll and Peto[3] have estimated the percentage that might be avoidable at about 6%. Adding this percentage to the 1% of deaths that would be avoidable by control of cervical cancer yields a total estimate of 7%.

WAYS IN WHICH DIET MIGHT AFFECT CANCER

There has been strong but indirect evidence that most common cancers could be reduced by changes in dietary practices. However, there is no precise, reliable evidence as to exactly what changes are necessary. The mechanisms whereby dietary factors influence cancer risks must be understood. Certainly the mechanisms by which dietary factors affect cancer are important, but identifica-

Table 1-7. Currently Promising Hypothetical or Actual Ways or Means Whereby Diet May Affect the Incidence of Cancer[a]

Possible ways or means	Example
Ingestion of powerful, direct-acting carcinogens or their precursors	Carcinogens in natural foodstuffs (plant products) Carcinogens produced in cooking Carcinogens produced in stored food by microorganisms (bacterial and fungal)
Affecting the formation of carcinogens in the body	Providing substrates for the formation of carcinogens in the body (e.g., nitrates, secondary amines) Altering intake or excretion of cholesterol and bile acids (hence the production of carcinogenic metabolites in the bowel) Altering the bacterial flora of the bowel (hence the capacity to form carcinogenic metabolites)
Affecting transport, activation, or deactivation of carcinogens	Altering concentration in, or duration of contact with, feces (fiber) Altering transport of carcinogens to stem cells (alcohol)? Induction or inhibition of enzymes (which effect carcinogen metabolism or catabolism) Deactivation, or prevention of formation, of short-lived intracellular species (e.g., by use of selenium, vitamin E, or otherwise trapping free radicals; by use of β-carotene or otherwise quenching singlet oxygen; by use of other antioxidants
Affecting "promotion" of cells (that are already initiated)	Vitamin A deficiency (clinical or subclinical) Retinal binding protein (hormonal and other factors determine blood RBP, although vitamin A intake may not affect it much Otherwise affecting stem cell differentiation (carotenoid? determinants of lipids "profile"?)
Overnutrition	Age at menarche Adipose tissue-derived estrogens Other effects

[a]Source: Doll and Peto.[3]

tion of the dietary factors is perhaps even more crucial. Some of the ways in which diet might act and are potentially significant in relationship to the development of cancer are listed in Table 1-7. As the science of nutrition and cancer progresses, the list of important protective factors and causes may replace the present list of possibly significant mechanisms (Table 1-7).

Ingestion of Powerful Direct-Acting Carcinogens

Carcinogens in Natural Foodstuffs

Perhaps the easiest and most obvious dietary mechanism of cancer is the direct ingestion of small amounts of substances identified in laboratory animals as powerful direct-acting carcinogens, and their conversion into carcinogens through metabolism by the body. These substances include cycasin in the cycad nut, pyrrolizidine alkaloids in *Senecio* and other plant genera, extracts of coltsfoot, safrole in sassafras, and bracken fern. Only bracken fern has been related to cancer in humans. Japanese who eat bracken fern have about three times the risk of Japanese who avoid it.[15] Bracken fern is commonly only consumed in Japan, and therefore the naturally occurring carcinogens known thus far cannot be regarded as a significant cause of cancer in the United States. A thorough search for foodstuffs containing naturally occurring carcinogens is not complete, while the search for cocarcinogens and promoters is even less complete.

Many natural foodstuffs can be tested for their influence on cancer rates in animals; for example, uncooked soya flour predisposes rats to pancreatic cancer.[16] Any observed effects may be due to the gross disturbances of the diet rather than to carcinogens in minute amounts. Short-term tests may help draw attention to possible carcinogens, such as quercetin, a mutagenic[17] natural substance that may cause cancer in animals.[18] The precursors of quercetin have been found in tea, red wine, bracken fern, and particularly onions.[19] Even though short-term tests may overlook some carcinogens, especially those that do not bind directly to the genetic material of the cells, laboratory discoveries of active agents may give clues for a useful epidemiological study. In any case, it is not clear whether any powerfully active substances are present in sufficient amounts in the natural components of the American diet.

Carcinogens Produced During Cooking

Cooking may be another possible source of carcinogens. It has been known for some time that benzpyrene other polycyclic hydrocarbons can be formed by pyrolysis when meat or fish is broiled or smoked or when any food is fried repeatedly in the same fat.

Sugimura *et al.* demonstrated that pyrolysis of food such as that of charcoal-broiled steaks also produces powerful mutagens that cannot be accounted for by the production of benzpyrene alone.[20] During the cooking process, food is not usually pyrolyzed, but in some cases may be caramelized. The chemical changes occurring during this more normal cooking procedure involve temperatures of only 100°–200°C. There is evidence that several different chemicals are produced that can damage or fragment cellular genetic material in cultured cells and in the mouse intestinal tract.[21]

Many investigators have sought to relate the consumption of various cooked foods to the development of gastric cancer, but none have succeeded. Dungal and Sigurjonsson found evidence that suggests that smoked foods are related to gastrointestinal cancer, however, it is not conclusive.[22] Americans eat more broiled food than others, but gastric cancer is rapidly decreasing in incidence in the United States. Broiling may be associated with some types of cancer other than gastric cancer, but this has not been proved.

Carcinogens Produced in Stored Foods by Microorganisms

Food storage is a less obvious source of carcinogens by the action of microorganism and was entirely overlooked until the 1960s. It is likely that aflatoxin, a product of the fungus *Aspergillus flavus,* which frequently contaminates peanuts and other staple carbohydrate foods stored in hot and humid climates, is an important factor in the production of liver cancer in certain tropical countries. In several animal species, it is among the most powerful liver carcinogens known. Because the enzymes needed to produce the particular metabolic products that appear to be responsible for its carcinogenic activity, aflatoxin is also likely to be carcinogenic in humans. It is apparent that the incidence of primary liver cancer, which is the most common type of cancer in inhabitants of large areas of Africa, including Mozambique, Swaziland, and Kenya, as well as Thailand and China is approximately proportional to the amount of dietary aflatoxin.[23] In addition, liver cancer occurs more commonly in people whose livers are chronically infected with hepatitis B virus. Possibly where aflatoxin is present in large quantities in the diet, both aflatoxin and hepatitis B virus contribute to the liver cancer and each may have a synergistic effect on the other. The differences of individual diets and the short half-life of aflatoxin within the human body make it unlikely that a direct relationship will be established between aflatoxin and liver cancer. However, if the aflatoxin concentration of various foods were reduced in tropical areas, the disease would likely begin to disappear within 10–20 years.

Primary cancer of the liver is rare in the United States (less than 1% of cancer deaths in people under 65 years of age). At older ages, the diagnosis is often inaccurate because cancers that have metastasized to the liver may have beem miscertified as primary liver cancers. It may therefore be questionable to use rigorous methods to eliminate all aflatoxin from the diet, because the return may not justify the effort. Certainly, it would seem prudent to make reductions in aflatoxin especially in retail nuts and nut products as well as dairy products that might be affected via contaminated cattle feed if these levels could be achieved without disproportionate expense.

Although aflatoxin may not be an important danger to Americans, the discovery of aflatoxin may indicate that other mycotoxins exist in food and be carcinogenic. No other agents have been clearly demonstrated to be carcinogenic in any country, but fusarial infection of stored food may contribute to the high incidence of esophageal cancer in parts of China. This, of course, could mean a similar agent could exist in the United States or other countries. There could be dangers of fungal contamination by Aspergillus, Penicillium, or Fusarium.

Substances Affecting the Formation of Carcinogens in the Body

Providing Substrates for the Formation of Carcinogens in the Body

One possible mechanism that has aroused considerable interest is the formation of N-nitroso compounds in the body. N-nitroso compounds are among the most powerful chemical carcinogens in laboratory animals, and the production of even small amounts in the human body could be important. N-nitroso compounds are present in small amounts in the resting gastric juice and may also be formed in the digestive tract or possibly in the infected bladder by a reaction between nitrites and certain nitrosable compounds such as secondary amines or N-substituted amides. This nitrosation is enhanced by formaldehyde or by thiocyanate ions. The nitrosation requires either a mildly acid medium or bacterial assistance, but is inhibited by the presence of antioxidants (e.g., vitamin C) in the stomach.

This pathway of synthesizing carcinogens *in vivo* is of particular interest because neither nitrites nor nitrosable compounds can easily be avoided in the diet. Compounds are found especially in fish and meat, they may be ingested as pesticide residues or drugs, and nitrosable compounds may be formed in the colon from amino acids. Nitrite found in food may be derived from preservative color or a color and flavor enhancer; nitrate may be formed in the body by its bacterial action on nitrates in the salivary ducts, the hypoacid stomach, the infected bladder, and possibly on nitrates or nitrogen in the gut. Apparently the most important source of nitrite is from the *in vivo* production from nitrate, which is ingested in vegetables and to a smaller extent in drinking water or in foods to which nitrate has been added as a preservative. The formation of N-nitroso compounds might be altered in many ways. It is not known, however, whether or not the amounts produced correlate with the incidence of cancer or if within populations they correlate with the risk to the individual.

It is possible that cancer of the esophagus and stomach may be related to nitrosamine formation, but in neither have positive findings emerged.[24] No clear positive associations were found when drinks and foodstuffs associated with cancer of the esophagus were examined for nitrosamine content. Some relationships have been suggested between gastric cancer and nitrate content of the diet, especially in Latin American, but have not been consistent. There is a well-known example of high gastric cancer in an English town in which the supply had an unusually high concentration of nitrate.[25] However, a high percentage of the resident population were employed as coal miners whose gastric cancer rates are likely to be high.[26] Therefore, it cannot be definitely determined whether or not high nitrates in the water supply or occupational or other factors are responsible for the high gastric cancer death rate.

Vegetables are usually the main source of dietary nitrates. Instead of causing gastric cancer, vegetable nitrates may actually protect against the development of gastric and other types of cancer (see MacLennan et al.[27] and many other studies). There is apparently little evidence that dietary nitrates, nitrites, or nitrosable compounds contribute to gastric or other types of cancer. Perhaps this is because gastric cancer is decreasing rapidly in most countries and other factors may be involved, which are masking the effect of nitrates. Perhaps the failure to relate nitrates to gastric cancer may be that there is inadequate evidence of carcinogenicity of nitrosamines in humans.

Altering Intake or Excretion of Cholesterol and Bile Acids

Certain fats might contribute to the production of carcinogens in the body by increasing the amounts of bile acids and cholesterol metabolites that come into contact with the gastrointestinal tract. Reddy et al. reviewed the substantial amount of evidence that supports this suggestion. Larger amounts of these substances, especially deoxycholic and lithocholic acids, are found in the feces of populations on a Western-type diet in whom colorectal cancer is more common than in populations on characteristic Asian or African diets in whom colorectal cancer is rare.[28] Larger amounts of deoxycholic and lithocholic acids are also found in the stools of patients with adenomatous polyps in the colon than in those of patients with other diseases or of healthy controls. The amounts of deoxycholic and lithocholic acids can be increased experimentally in humans by high-fat, high-meat diets. In laboratory animals high-fat diets (with a variety of different fats) increase the fecal excretion of the same group of bile acids and increase the incidence of colon cancer induced by a variety of colon carcinogens, including methylnitrosourea and 1,2-dimethylhydrazine. Cholestyramine, a nonabsorbable resin that increases the excretion of bile also has the same effects on cancer incidence. Cruse *et al.*[29] found that bile acids fed or administered intrarectally for a long period to animals have a synergistic effect with small doses of carcinogens on the incidence of large intestine tumors.

In spite of these observations and experiments, it is not known what relevance fecal cholesterol has to human cancer. Levels of any form of cholesterol in the blood cannot be correlated with the risk of contracting cancer. Studies indicate that people with low cholesterol levels have a greater mortality from a variety of cancers. It is not known whether the association is an artifact due to the effect of an undiagnosed cancer on the body's metabolism or whether it is real. If the association is real, it may be coincidental, not causal. A coincidental association between the blood levels of cholesterol and vitamin A could exist because both substances are synthesized through acetate and the mevalonic acid pathway. Vitamin A seems to have marked cancer-protecting effects in animals and humans. These effects are outlined in Chapter 4. An association could be made, since biologically active fat-soluble substances share with cholesterol, a common vehicle of transport in the blood and of uptake by many types of tissue cells. The transport system consists of fatty low-density lipoprotein particles that contain cholesterol, vitamin E, β-carotene, and other types of provitamin A.

Altering the Bacterial Flora of the Bowel

It is likely that cholesterol and bile acids are relevant to colon cancer and that they are acted on by the bacteria in the colon to produce carcinogens that either act locally or elsewhere in the body. A large number of chemical reactions can be affected by these bacteria. Alterations of these chemical reactions may affect a variety of disease processes that can be altered by any factor that ascertains which bacteria fluorish in the large intestine and in what relative proportions. The metabolism and interactions of a large number of intestinal bacteria may be quite complex and therefore the dietary components that affect the intestinal flora are poorly understood.

Substances Affecting Transport, Activation, or Deactivation of Carcinogens

Altering Concentration in/or during Contact with Feces

Dietary fiber may affect the bacterial flora. Diseases of the intestine that are common in developed countries are rare in rural Africa and India where unprocessed food is consumed and the stools tend to be soft, bulky, and frequent.[30] Many early epidemiological studies refer to crude fiber, and considerable work has been done recently to characterize the various components of dietary fiber.

Trowell defined dietary fiber as the remnants of the cell wall that are not hydro-lyzed by human alimentary enzymes.[31] In this sense Trowell's fiber is about five times as abundant as crude fiber. For example, whole wheat contains lignins that pass through the bowel unchanged, cellulose which is about 50% degraded by bacteria in the large bowel and those which are largely degraded (85%) including hexose, pentose, and uronic acid polymers.

The latter fiber appears to have different effects. The production of soft, bulky stools is thought to be mainly due to the pentose polymers which increase the population of certain intestinal bacteria. At first, it was thought that pentose polymers act through their capacity to bind water, but by increasing the popula-tion of certain intestinal bacteria much bulk was added, as a large part of the bulk of a typical stool consists of intestinal bacteria.

The various components of fiber in certain foods are listed in food tables. Bingham *et al.* used these tables to correlate the mortality from colonic and rectal cancer in different areas of Great Britain with each fiber component. A close inverse correlation was observed between the pentose-fiber content of the diet and colon cancer mortality, but not of the rectum. However, there was no correlation with any of the other types of fiber once the pentose fiber content was considered.[32] No good correlation was observed with dietary fiber as a whole, nor with vitamin C, fat, or beef. It will be difficult to interpret these findings until the contributions from each component of dietary fiber has been assessed in case-control or other studies on individuals rather than on whole populations.

Unrefined cereal fiber has an abundant amount of pentose polymers, and they are present to a lesser extent in various vegetables (but not in potatoes). Several case-control studies have suggested that patients with large bowel cancer tend to have a below-average consumption of certain such vegetables. The pen-tose polymer content of cereals could account for the correlation observed in Scandinavia between bulky stools and low colorectal cancer incidence. Similarly in rural Finland, where large amounts of unrefined rye bread are eaten, the stools are bulky and the incidence of colorectal cancer is low. The opposite is true in Copenhagen, where the chief difference from the Finnish diet seems to be a much smaller consumption of unrefined cereals.

If some component of dietary fiber reduces the incidence of colorectal cancer, it might be acting by decreasing the length of time stools remain in the bowel thereby decreasing the time of contact between the carcinogen and the bowel. Dietary fiber may also decrease concentrations of carcinogen in the stools through an increase in bulk, or perhaps dietary fiber alters the total numbers or proportions of different bacterial species in the bowel, part of which may pro-duce or destroy carcinogenic metabolites.

Altering Transport of Carcinogens to Target Cells

Certain factors including alcohol have been suspected of affecting the trans-port of carcinogens.

Induction or Inhibition of Enzymes

In experimental laboratory animals carcinogens can be activated or deactivated by certain enzymes. In some cases the activation or deactivation can be affected by seemingly innocuous agents that may induce or inhibit certain enzymes in the target tissue. Wattenberg and Loub have suggested this role for indoles in *Brassica* and other vegetables.[33] Although theoretically important mechanisms may be important for humans, none has been demonstrated. This effect might be found in populations where there is a single chemical carcinogen. In some African countries, aflatoxin dominates the list of preventable causes of cancer, so that in this case only a relatively small number of enzymes are of great importance.

Deactivation or Prevention of Formation of Short-Lived Intracellular Active Species

Many carcinogens must be oxidized before they can damage the cells of the body, yielding "metabolically activated intermediates." In some cases oxidative enzymes carry out the oxidative process. In other cases "simple" addition of ordinary oxygen results in *in vivo* oxidation and peroxidation, which generates short-lived intermediates such as (1) oxidative free radicals, or (2) excited molecular oxygen. Therefore, the dangers from certain carcinogens might be reduced if increased levels of antioxidants, free radical traps, or quenchers of molecular excitation were available to tissues.

One of the main intracellular systems, but not necessarily the most important, is that which traps free radicals and peroxides. This involves collaboration between vitamin E and a selenium-containing enzyme, glutathione peroxidase, which accounts for most of the selenium in humans. Glutathione *S*-transferase is also probably important in reducing organic peroxides. Both selenium and vitamin E are known to protect laboratory animals against carcinogens under suitable experimental circumstances. Selenium levels are also known to be decreased in cancer patients; however, there is a possibility that the tumors disturbed their appetite or general metabolism. Even though geographic correlations are not strong evidence for a true protective effect, selenium intakes vary widely from place to place within the United States and Canada and inverse correlations with cancer risk have been reported. At high levels selenium is toxic and should be used with caution.

Clinical deficiency of vitamin E is so rare that epidemiological study is difficult. Those who habitually self-medicate with vitamin E absorb more than ten times as much vitamin E as people who do not self-medicate. Large prospective studies of cancer onset in relation to vitamin E are under way.

β-Carotene and other carotenoids under certain circumstances can become excited molecules and are among the most efficient molecules discovered for quenching the energy of "single-excited oxygen." β-Carotene is found in high concentration in carrots and in many dark green leafy vegetables. β-Carotene and many other carotenoids are found in many other plant products in the American diet. There is considerable interest in β-carotene because it is the precursor in poor countries of much of the vitamin A in the normal human diet. One molecule of β-carotene can be converted in the intestine into two molecules of vitamin A. Much of the β-carotene in the diet is absorbed directly from the gut and circulates unchanged throughout the body. Because of this provitamin A activity, there have been several epidemiologic studies of the β-carotene levels in the blood or diet of cancer patients as well as healthy people who subsequently develop cancer. Numerous studies have indicated a trend toward a protective effect.

For public health purposes it may be more important to identify causes rather than mechanisms. Certainly it would be more important to prove that β-carotene is able to reduce cancer risks among apparently healthy people. The mechanism of action of β-carotene is more complex and could be due to several factors: quenching of single oxygen, acting as precursor of vitamin A, acting through a direct hormone-like mechanism by affecting immune functions, or by trapping free radicals.

Affecting "Promotion" of Cancer Cells

Vitamin A Deficiency

Vitamin A (retinol) and its esters and analogues (retinoids) can reduce the probability that partially altered cells will become fully transformed and will successfully change into a pathological tumor in cell cultures and in experimental animals. Two small human blood studies have shown that there is a significant inverse correlation between blood vitamin A and the risk of subsequent cancer. Little is known about how the body controls the blood levels of vitamin A. Otherwise the amount of vitamin A in the blood could be controlled by dietary means. In vitamin A deficiency, which is rare in developed countries, the simple solution of adding vitamin A would have little effect on the level of vitamin A in the blood. Therefore, vitamin A supplementation probably would not substantially affect cancer risks in developed countries such as the United States.[34] However, it suggests that in underdeveloped countries the consequence of chronic vitamin A deficiency may be an increased cancer risk. In underdeveloped countries the normal source of vitamin A is the intestinal oxidation of β-carotene, which is a molecule that may alternately reduce cancer risks in other ways. Because both vitamin A and β-carotene are present in the blood, it is also difficult to determine which of the two factors had the anticancer effect.

Retinol-Binding Protein

Retinol-binding protein functions mainly in of transporting vitamin A (retinol) in the bloodstream and seems to be the major control factor of blood vitamin A level. Factors that affect the rate of synthesis or degradation might affect blood vitamin A levels and therefore the risk of cancer. Estrogens are known to affect blood vitamin A levels substantially in animals that have been nourished adequately. Women who use oral contraceptives have elevated blood vitamin A levels. However, there is not much evidence for cancer avoidance (except possibly the ovary) resulting from oral contraceptives. Both postmenopausal and diet-derived estrogens may well increase the risk of endometrial cancer.

Affecting Cellular Differentiation

Vitamin A and its derivatives are of interest both because of their anticarcinogenic properties and because cell differentiation can be modified and reversed. Three promising dietary factors that have an effect on cell differentiation: protease inhibitors (which if eaten, may diffuse throughout the body); hormonal factors (e.g., retinol); and their endocrine determinants. Almost all hormonal factors could be affected by diet and could affect the risk of cancer.

The phospholipids also may affect cell differentiation. Phospholipids comprise the outer walls of cells and their "profile" in degree of saturation and exact chemical structure depends on the nature of the components of dietary fat and could have a marked effect on the various prostaglandins of which they are precursors. The prostaglandins may in turn substantially affect cellular behavior.

Overnutrition

The variation of the macrocomponents of the diet of laboratory animals may have profound effects on the risks of spontaneous or induced tumors. The role of overnutrition may be important although the mechanisms are unclear. Tannenbaum's experiments on mice first showed the importance of restricting the intake of macronutrients.[35] Restricting the intake of food without modifying the proportion of the individual constituents could halve the occurrence of breast and lung spontaneous tumors as well as a variety of cancers produced experimentally by known carcinogens. The underfed mice only grew to half the size of those fully fed. In spite of their size the smaller mice were active and sleek, appeared to be healthier, and generally lived longer than the larger mice. These experiments have been repeated several times with the same or even more striking results. Roe and Tucker (1974) reported a high spontaneous incidence of nonfatal mammary tumors (64%) in a group of mice who were continuously ad libitum.[36] The diet-restricted group was fed only 6 gm/day in frequent small amounts, and with intermittent feeding. Only 8% of those intermittently fed mice developed spontaneous mammary tumors.

Overweight has been associated with cancer risk. Lew and Garfinkel studied 750,000 American men and women for 13 years and calculated mortality ratios from various types of cancer by weight index[37] (Table 1-8). In view of the striking effects the nutritional factors have on overall animal cancer rates, the association of obesity with cancer is not particularly impressive. Among women there is a consistent trend toward increasing total risk with increasing body weight. The trend among men is more irregular. There is a contrasting trend with

Table 1-8. Mortality Ratios from Various Types of Cancer, by Weight Index[a]

Site of cancer	Patients' sex	Mortality ratio for weight index (ranges)[b]						
		<0.80 (Thin)	0.80– 0.89	0.90– 1.09	1.10– 1.19	1.20– 1.29	1.30– 1.39	≥1.40 (Large)
Endometrium	F	0.89	1.04	1.00	1.36	1.85	2.30	5.42
Gallbladder, plus biliary passages	F	0.68	0.74	1.00	1.59	1.74	1.80	3.58
Cervix	F	0.76	0.77	1.00	1.24	1.51	1.42	2.39
Kidney	F	1.12	0.70	1.00	1.09	1.30	1.85	2.03
Stomach	M	1.34	0.61	1.00	1.22	0.97	0.73	1.88
	F	0.74	0.95	1.00	1.07	1.28	1.26	1.03
Colon, rectum	M	0.90	0.86	1.00	1.26	1.23	1.53	1.73
	F	0.93	0.84	1.00	0.96	1.10	1.30	1.22
Lymphoma	F	0.83	1.14	1.00	1.06	1.00	0.92	1.13
Brain	F	0.86	0.89	1.00	0.95	1.52	0.69	1.01
Leukemia	F	0.73	1.00	1.00	1.01	0.88	0.85	1.24
Breast	F	0.82	0.86	1.00	1.19	1.16	1.22	1.53
Prostate	M	1.02	0.92	1.00	0.90	1.37	1.33	1.29
Lung	M	1.78	1.38	1.00	0.85	1.04	1.00	1.27
	F	1.49	1.20	1.00	1.10	1.06	1.06	1.22
Ovary	F	0.86	0.98	1.00	1.15	0.99	0.88	1.63
Pancreas	M	1.20	0.82	1.00	0.91	0.88	0.76	1.62
	F	1.17	1.06	1.00	1.36	1.43	1.18	0.61
All cancers	F	0.96	0.92	1.00	1.10	1.19	1.23	1.55
	M	1.33	1.13	1.00	1.02	1.09	1.14	1.33

[a]Source: Doll and Peto.[3]
[b]Actual weight divided by the average weight of people of similar height and sex. Values in the range 0.90–1.09 are close to average weight.

respect to lung cancer with thin men and women having the greatest lung cancer risks. There was a marked increase in women in the mortality ratio from endometrial, gallbladder, cervical, and kidney cancer among the heaviest group of women.

Armstrong believes that overnutrition would be a major factor in the development of cancer of the endometrium, because the disease can be produced by excessive exposure to estrogen.[38] The only natural estrogens to which women are exposed after the menopause are made from adrenal hormones in adipose tissue. If estrogens are not prescribed medically after the menopause, the level of estrogens in the blood is directly proportional to the degree of adiposity.

Except for cancer of the endometrium, no other type of cancer has been definitely related to overnutrition. However, a high standard of nutrition in childhood also advances the age of menarche which, because of the association that exists between early menarche and breast cancer risk, should also increase the subsequent risk of breast cancer.

There are several findings that encourage the belief that many common types of cancer are determined by individual dietary components or their general balance. Colorectal and breast cancer are generally associated with a high standard of living, which probably includes a high proportion of fat or meat. The national consumption of fat and meat per head of population correlates highly with breast and colorectal cancer. However, these cancers are uncommon in vegetarians, Seventh-Day Adventists, and Mormons, who consume low-fat diets or diets containing little or no meat.

Diet and Future Cancer Trends

Future controlled laboratory research as well as the epidemiologic trends of cancer risks should show that a high proportion of cancers of the stomach and large bowel, uterus (endometrium), gallbladder, and the liver in tropical countries is linked to dietary practices. Diet may prove to also have an effect on the incidence of cancers of the breast and pancreas, and the anticarcinogenic effects of various micronutrients may be shown to have an effect on the incidence of cancers in many other tissues.

If these relationships are established, it may be possible to reduce the cancer death rates in United States by as much as the average 35% estimated by Doll and Peto.[3] This estimate included stomach and large bowel, 90%; endometrium, gallbladder, pancreas, and breast, 50%; lung, larynx, bladder, cervix, mouth, pharynx, and esophagus, 20%; and other types of cancer, 10%. There is an unlikely possibility that no useful dietary modifications can be found that can reduce the total cancer death rates in United States by more than 10%, but it is also possible with good dietary research breakthroughs that as much as a 70%

Table 1-9. Changes in Food Selection and Preparation Suggested by U.S. Dietary Goals[39]

Increase consumption of fruits and vegetables and whole grains.

Decrease consumption of refined and other processed sugars and foods high in such sugars.

Decrease consumption of foods high in total fat, and partially replace saturated fats, whether obtained from animal or vegetable sources with polyunsaturated fats.

Decrease consumption of animal fat, and choose meats, poultry, and fish that will reduce saturated fat intake.

Except for young children, substitute low-fat and nonfat milk for whole milk, and low-fat dairy products for high-fat dairy products.

Decrease consumption of butterfat, eggs, and other high-cholesterol sources. Some consideration should be given to easing the cholesterol goal for premenopausal women, young children, and the elderly in order to obtain the nutritional benefits of eggs in the diet.

Decrease consumption of salt and foods high in salt content.

reduction might ultimately be achievable, although this percentage cannot be expected in the next few years.

Dietary Goals for the United States

Nutritional scientists selected by the Senate Committee on Nutrition and Human Needs have formulated a set of proposed Dietary Goals for the United States.[39] The goals encompass some of the major areas of nutrition research and speculation and introduce the issues of public nutrition policy as well as the proper role of the federal government in the dietary behavior of the public.

The goals were designed with the so-called "killer diseases" in mind: specifically, coronary heart disease, cerebrovascular disease, hypertension, diabetes, and cancer. Significant reductions in the total dietary fat, cholesterol, refined sugar, and salt, and increases in the use of polyunsaturated fat, fiber, complex carbohydrates, and natural fruit sugars are recommended (Table 1-9).

Because 27 million Americans suffer from heart or blood vessel disease and another 20% have hypertension, there is a need for a dietary change in our society. There is no evidence that the proposed diet will do harm. However, there is a difference of opinion regarding what constitutes a practical application of the goals, which seem to be reasonable and appropriate modifications of the modern diet. These recommendations support those that nutritionists have been making for some time—a decrease in foods of nutrient density in favor of more whole grains, moderation of fat and sugars, and increased vegetable protein.

Table 1-10. Dietary Goals for the United States[39]

To avoid overweight, consume only as much energy (calories) as
  expended; if overweight, decrease energy intake and increase energy
  expenditure.
Increase consumption of complex carbohydrate and "naturally occurring" sugars from about 28% of energy intake to about 48% of
  energy intake.
Reduce the consumption of refined and processed sugars by about 45%,
  so that it accounts for about 10% of total energy intake.
Reduce overall fat consumption from approximately 40% to about 30%
  of energy intake.
Reduce saturated fat consumption to about 10% of total energy intake;
  balance that with polyunsaturated and monounsaturated fats, which
  should account for about 10% of energy intake each.
Reduce cholesterol consumption to ~300 mg/day.
Limit the intake of sodium by reducing the intake of salt to ~5 gm. a
  day.

When these recommendations are translated into actual dietary practice, it becomes apparent that food choices will seem quite different to the American public (Table 1-10). The increase in complex carbohydrates from 28 to 48% of total calories translates into amounts of potatoes, cereals, pastas, legumes, and breadstuffs that upset American consumers who have previously allowed themselves to be persuaded that all carbohydrates are evil. To educate the public to accept school lunches containing almost twice as much starch will be a difficult task for nutritionists. Again, it will be difficult to expect consumers to adopt a level of salt intake that is approximately one-half the present level, and a sugar intake well below levels prevailing in 1900. These recommendations are similar to those made some years previously by the American Heart Association.

The changes affecting cancer are those that suggest decreased consumption of animal fat and increased consumption of fiber. There are direct animal and epidemiological relationships between fat consumption and colon and breast cancer (Chapter 2) and inverse relationships between fiber consumption and colon cancer in humans and animals (Chapter 3).

MECHANISMS OF CANCER FORMATION

Causes of Human Cancer

Modern technology and industrial development has led to a number of carcinogenic food additives, pesticides, insecticides, and industrial chemicals

Table 1-11. Recognized Causes of Human Cancer[3]

	Circumstance	Site of cancer
Aflatoxin	Consumption of unprotected food in tropics	Liver
Alkylating agents		
Cylophosphamide	Medical treatment	Bladder
Melphalan	Medical treatment	Marrow (leukemia)
Anabolic steroids	Medical treatment	Liver
Aromatic amines[a]	Manufacture of chemicals, coal-gas rubber articles	Bladder
Arsenic	Manufacture of pesticides Mining (some mines) Medical treatment	Skin, bronchus
Asbestos	Manufacture of or work with asbestos articles	Bronchus, pleura, peritoneum
Benzene	Work with glues, varnishes, etc.	Marrow (leukemia)
Bis(chloromethyl) ether	Manufacture of ion-exchange resins	Bronchus
Cadmium	Refining	Prostate
Chlornaphazine	Medical treatment	Bladder
Chrome ores	Manufacture of chromates	Bronchus
Ethanol	Consumption	Mouth, pharynx, larynx, esophagus
Immunosuppression[b] (azathioprine plus prednisone)	Medical treatment	Non-Hodgkin's lymphoma, skin (squamous carcinoma) various other rare sites
Ionizing radiations	Mining (some mines) Use of X-rays, radium Medical treatment Luminous dial painting Manufacture of isopropylene	All sites Nasal sinuses
Mustard gas[b]	Manufacture	Bronchus, larynx, nasal sinuses
Nickel ores	Refining	Bronchus nasal sinuses
Estrogens diethylstilbestrol premarin, etc.[b]	Exposure in utero Medical treatment	Vagina (adenocarcinoma) Corpus uteri
Phenacetin	Medical treatment	Renal pelvis
Polycyclic hydrocarbon[c]	Work involving exposure to combustion products of coal and certain mineral oils; use of kangri	Skin, rectum, bronchus
Quid composed of mixture of betel and lime	Chewing	Mouth
Soots, tars, and oils	Work involving exposure	Skin, scrotum, and lungs
Steroid contraceptives[b]	Social use	Liver (benign)

(continued)

Table 1-11. (*Continued*)

	Circumstance	Site of cancer
Tobacco smoke	Smoking, particularly cigarettes	Bronchus, mouth, pharynx, larynx, esophagus, bladder, pancreas
Ultraviolet light	Exposure to sunlight	Skin, including melanoma
Wood dust	Manufacture of hardwood furniture	Nasal sinuses (especially adenocarcinoma)
Vinyl chloride[b]	Manufacture of polyvinyl chloride (PVC)	Liver (angiosarcoma)
?	Some industrial uses of rubber	Bronchus
?	Some work in leather and shoe industry	Nasal sinuses
?	Heavy urinary infection with schistosomiasis	Bladder

[a] 4-Amino-diphenyl, benzidine, 1,2-naphthylamine.
[b] Carcinogenicity recognized by animal experiments before human hazard detected.
[c] Benzo(a)pyrene and various others.

introduced commercially during the last 40 years. To the chemicals used in the workplace one should add a growing list of naturally occurring chemicals, drugs used in medicine as well as UV light. Chemicals known to cause cancer are listed in Table 1-11. These together with ultraviolet light, which is the single most prevalent cause of cancer, accounts for about 50% of the cases observed in the United States, Canada, and several other Western countries.

The remaining cancers—those of the breast, colon, uterus, prostate as well as a substantial percentage of those in the urinary bladder and pancreas—are related to chemical contamination of air, food, and water as well as dietary influences. This multitude of chemical carcinogens and dietary influences affect development of cancer in different ways. In recent years new knowledge of the mechanisms of carcinogenesis has been developed. The carcinogenesis mechanism has been a controversial issue for over 100 years, but multidisciplinary approaches have provided an adequate scientific basis for the concept that neoplasia may result from a somatic mutation involving a change of normal cells at the level of the genetic material.

It is now apparent that the development of cancer in human beings in various sites takes many years and that progressive tissue as well as cellular changes can be observed during the so-called latent period. New cell populations often appear that most probably represent stages or steps in the cellular evolution from the initial carcinogenic event, i.e., preneoplastic and premalignant cells. In laboratory animals research has concentrated mainly on the early events and have suggested the existence of common patterns of early preneoplastic changes in several organ systems in many species. In contrast, research on human beings has concentrated largely on the later events of carcinogenesis and has confirmed the stages of atypical hyperplasias, dysplasia, and carcinoma *in situ* as likely precancerous steps in many organs late in the process.

Chemical carcinogens, accounting for most human cancers, have been classified by Weisburger and Hohn into eight classes (Table 1-12), which in turn belong to two main groups: genotoxic carcinogens, which include the direct-acting carcinogens; procarcinogens; and the inorganic carcinogens.[40] The other main group operates through epigenetic mechanisms and includes solid-state carcinogens, hormones, immunosuppressors, cocarcinogens and promotors.

Genotoxic Mechanisms

Genotoxic changes seem to arise through several different mechanisms. First, genetic material can be altered through direct attack by radiation, chemicals, or viruses. In the case of radiation and chemicals genetic material is damaged at a number of loci along the DNA chain. Some carcinogens react with guanine in RNA and DNA combining with these bases at the carbon-8 position. However, some carcinogens react at the nitrogen-7 or oxygen-6 position. When there is combination of a carcinogen with guanine, this base twists around so it can no longer pair properly with other bases. Both alkylating and acylating agents can act in this manner. Alkylating agents including nitrogen mustards, choloromethyl ethers, diazomethane, and activated epoxides can add alkyl groups to guanine and other similar molecules. Acylating agents including dimethyl carbamyl chloride, β-propiolactone, and propane sulfone can add acyl groups to molecules such as guanine. Other carcinogens can enter between the base pairs of DNA, thereby causing the double helix to uncoil, while still others can insert along the long axis of the DNA, perpendicular to the bases. Some carcinogens such as dimethylnitrosamine bind to proteins and add a methyl group to histidine residues.

These chemical changes of the DNA are converted to permanent alterations by means of the mispairing of bases during replication of the damaged regions of DNA. These changes probably represent a process called initiation. The chemicals that react with DNA can be classified into two categories, direct acting or procarcinogens, which require metabolic activation before they are able to react with DNA.

Table 1-12. Classification of Carcinogenic Chemicals[a]

Type	Mode of action	Example
Genotoxic		
Direct-acting	Electrophile, organic compound genotoxic, interacts with DNA	Ethylene imine, bis(chloromethyl)ether, alkynitrosourea
Procarcinogen	Requires conversion through metabolic activation by host or *in vitro*	Vinyl chloride, benzo(a)pyrene, 2-naphthylamine, dimethylnitrosamine, 2-acetylaminofluorene
Inorganic carcinogen	Not directly genotoxic, leads to changes in DNA by selective alteration in fidelity of DNA replication	Nickel, chromium
Epigenetic		
Solid-state carcinogen	Precise mechanism unknown; usually affects only mesenchymal cells and tissues; physical form vital	Polymer or metal foils, asbestos
Hormone	Usually not genotoxic; mainly alters endocrine system balance and differentiation; often acts as promoter	Estradiol, diethylstilbestrol
Immunosuppressor	Usually not genotoxic; mainly stimulates "virally induced," transplanted, or metastatic neoplasms	Azathioprine, antilymphocytic serum
Cocarcinogen	Not genotoxic or carcinogenic, but enhances effect of initiators	Phorbol esters, pyrene catechol, ethanol, *n*-dodecane, SO_2
Promoter	Not genotoxic or carcinogenic, but enhances effect of initiators	Phorbol esters, phenol anthraline, bile acid, tryptophan metabolites, saccharin

[a]Source: Weisburger *et al.*[40]

Direct Acting

The best known form of reactive moieties generated from several different types of carcinogens is the "electrophilic reactant" (Fig. 1-6). The electrophilic reactants are positively charged molecules that react well with sites of electron densities in many different cellular components, including DNA, RNA, and protein. A small number of chemical carcinogens, such as nitrosamide, e.g.,

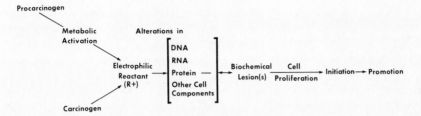

Figure 1-6. Steps in the initiation of carcinogenesis with chemicals. (By permission of the *New England Journal of Medicine* 1981, *305:*1379–1389.)

alkyl nitrosourea, ethyleneimine, bis(chloromethyl)ether, and nitrogen mustard are known to be active by themselves and do not seem to require metabolic conversion to more reactive metabolites.

Procarcinogen

Other types of carcinogenic initiators are called procarcinogens because they require metabolic conversion. The first type of metabolic activation discovered was the conversion of an aromatic amine, 2-acetylaminofluorene by *N*-hydroxylation to an *N*-OH derivative. More recently, much research has been done to clarify the activation of benzpyrene and other carcinogens. In the case of benzpyrene and probably other polycyclic aromatic hydrocarbons, the initial site of epoxidation may undergo hydration to form a dihydrodiol through a reaction catalyzed by epoxide dehydratase (Fig. 1-7). This derivative is all inactive, but in

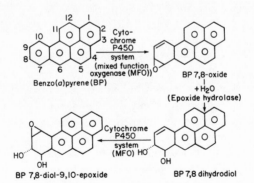

Figure 1-7. Current view of the activation of benzpyrene (BP) to benzpyrene 7,8-dihydrodiol, 9,10 epoxide through the mixed-function oxygenase (MFO) system (cytochrome P-450 system) and epoxide hydrolase. (By permission of the *New England Journal of Medicine* 1981, *305:* 1379–1389.)

turn, can be converted to another epoxide at a second site to form a dihydrodiol epoxide. The dihydrodiol epoxides are considered the most likely ultimate carcinogens for at least some of the polycyclic aromatic hydrocarbons. Aflatoxin β-1, which is one of the more important carcinogens in humans, is also subject to activation through epoxidation. Aflatoxin β-1 undergoes oxidation at its 2,3-position, and this derivative, the 2,3-oxide, appears to be one form of ultimate carcinogen of this mycotoxin. Vinyl chloride is also known to be activated through epoxidation.

The most active system for the majority of known conversions in the cell is the "mixed-function oxygenase" system, which consists of several cytochromes P450, reduced nicotinamide-adenine dinucleotide phosphate cytochrome reductase and lipid. This inducible system is located mainly in the microsomal fraction of the cell (endoplasmic reticulum), although there may be a second comparable system in the nucleus.

In addition to these oxidative systems, reducing systems also exist for some procarcinogens, such as the aromatic or heterocyclic nitro compounds. In the reducing system diaphorase or other reduced nicotinamide-adenine dinucleotide reductases are widely distributed among different cells and are known to be effective in reducing the nitro group to the hydroxy-amino-derivative.

The liver is the most active and versatile organ in the metabolism of procarcinogens. The liver and certain other organs can detoxify potential carcinogens or activate them. The ultimate fate of a potential carcinogen demands mainly on the balance between activation and inactivation, a balance that is easily altered in major ways by drugs and other chemicals, age, nutrition, and hormones, as well as genetics. For example, the carcinogenicity of several aromatic amines of the liver can be completely prevented by exposure to phenobarbital or 3-methylcholanthrene, agents that induce many liver enzymes. This phenomenon may be of practical importance to many people in the Western world because they have been exposed to agents such as dieldrin, aldrin, polychlorinated biphenyls, and dioxins. These agents as a group are known to be effective enzyme inducers in the liver. In addition, many other drugs induce microsomal or other enzymes in the liver or in other tissues.

The organ or tissue distribution of the carcinogen-metabolizing enzymes may be involved in the organ specificity of carcinogens. The absolute activities of the various enzymes and especially their relative balance may play important roles in determining which organ will be a target for a particular carcinogen. One interesting example of this modulation is the liver–kidney interrelationship with dimethylnitrosamine. Ordinarily this potent carcinogen induces liver cancer when absorbed through the gastrointestinal tract. If the animal is fed a low-protein diet, the hepatic activation and metabolism pathways are reduced. This reduction allows more of the carcinogen to be available for action on the kidney and also changes the dominant cancer pattern from the liver to the kidney.

Viruses

Viruses are able to insert specific DNA segments into the host cell, either through reverse transcriptase of RNA sequences, or through the operation of specific polymerases and therefore cause production of an abnormal DNA containing new information. Other mechanisms, such as the faulty operation of DNA polymerase during DNA synthesis, may result in an inaccurate transcription of the parent DNA segment, a process that can produce abnormal DNA.

Inorganic Carcinogens and Other Factors

Carcinogen metal ions, like the viruses, can also cause the faulty operation of the DNA polymerase during DNA synthesis resulting in inaccurate transcription of the parent DNA segment. Abnormal DNA can also result, especially during postreplicative DNA synthesis, through errors that were introduced by specific DNA polymerases concerned with DNA repair. During the replication of early tumor cells, the infidelity of DNA polymerases may lead to further abnormalities in the DNA that is produced. This may represent a means by which tumor cells progress to less differentiated, more malignant cancer types during their growth and development.

Epigenetic Mechanisms

Promotion

Production of an abnormal DNA in a genome by any of the above mechanisms is only the first step in a long series of biochemical events resulting in a malignant invasive neoplasm. Another important factor is the ability of an abnormal cell population to achieve a selective growth advantage in the midst of surrounding normal cells. The cell duplication process depends on a number of endogenous and exogenous controlling elements, two of which are both the promoters or inhibitors of growth, which could potentially either enhance or retard the growth process.

Numerous experiments indicate that promoters do not lead to the production of an invasive cancer unless there has been previous cell damage. Thus, in studying the causes of any specific human cancer, consideration should be given both to agents leading to an abnormal genome and to other agents that may be involved in the growth and development of the abnormal neoplastic cells and their further progression to clinical malignancy.

One of the first major phenomena in promotion is the selection of an appropriately altered cell to produce a focal proliferation. As observed *in vivo* in experimental models, cell proliferation is an essential step in promotion. Many biochemical changes seen in the different phases of the cell cycle, such as an increase in ornithine decarboxylase activity, will be seen in promotion. It is still to be determined whether one or more of such changes in enzymes such as ornithine decarboxylase, or changes in the cell membrane, DNA organization, or other factors have a special role in the promotion mechanism over and above that related to the cell cycle itself.

Synergism or promotion is important in human exposure to asbestos, nickel, or uranium, for example, may be associated with only a relatively low risk of lung cancer. However, when these factors are coupled with cigarette smoking, the risk becomes extremely great—much greater than that associated with smoking alone.

Progression

Focal proliferative lesions resulting from a promoting environment, such as nodules, papillomas, or polyps, undergo several additional changes before malignant behavior is observed. In many organs, including the bronchial tree in the smoker, one can observe several types of precancerous lesions, such as atypical hyperplasias, dysplasias, and carcinoma *in situ*. How these lesions relate to each other is not clear, but an important property of many of these changes is reversibility. In experimental animal models and in human beings there are some focal proliferative lesions, such as hyperplastic nodules in the liver (and their possible human equivalent, liver "adenomas," polyps in the colon, and papillomas in the skin can undergo regression or remodeling with normal differentiation. Vitamin A analogues such as *cis*-retinoic acid can prevent or delay cancer development possibly by reversing the focal proliferative process.

Transformation

An interesting development is the discovery of a process called transformation in which DNA or chromatin is transferred to susceptible cell lines. DNA from several types of cells transformed *in vitro* or *in vivo* with different carcinogrens has been shown to induce transformation. Even the DNA from normal cells can induce transformation. Using this type of test system, investigators might be able to explore the question of whether the information contributions of the DNA are positive (i.e., they code for an identifiable cellular component that is important for cell transformation) or negative (i.e., they are able to disorganize the host genome in a consistent manner).

**Table 1-13. Estimated New Cases and Deaths
for the Major Sites of Cancer: 1983[a,b]**

Site	No. of cases	No. of deaths
Lung	135,000	117,000
Colon–rectum	126,000	58,000
Breast	115,000	38,000
Prostate	75,000	24,000
Uterus	55,000[c]	10,000
Urinary	57,000	19,000
Oral	27,000	9,200
Pancreas	25,000	23,000
Leukemia	24,000	16,000
Ovary	18,000	12,000
Skin	17,000[d]	7,000

[a]Incidence estimates are based on rates from the National Cancer Institute SEER Program, 1973–1979.
[b]Figures rounded to nearest 1000.
[c]If carcinoma *in situ* is included, cases total over 99,000.
[d]Estimated new cases of nonmelanoma about 400,000.

CANCER TRENDS

New Cases

About 66 million Americans now living will contract cancer in their lifetime, or about 30% of the present population. Over the years cancer will strike
about three out of four families. There are more than five million Americans who
have a history of cancer, three million of them with diagnosis 5 or more years
old. Most of these three million can be considered cured.

In 1983 about 855,000 people were diagnosed as having cancer and about
444,000 died of cancer. The estimated number of new cases and deaths from the
major sites of cancer are listed in Table 1-13. Cancer incidence and deaths by site
and sex are estimated for 1983 in Figure 1-8. Age is also an important factor in
the cancer process with mortality increasing substantially with increasing age.
The nonrespiratory cancer death rates are increased more than fifty times for both
males and females (Figs. 1-9 and 1-10). The 440,000 who died in 1983
amounted to 1205 people per day or about one every 72 seconds. One of five
deaths from all causes in the United States, is from cancer. In 1982 an estimated
431,000 Americans died of cancer. In 1981 it was 423,000; in 1980 the number
was 414,000.

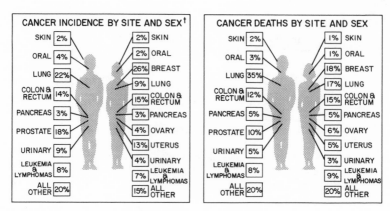

Figure 1-8. 1983 estimates of cancer incidence by site and sex. (By permission of the American Cancer Society.)

There has been a steady rise in the age-adjusted national death rate. In 1930 the number of cancer deaths per 100,000 population was 143. In 1940 it was 152. By 1950 the age-adjusted national death rate had risen to 158, and in 1978 the number had reached 176. The major factor in these increases has been cancer of the lung. Except for that form of cancer, which is increasing dramatically, age-adjusted cancer death rates for major sites are leveling off, and in some other cases declining (Fig. 1-11).

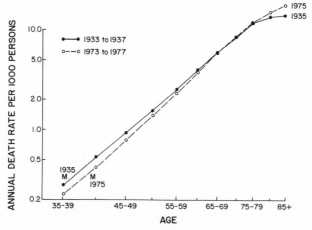

Figure 1-9. Nonrespiratory cancer death rates in the United States males by age, 1935 and 1975 (all races). (By permission of Doll and Peto 1981, *J. Nat. Cancer Inst. 66:* 1192–1308.)

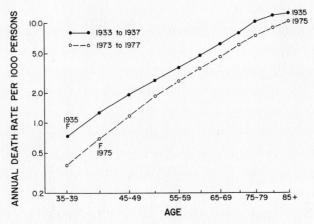

Figure 1-10. Non-respiratory cancer death rates in United States females by age, 1935 and 1975 (all races). (By permission of Doll and Peto 1981, *J. Nat. Cancer Inst. 66:* 1192–1308.)

Survival

About 320,000 Americans or three of eight patients who contracted cancer in 1983 will be alive five years after diagnosis. However, another 145,000 people with cancer died in 1983 who might have been saved by earlier diagnosis and prompt treatment. The importance of early diagnosis and treatment is outlined in Figure 1-12, which shows 5-year survival for Whites and Blacks on the

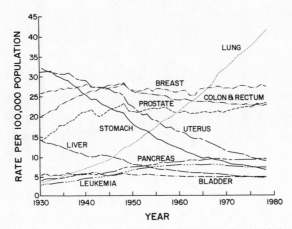

Figure 1-11. Cancer death rates by site—United States, 1930–1978. (By permission of the American Cancer Society.)

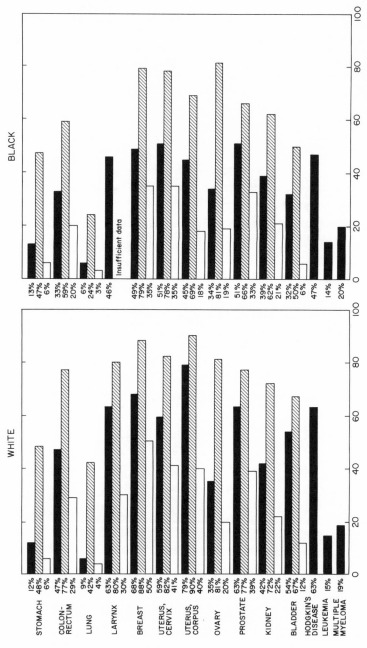

Figure 1-12. Five-year cancer survival rates for selected sites by race: (■) All stages; (▨) localized; (□) spread. (By permission of the American Cancer Society).

Table 1-14. Trends in Survival by Site of Cancer in Black and in White Populations: 1960–1963 to 1970–1973

Site	White			Black		
	1960–1963 Relative 5-year survival (%)	1970–1973 Relative 5-year survival (%)	Increase	1960–1963 Relative 5-year survival (%)	1970–1973 Relative 5-year survival (%)	Increase
Prostate	50	63	13	35	55	20
Kidney	37	46	9	38	44	6
Uterine corpus	73	81	8	31	44	13
Bladder	53	61	8	24	34	10
Colon–rectum	41	48	7	31	35	4
Uterine cervix	58	64	6	47	61	14
Breast	63	68	5	46	51	5
Ovary	32	36	4	32	32	0
Brain and central nervous system	18	20	2	19	19	0
Lung and bronchus	8	10	2	5	7	2
Stomach	11	13	2	8	13	5
Esophagus	4	4	0	1	4	3
Hodgkins' disease	40	67	27	—	—	—
Lymphocytic leukemia, acute	4	28	24	—	—	—
Lymphocytic leukemia, chronic	35	51	16	—	—	—
Non-Hodgkin's lymphoma	31	41	10	—	—	—
Larynx	53	62	9	—	—	—
Tongue	28	37	9	—	—	—
Melanoma of skin	60	68	8	—	—	—
Pharynx	24	28	4	—	—	—
Thyroid	83	86	3	—	—	—
Mouth	44	44	0	—	—	—

[a]Source: Biometry Branch, National Cancer Institute.

Table 1-15. Twenty-Five Year Trends in Male and Female Age-Adjusted Cancer Death Rates by Site per 100,000 Population: 1951–1953 to 1976–1978

Sex	Site	1951–1953	1976–1978	Percent changes	Comments
Male	All sites	171.9	215.7	+25	Steady increase mainly due to lung cancer
Female	All sites	146.4	136.1	−7	Slight decrease
Male	Bladder	7.2	7.2	a	Slight fluctuations; overall no change
Female	Bladder	3.1	2.1	−32	Some fluctuations; noticeable decrease
Male	Breast	0.3	0.3	a	Constant rate
Female	Breast	26.0	27.1	+4	Slight fluctuations; overall no change
Male	Colon–rectum	25.8	26.4	a	Slight fluctuations; overall no change
Female	Colon–rectum	24.8	20.0	−19	Slight fluctuations; noticeable decrease
Male	Esophagus	4.7	5.4	+15	Some fluctuation; slight increase
Female	Esophagus	1.2	1.5	a	Slight fluctuation; overall no change in females
Male	Kidney	3.4	4.7	+38	Steady slight increase
Female	Kidney	2.1	2.2	a	Slight fluctuations; overall no change
Male	Leukemia	7.9	8.8	+11	Early increase, later leveling off
Female	Leukemia	5.4	5.2	a	Slight early increase, later leveling off
Male	Liver	6.7	4.8	−28	Some fluctuations. Steady decrease in both sexes
Female	Liver	7.6	3.6	−53	
Male	Lung	25.5	69.3	+172	Steady increase in both sexes due to cigarette smoking
Female	Lung	5.0	17.8	+256	
Male	Oral	5.9	5.8	a	Slight fluctuation; overall no change in both sexes
Female	Oral	1.5	2.0	a	
Female	Ovary	8.1	8.6	+8	Steady increase, later leveling off
Male	Pancreas	8.6	11.2	+30	Steady increase in both sexes, than leveling off
Female	Pancreas	5.5	7.1	+29	Reasons unknown
Male	Prostate	21.0	22.6	+8	Fluctuations all through period; overall no change
Male	Skin	3.1	3.4	a	Slight fluctuations; overall no change in both sexes
Female	Skin	1.9	1.9	a	
Male	Stomach	22.8	9.3	−59	Steady decrease in both sexes; reasons unknown
Female	Stomach	12.3	4.3	−65	
Female	Uterus	20.0	8.7	−57	Steady decrease

aPercent changes not listed, as they are not meaningful.

basis of whether or not their tumors were localized or spread. In several types of cancer there are dramatic percentage differences in the survival between cancer patients whose tumors were localized or spread. Presumably an early diagnosis and treatment would be important in preventing tumor spread thereby saving an additional 145,000 people. Trends in survival are compared for the periods of 1960–1963 and 1970–1973 by site of cancer and race (Table 1-14). In most types of cancer there were gradual improvements for that decade, possibly because of earlier diagnosis and improved treatment.

Table 1-15 shows the 25-year trends in the male and female age-adjusted cancer death rates by site per 100,000 population 1951–1953 to 1976–1978. For the most part, there were no major changes in several of the death rates, but in a few cases there were significant changes in the 25-year trends.

The overall male age-adjusted cancer death rate showed a steady increase primarily due to lung cancer. Male lung cancers were increased 172%, whereas the female age-adjusted lung cancer rate was increased 256%. This dramatic increase is likely due to an increase of smoking. An international correlation has been made between the manufactured cigarette consumption per adult in 1950 as one generation entered adult life in 1950 and lung cancer rates as that generation entered middle age in the mid-1970s (Fig. 1-13).[3] The increase in the male death rate from kidney cancer may also relate to smoking. There has also been a

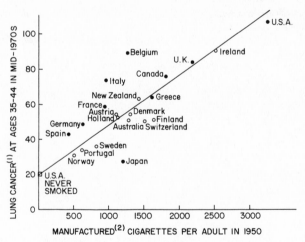

Figure 1-13. International correlation between manufactured cigarette consumption per adult in 1950 while one particular generation was entering adult life (in 1950) and lung cancer rates in that generation as it entered middle age (mid-1970s). (1) Lung cancer death certification per million adults aged 35–44 from WHO (1977, 1980). (2) Manufactured cigarettes per adult for the year 1950. (3) Estimated rates of lung cancer among nonsmokers in the United States. (●) Rates based on more than 100 deaths; (○) rates based on 25–100 deaths; (□) U.S. nonsmokers, 1959–1972. (By permission of Doll and Peto 1981, *J. Nat. Cancer Inst. 66:* 1192–1308.)

dramatic decrease in the stomach cancer death rates in both sexes. The reasons for this decrease are unknown. Stomach cancer is also decreasing throughout the developed world even though the case fatality rate is still about 90%. A large decrease has also been observed for cancer of the uterus. This decrease may well be related to the increased use and acceptance of the Papnanicolaou smear. This decrease may also be related to the decrease in deaths from female bladder cancer. Some deaths from bladder cancer in females in the 1950s may have actually had their major source in the uterus and were miscoded.

REFERENCES

1. Higginson, J., and Muier, C. S., 1979. Environmental carcinogenesis: Misconceptions and limitations to cancer control. *J. Natl. Cancer Inst. 63:*1291–1298.
2. Higginson, J., 1979. Cancer and environment: Higginson speaks out. *Science 205:*1363–1366.
3. Doll, R., and Peto, R., 1981. The causes of cancer: Quantitative estimates of avoidable risks of cancer in the United States today. *J. Natl. Cancer Inst. 66:*1192–1308.
4. Wynder, E. L., and Gori, B. B., 1977. Contribution of the environment to cancer incidence. An epidemiologic exercise. *J. Natl. Cancer Inst. 58:*825–832.
5. Weisburger, J. H., Hegsted, D. M., Giori, G. B., and Lewis, B., 1980. Extending the prudent diet to cancer prevention. *Prev. Med. 9:*297–304.
6. Hirayama, T., 1981. Non-smoking wives of heavy smokers have a higher risk of lung cancer: A study from Japan. *Br. Med. J. 282:*183–185.
7. Trichopoulos, D., Kalandidi, A., Sparros, L., and MacMahon, B., 1981. Lung cancer and passive smoking. *Int. J. Cancer 27:*1–4.
8. Hammond, E. C., and Seidman, H., 1980. Smoking and cancer in the United States. *Prev. Med. 9:*169–173.
9. Enstrom, J. E., 1979. Cancer mortality among low-risk populations. *UCLA Cancer Center Bull. 6:*3–7.
10. Jick, H., Walker, A. M., and Rothman, K. J., 1980. The epidemic of endometrial cancer: A commentary. *Am. J. Public Health 70:*264–267.
11. Hoover, R., Gray, L. A., Cole, P., and MacMahon, B., 1976. Menopause estrogens and breast cancer. *N. Engl. J. Med. 295:*401–405.
12. Jick, H., and Smith, P. G., 1977. Regularly used drugs and cancer. In H. H. Hiatt, J. D. Watson, and J. A. Winsten (Eds.) *Origins of human cancer.* Cold Spring Harbor, New York: Cold Spring Harbor Laboratory.
13. Smith, P. G., Kinlen, L. J., White, G. C., Adelstein, A. M., and Fox, A. J. 1980. Mortality of wives of men dying with cancer of the penis. *Br. J. Cancer 41:*422–429.
14. Rimington, J. 1971. Smoking, chronic bronchitis, and lung cancer. *Br. Med. J. 2:*373–375.
15. Hirayama, T. 1979. Diet and cancer. *Nutr. Cancer 1:*67–81.
16. McGuinness, E. E., Morgan, R. G., Levison, D. A., Frape, D. L., Hopwood, D., and Wormsley, K. G. 1980. The effects of long-term feeding of soya flour on the rat pancreas. *Scand. J. Gastroenterol. 14:*497–502.
17. Tamura, G., Gold, C., Ferro-Luzzi, A., and Ames, B. N. 1980. Fecalase: A model for activation of dietary glycosides to mutagens by intestinal flora. *Proc. Natl. Acad. Sci. (USA) 77:*4961–4965.
18. Bryan, G. T. 1980. Quercetin, a rat intestinal and bladder carcinogen in bracken fern. *Cancer Res. 40:*3468–3472.

19. Sugimura, T., and Nagao, M. 1979. Mutagenic factors in cooked foods, *CRC Crit. Rev. Toxicol.* 6:189–209.
20. Sugimura, T., Nagao, M., Kawachi, T., Honda, M., Yahagi, T., Seino, Sato, S., Matsukura, N., Matsushima, T., Shirai, A., Sawamura, M., and Matsumoto, H. 1977. Mutagen-carcinogen in food, with special reference to highly mutagenic pyrolytic products in broiled foods. In H. H. Hiatt, J. D. Watson, and J. A. Winsten (Eds.) *Origins of human cancer*. pp. 1561–1577. Cold Spring Harbor, New Jersey: Cold Spring Harbor Laboratory.
21. Spingarn, N. E., Slocum, L. A., and Weisburger, J. H. 1980. Formation of Mutagens in cooked foods. II. Foods with high starch content. *Cancer Lett.* 9:7–12.
22. Dungal, N., and Sigurjonsson, J. 1967. Gastric cancer and diet. A pilot study and dietary habits in ten districts differing markedly in respect of mortality from gastric cancer. *Br. J. Cancer* 21:270–276.
23. Linsell, C. A., and Peers, F. G. 1977. Field studies on liver cell cancer. In H. H. Hiatt, J. D. Watson, and J. A. Winsten (Eds.) *Origins of human cancer*. pp. 549–556. Cold Spring Harbor, New York: Cold Spring Harbor Laboratory.
24. Fraser, P., Chilvers, C., Beral, V., and Hill, M. J. 1980. Nitrate and human cancer: A review of the evidence. *Int. J. Epidemiol.* 9:3–11.
25. Hill, M. J., Hawksworth, G. M. and Tattersall, G. 1973. Bacteria, nitrosamines and cancer of the stomach. *Br. J. Cancer* 28:562–567.
26. Davies, J. M. 1980. Stomach cancer mortality in Workshop and other Nottinghamshire mining towns. *Br. J. Cancer* 41:438–445.
27. MacLennan, R., DaCosta, J., Day, N. E., Law, C. H., Ng, C. H., and Shanmugaratnam, K. 1977. Risk factors for lung cancer in Singapore Chinese, a population with high female incidence rates. *Int. J. Cancer* 20:854–860.
28. Reddy, B. S., Cohen, L. A., McCoy, D., Hill, P., Weisburger, J. H., and Wynder, E. L. 1980. Nutrition and its relationship to cancer. *Adv. Cancer Res.* 32:237–245.
29. Cruse, J. P., Lewin, M. R., Ferulano, G. P., and Clark, C. G. 1978. Cocarcinogenic effects of dietary cholesterol in experimental colon cancer. *Nature* 276:822–824.
30. Burkitt, D. 1969. Related disease-related cause. *Lancet* 2:1299–1231.
31. Trowell, H. 1972. Ischemic heart disease and dietary fiber. *Am. J. Clin. Nutr.* 25:926–932.
32. Bingham, S., Williams, D. R., Cole, T. J., and James, W. P. T. 1979. Dietary fibre and regional large-bowel cancer mortality in Britain. *Br. J. Cancer* 40:456–463.
33. Wattenberg, L. W., and Loub, W. D. 1978. Inhibition of polycyclic aromatic hydrocarbon-induced neoplasia by naturally occurring indoles. Cancer Res. 38:1410–1413.
34. Peto, R., Doll, R., Buckley, J. D., and Sporn, M. B. 1981. Can dietary beta-carotene materially reduce human cancer rates? *Nature* 290:201–208.
35. Tannenbaum, A. 1940. Initiation and growth of tumors; introduction; Effect of underfeeding. *Am. J. Cancer* 38:335–350.
36. Roe, F. J., and Tucker, M. J. 1974. Recent developments in the design of carcinogenicity tests on laboratory animals. *Proc. Eur. Soc. Study Drug Toxicity 15:*171.
37. Lew, E. A., and Garfinkel, L. 1979. Variations in mortality by weight among 750,000 men and women. *J. Chronic Dis.* 32:563–576.
38. Armstrong, B. K. 1977. The role of diet in human carcinogenesis with special reference to endometrial cancer. In H. H. Hiatt, J. D. Watson, and J. A. Winsten (Eds.) *Origins of human cancer*. pp. 557–565. Cold Spring Harbor, New York: Cold Spring Harbor Laboratory.
39. Select Committee on Nutrition and Human Needs, U.S. Senate. 1977. *Dietary goals for the United States*. 2nd ed. Washington, D.C., U.S. Government Printing Office.
40. Weisburger, J. H., and Horn, C. 1982. Nutrition and cancer: Mechanisms of genotoxic and epigenetic carcinogens in nutritional and carcinogenesis. *Bull. N.Y. Acad. Sci. 58:*296–312.

Chapter 2

Macronutrients and Cancer

LIPIDS

Epidemiological Evidence

Fats

Of all dietary factors associated epidemiologically with cancer of various sites, fat has been studied the most thoroughly and has produced the greatest number of direct associations. Dietary fat is highly correlated with consumption of other nutrients present in the same foods, especially protein, in Western diets. Therefore, it is not always possible to attribute these associations to intake *per se* with absolute certainty.

Breast Cancer

*Correlation Studies/*Several international correlation studies show direct associations between per-capita fat intake and breast cancer incidence or mortality. In general, these correlations were greater for total fat than for several other dietary factors studied, e.g., animal protein, meat, specific fat components, and oils.

Intracounty data sets have been used to compare dietary fat and breast cancer in other correlation studies (Fig. 2-1).[1] When the per-capita intake of various foods was compared by state within the United States with the corresponding breast cancer mortality rates, Gaskill *et al.* found a significant direct correlation with fat intake when results from all states studied were combined. These correlations disappeared, however, when the Southern states were excluded from the study or when they controlled for age at first marriage (as a reflection of age at first pregnancy) or for median income. The results of this study also suggested that dairy products as a class increased the risk of breast cancer. In another study, Hems observed that time trends for breast cancer mortality in England and Wales from 1911 to 1975 correlated best with the corresponding per-capita intake patterns for fat, sugar, and animal protein one

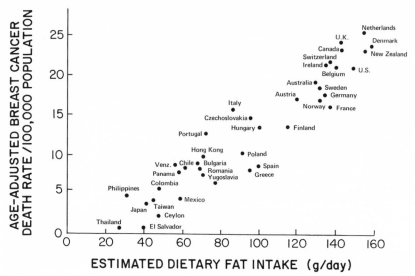

Figure 2-1. Correlation between per capita consumption of dietary fat and age-adjusted mortality from breast cancer. (By permission of Carroll 1975, *Cancer Res. 35:* 3374–3383.)

decade later.[3] In studies based on personal interview data, Kolonel *et al.* correlated the ethnic patterns of breast cancer incidence in Hawaii and the individual consumption of fat.[4] Significant associations with total fat, animal fat, and both saturated and unsaturated fat were found by these investigators.

Controlled Studies/Three controlled studies support the role of dietary fat as an important risk factor in breast cancer. A direct association between the frequency of consumption of high-fat foods and breast cancer in a study of 77 breast cancer cases and matched controls among Seventh-Day Adventists in California was reported by Phillips.[5] A weak direct association, but no evidence of a dose response, between total fat consumption (based on quantitative dietary histories) and breast cancer in a study of 400 cases and 400 matched neighborhood controls in Canada has been observed by Miller *et al.*[6]

The weakly positive association may partly reflect the fact that recent food consumption was measured, rather than dietary intake patterns earlier in life, which may have been the more important exposure period. For example, the changing breast cancer incidence among Japanese migrants to the United States and their descendents suggests that early-life exposures are an important factor in breast cancer risk.

In a third controlled study, Lubin *et al.* reported significant increasing trends in relative risk with more frequent consumption of beef and other red meat, pork, and sweet desserts.[7] When the computed mean daily nutrient intake was analyzed, the results supported a link between breast cancer and consumption of animal fat and protein. Nomura *et al.* compared the diets of husbands of women with and without breast cancer. These men were participants in a prospective cohort study of Japanese men in Hawaii.[8] The results indicated a direct association between the high-fat diets of the husbands and breast cancer in their wives, who were assumed to have eating patterns similar to their husbands.

Prostate Cancer

Correlation Studies/Epidemiological associations with fat intake have also been observed for prostatic cancer. Mortality data from international sources, but not incidence data, showed strong direct correlation of per-capita total fat intake and prostatic cancer.[9] Similar results were reported in a study based on a rank correlation with mortality in 41 countries.[10] In Hawaii, the consumption of both animal and saturated fat was highly correlated in four ethnic groups with the incidence of prostate cancer.[4] Blair and Fraumeni correlated prostate cancer mortality with dietary variables in the mainland United States.[11] They found that countries with a high risk for prostate cancer among Whites had correspondingly greater per capita fat intakes among the same population. In addition, one of the most notable dietary changes in Japan since 1950 is an increased per capita fat intake, and this change parallels a striking increase in mortality from prostate cancer.[12]

Controlled Studies/Two controlled studies associate prostate cancer with dietary fat. Rotkin found in an ongoing study based on 111 cases with prostate cancer and 111 matched hospital controls that the prostatic cancer cases consumed high-fat foods with greater frequency than did the controls.[13] Schuman *et al.* reported more frequent consumption of foods high in animal fat content by patients than by controls.[14]

Cancer of the Other Reproductive Organs. Associations have also been found between dietary fat and cancer of other reproductive organs, including the testes, corpus uteri, and the ovary. Direct correlations between the per-capita intake of total fat and the incidence of cancer of the testes and corpus uteri and mortality from ovarian cancer were reported by Armstrong and Doll.[9] In another study, mortality from ovarian cancer was correlated with international data on fat intake.[15] Kolonel *et al.* observed a direct association between ethnic patterns of total, animal, saturated, and unsaturated fat consumption in Hawaii and the incidence of cancer of the corpus uteri.[4]

Gastrointestinal Tract Cancer

Correlation Studies/Carroll and Khor observed strong correlations between the per capita consumption of dietary fat and age-adjusted mortality from cancer of the intestine (except rectum) in several countries (Fig. 2-2).[16]

Controlled Studies/Associations have also been made between dietary fat
and cancer at several sites in the gastrointestinal tract. In one controlled study,
which associated stomach cancer with dietary fat, more frequent consumption of
fried foods and greater use of animal fats in cooking were observed in gastric
cancer cases than in controls.[17] In a subsequent study of 168 gastric cancer cases
matched to hospital controls, Graham *et al.* failed to confirm this finding.[18]

Although time-trend data in Japan[12] and one international correlation
study[19] showed associations of fat intake with pancreatic cancer, most epidemiological studies relate to cancers of the large bowel. On the basis of international data, Armstrong and Doll reported direct correlations between colon and
rectal cancer incidence and mortality and per capita intake of total fat.[9] A strong
correlation was also found between mortality from cancer of the large intestine
(excluding rectum) and the per capita total fat intake; an almost equally strong
correlation was found between mortality from cancer of the rectum and intake of
total fat and animal fat.[20]

Enig *et al.* reviewed their data from an earlier study and revised their earlier
conclusion that colon cancer was directly correlated with intake of total, saturated, and vegetable fat, but not with animal fat.[21] In another study, in which the
average intake of nutrients by populations in different regions of Great Britain
was calculated, there was no significant association of fat intake with mortality

INTESTINE (EXCEPT RECTUM)

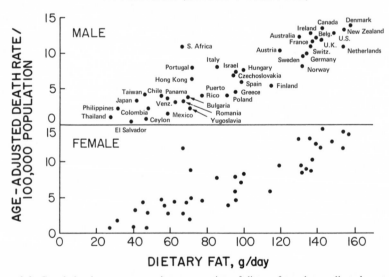

Figure 2-2. Correlation between per capita consumption of dietary fat and age-adjusted mortality
from cancer of the intestine (except rectum). (By permission of Carroll 1975, *Prog. Biochem.
Pharmacol. 10:* 308–353, and S. Karger, Basel.)

from colon and rectal cancer. There was also little difference in fat intake between the population of Utah, which has a low risk for colon cancer, and that of the United States as a whole.[22]

There is a striking contrast between the strong international correlations and the lack of associations within countries. It is likely that the regional food intake data within a country are based on individual consumption data and thus may be too similar to show any strong associations of risk of colon or rectal cancer. In contrast, the variation in fat intake among countries is much greater, thereby demonstrating the association more clearly.

The diets of adult men in two Scandinavian populations with different risks for colon cancer (high risk for Danes in Copenhagen and low risks for Finns in Kuopio) were compared by MacLennan et al.[23] These studies were based on food diaries and indicated that the consumption of fat was similar for both groups, but with differences in fiber intake. The diets of this low-risk Finnish population were compared with diets of a high-risk population in New York by Reddy et al.[24] Reddy and colleagues observed no difference between groups in total fat intake, but noted that a higher proportion of total fat was consumed as dairy products by the Finns and as meat by the New Yorkers. This may indicate that the possibility that the source as well as the quantity of dietary fat may be important.

Phillips found a direct association between colon cancer and frequent consumption of high-fat foods by Seventh-Day Adventists in a case-controlled study conducted in parallel with a breast cancer study.[5] Dales et al. studied cancer cases and hospital controls among Blacks in California[25] and observed a direct association between the risk of colon cancer and the frequent consumption of foods high in saturated fat. Association was greatest in diets high in saturated fat and low in fiber content. Among large bowel cancer cases there was higher total fat consumption, estimated from frequency data, than among controls in a study conducted in Puerto Rico.[26]

Nutrient intake estimates were made from dietary histories in a controlled study conducted by Jain et al. in Canada.[27] A direct association, including a dose response, was reported between a risk of both colon and rectal cancer and fat consumption, especially saturated fat. Even after adjustments for other nutrients in the diets, persistent elevated risks were observed for fat intake.

Relationship to Meat Consumption

Colon Cancer/Because meat can be an important source of dietary fat, especially saturated fat, several reports on meat consumption may be important. Howell reported a high correlation between colon cancer mortality and meat intake, especially beef, based on international per capita intake data.[28] Haenszel et al. reported a direct association between the frequency of meat consumption, especially beef, and large bowel cancer among Japanese patients and hospital controls in Hawaii.[29] However, this observation could not be confirmed in several studies confirmed in Buffalo, New York, in Japan, and in parallel cohorts followed prospectively in Minnesota and Norway. In addition, Enstrom observed that trends in beef intake in the United States do not correlate with trends in the incidence of mortality from colorectal cancer.[30]

Pancreatic Cancer/Pancreatic cancer has also been associated with meat consumption. Ishii *et al.* found a direct association between meat consumption by men and mortality from pancreatic cancer in a controlled study conducted in Japan.[31] Results were based on responses to mailed questionnaires, most of which were completed by relatives of deceased persons. A relative risk of 2.5 for daily meat intake and incidence of pancreatic cancer in a prospective cohort study of 265,118 Japanese has been reported by Hirayama.[12]

Cholesterol

Diets high in fat have been associated with atherosclerosis—a condition that has also been associated with elevated serum cholesterol levels. This association has led to interest in studying the relationship of serum cholesterol levels as well as cholesterol intake to the incidence of cancer. Most of the studies were initially designed to examine the association between cholesterol and cardiovascular disease and were not originally intended to measure cancer incidence or mortality. These studies have resulted in a number of different reports on the associations that were found.

Correlation Studies. When per-capita food intake data from 20 industrialized nations was analyzed, Liu *et al.* found a strong direct correlation between the per capital intake of total fat and cholesterol and the mortality rate for colon cancer, but an inverse correlation for fiber intake.[32] These investigators suggested that the data support a causal relationship between dietary cholesterol and colon cancer.

Pearce and Dayton conducted an 8-year clinical trial in which groups of 422 and 424 men were fed a conventional diet or a diet containing high levels of polyunsaturated fat (to lower levels of cholesterol), respectively.[33] In the groups on the experimental diet, the incidence of cancer deaths was higher. In a similar experiment conducted in Finland, Miettinen *et al.* found more carcinomas in the test group.[34] Another study group, which examined cancer incidence in men from five controlled trials of cholesterol-lowering diets, demonstrated little difference in relative risks.[35]

Serum Cholesterol and Cancer

Clinical Associations/Rose *et al.* observed that initial levels of serum cholesterol in colon cancer patients was lower than expected. However, serum cholesterol levels were higher in patients with cancer of the stomach, pancreas, liver, bile ducts, and rectum than in controls.[36] A similar correlation between colon cancer and low levels of serum cholesterol has been reported by Bjelke.[37] After measuring total serum cholesterol levels in 186 controls and 122 subjects with malignant tumors, Nydegger and Butler observed lower cholesterol levels in the cancer patients.[38]

In another study, clofibrate, a hypolipidemic agent, or a placebo was administered to more than 10,000 volunteers between 30 to 50 years of age with the highest serum cholesterol levels.[39] There were a disproportionately large number of neoplasms of the gastrointestinal tract and a few more neoplasms of the respiratory tract, but there were too few cancer deaths to demonstrate a statistically significant difference among the test groups.

The relationship between serum cholesterol concentration and mortality in New Zealand Maoris has been studied over a period of 11 years by Beaglehole *et al.*[40] They reported a significant inverse relationship between serum cholesterol concentrations and cancer mortality. Rose and Shipley observed in a 7.5-year follow-up study of London civil servants that mortality from cancer at all sites was related to a progressive decline in plasma cholesterol levels.[41] Cancer deaths were grouped into those that occurred less than 2 years after the subjects entered the study and those that occurred from 2 to 7.5 years later. The group with the lowest plasma cholesterol levels in which deaths occurred within 2 years had an age-adjusted mortality rate more than double that of those with the highest cholesterol level. However, cancer deaths among those followed for more than 2 years occurred at the same rate, regardless of the plasma cholesterol level at entry into the study. The decline in cholesterol levels was possibly a metabolic consequence of cancer that, while unsuspected, was already present when the subjects entered the study. Similar results were also observed by an international collaborative group.[42]

In the Framingham Heart Study, in which more than 5000 subjects were studied for 24 years, an inverse relationship was observed between serum cholesterol levels and cancer of the colon and other sites in men, but not in women.[43] Kark *et al.* related serum cholesterol levels to cancer incidence in more than 3000 subjects followed for as long as 14 years in Evans County, Georgia.[44] After entry into the study, patients diagnosed as having cancer at any site for at least 1 year had entry serum cholesterol levels significantly lower than levels in non-cancer patients. This association was also the same for Black and White females as well as for Black and White males, but was stronger in males of both races. Kark *et al.* also investigated whether the presence of cancer may have been responsible for the lower serum cholesterol levels. Patients were divided into three groups according to when evidence of cancer was first observed after entry into the study: within 1 year, from 1 to 6 years, and from 7 to 13 years. In this study initial serum cholesterol levels were higher in the first group than in the other two groups, but no differences were observed between the latter two groups. Little difference in cholesterol levels in cancer cases and controls was seen when various cancer sites were grouped together. However, Kark *et al.* did report low serum cholesterol levels in lung cancer patients. In contrast, Stamler *et al.* observed that serum cholesterol levels were higher in lung cancer cases than in controls.[45]

In the Honolulu Heart Study, cholesterol levels were determined in 7961 men followed for 9 years.[46] There were 598 deaths. Direct associations of baseline serum cholesterol levels were observed with mortality from coronary heart disease, but the baseline serum cholesterol was inversely associated with total cancer mortality and with mortality from cancer of the esophagus, colon, liver, and lung as well as with malignancy of the lymphatic and hematopoietic system.

Korarevic *et al.* related baseline serum cholesterol in Yugoslavia to mortality in 11,121 males over a 7-year period.[47] The inverse association between cancer deaths and serum cholesterol levels is not statistically significant. In the Puerto Rico Heart Health Programme study, 9824 men were followed for 8 years.[48] Serum cholesterol levels measured at the first examination were found to vary inversely with subsequent cancer mortality. In a Swedish study of 10,000 men followed for an average of 2.5 years, Peterson *et al.* found that deaths from neoplastic disease and other noncoronary heart disease peaked at low levels of serum cholesterol.[49]

Several positive studies were assessed by Lilienfeld[50] and others, who concluded that the observed inverse correlations do not substantiate any direct cause-and-effect relationship between low blood cholesterol levels and cancer.

Lack of Clinical Association/ A study in Norway, indicated no overall relationship between serum cholesterol levels and total cancer incidence.[51] Dyer *et al.* found that serum cholesterol was not associated with the overall risk of death from cancer in three epidemiological studies of Chicago men.[52] When cancer deaths were studied by site, a significant inverse association was demonstrated between serum cholesterol and deaths from sarcoma, leukemia, and Hodgkin's disease in the nearly 2000 men studied for 17 years. However, no significant associations were found for deaths from lung cancer, colorectal cancer, cancer of the oral cavity, pancreatic cancer, or all other cancers combined. This study suggested a direct association for breast cancer in women.

Controlled Study. Only one controlled study was specifically designed to evaluate serum cholesterol levels in cases of colon cancer and matched controls.[53] In 133 pairs matched by age and sex, serum cholesterol levels were lower for cancer cases than for controls. By contrast, when the tumor stage was related to tumor stage, significant differences in cholesterol levels were observed only between cancer cases with advanced tumors and the controls. In addition, only women, not men, had significantly lower serum cholesterol levels with advancing disease. This lack of association in early disease supports the concept that low serum cholesterol levels in colon cancer patients could be the result of a metabolic change that accompanies tumor growth.

Dietary Cholesterol and Cancer. The association of dietary levels of cholesterol and breast cancer was studied by Miller *et al.*[6] They found no significant differences in the estimated cholesterol consumption between cases and controls. In another controlled study, Jain *et al.* found that cholesterol intake for males with rectal cancer and for females with colon and rectal cancer was higher than for controls.[27] Even though the relative risk for dietary cholesterol was significant at higher intakes for all male and female cancer cases, as compared with all controls, this relative risk was substantially less than the estimates of risk for other nutrients associated with intake of fat, especially saturated fat.

An apparent conflict in the evidence seems to exist, i.e., that there is an increased risk of cancer of the colon and other sites associated not only with dietary cholesterol (in conjunction with a simultaneous intake of other, possibly more important lipid components), but with low serum cholesterol levels as well. Possibly high intake of dietary fat or cholesterol, or both, by persons whose metabolism maintains low serum cholesterol results in reduced biosynthesis of cholesterol as well as a high rate of excretion for cholesterol breakdown products in the intestine. These breakdown products could become substrates for the intraluminal products of carcinogens by intestinal bacteria. However, in metabolic studies of hospitalized patients, low serum cholesterol is usually accompanied by excretion of low levels of bile acid as well. This latter observation is not consistent with the mechanisms normally postulated for carcinogenic effect of dietary lipids.

Relationship of Fecal Steroid Excretion to Bowel Carcinogenesis

The possibility that metabolites in the colon could be responsible for malignancy has stimulated several investigators to study the level and types of steroids in the feces of populations at low or high risk for colon cancer, as well as in animals fed colon carcinogens together with various dietary regimens. The levels of neutral and acidic fecal steroids correspond to the amount of fat intake. In general, studies of the ratios of primary to secondary bile acids or the ratio of cholesterol to its metabolic products (i.e., coprostanol and coprostanone) have not revealed any differences among the populations studied.

Epidemiological Studies. Comparisons of the high- and low-risk populations, e.g., three socioeconomic groups in Hong Kong,[54] Finland, and New York,[55] suggest that the concentration of bile acids is elevated in feces of groups at greater risk. Nomura *et al.* observed that the Japanese, who are at high risk for colon cancer, have a higher concentration of cholesterol and total animal steroids in their fecal specimens than do the people of Akita, Japan, who are at low risk.[56]

Reddy and Wynder demonstrated a strong correlation between the level of neutral steroids and bile acids in a given population, their general level of fat intake, and their risk from colon cancer.[57] The daily fecal neutral steroid and the daily fecal bile acid was measured in Americans (high risk), American vegetarians, American Seventh-Day Adventists, and the Japanese and Chinese (low risk) (Figs. 2-3 and 2-4). Further studies of colon cancer patients and high-risk groups, i.e., patients with adenomatous polyps, suggest that the main correlation was with bile acid. In addition, studies on patients with familial polyposis, a genetic disorder, showed a greater excretion of unmetabolized fecal cholesterol than in other high-risk groups or healthy controls.

Hill *et al.* first associated colon cancer mortality and fecal excretion of bile acids as well as the fecal degradation of cholesterol and its metabolites.[58] On the bases of structural and steric similarities, they believed that bile acids might be changed to the carcinogen 3-methylcholanthrene by anaerobic gut bacteria. Their theory was based on the earlier synthetic chemical conversion of cholic acid and deoxycholic acid to 3-methylcholanthrene. The chemical reactions in these studies occur naturally, i.e., by oxidation, hydrogenation, cyclization, and dehydrogenation, even though synthetic laboratory conditions for the synthesis are not conditions encountered in the normal biological setting.

Several investigators evolved the concept that fecal bile acid and metabolites of cholesterol may function as cocarcinogens, carcinogens, or promoters in

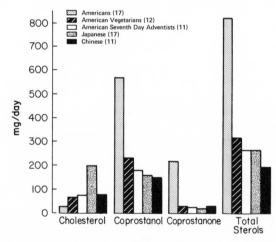

Figure 2-3. Daily fecal neutral sterol excretion in different population groups. Coprostanol, coprostanone, and total sterols are significantly ($p < 0.01$) higher in Americans on a mixed Western diet compared to other groups. (By permission of Reddy 1973, *J. Nat. Cancer Inst. 50:* 1437–1442.)

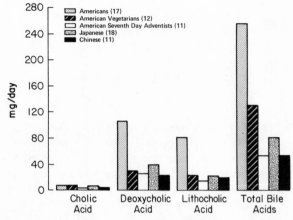

Figure 2-4. Daily fecal bile acid excretion in different population groups. Deoxycholic acid, lithocholic acid, and total bile acids are significantly higher in Americans on a mixed Western diet compared to other groups. (By permission of Reddy 1973, *J. Nat. Cancer Inst. 50:* 1437–1442.)

tumorigenesis of the large bowel. However, no active carcinogen derived from bile acids has been isolated from human or animal feces.

Studies in Animals. Reddy *et al.* demonstrated that a fourfold increase in dietary fat (from 5% to 20%) fed to rats increased the 24-hr fecal excretion of neutral and acid sterols by 30% to 40%, based on body weight.[59] A greater bacterial conversion of primary to secondary bile acids occurred more extensively in rats fed the high-fat diet than in those fed the low-fat diet.

The possible promoting effects by bile acids on bowel tumorigenesis have been tested by Narisawa *et al.* and Reddy *et al.*[60,61] In these studies, *N*-methyl-*N*-nitro-*N*-nitrosoguanidine (MNNG), which is a direct-acting carcinogen, was administered intrarectally to either conventional or germfree rats for 2 weeks. During the next 16 weeks, 20-mg doses of either sodium cholate, sodium chenodeoxycholate, or sodium lithocholate in 0.5 ml peanut oil were administered intrarectally to rats three times a week. The total number of large bowel tumors in both conventional and germfree rats given intrarectal instillations of bile acids was greater in the rats given MNNG without bile salts. However, the quantity of bile salts administered intrarectally was 20 to 60 times greater than that normally excreted in the feces during a 24-hr period.

The effects of bile acid on colon tumors induced by nitrosomethylurea (NMU) by feeding rats laboratory chow pellets with and without added bile acid have been studied by Cohen *et al.*[62] These workers observed that 0.2% cholic acid, but not chenodeoxycholic acid, increased the number of NMU-induced colon tumors compared with the number of rats fed nonsupplemented pellets.

With the dimethylhydrazine (DMH) model, no effect was observed on colon tumorigenesis in rats fed 0.3% cholic acid in a semisynthetic diet.[63] Feeding cholestyramine to rats given azoxymethane (AOM) for tumor induction increased the average number of tumors in the large bowel but not in the small bowel.[64] Chomchai *et al.* found that the increased quantities of bile acids in the colonic lumen were associated with the increase in AOM-induced colon tumors in rats.[65]

The possible tumor-promoting effects of bile acids are supported to some extent by reports that bile acids affect cell kinetics in the intestinal epithelium. If the biliary and pancreatic secretions are diverted from the intestine, there is a decrease in DNA synthesis and cell proliferation. On the other hand, administration of bile acids increase cell proliferation in liver bile ducts and the biliary tract epithelium.

After intestinal resection with diversion of the pancreatic and biliary ducts to the terminal ileum, Williamson *et al.* showed that bile initiated ileal hyperplasia in rats.[66] In addition, intraluminal infusion of an equal mixture of cholic, deoxycholic, and chenodeoxycholic acids twice daily for 5 days resulted in severe hyperplastic changes in the colonic mucosa.[67]

Bile salts readily interact with cellular membranes, which results in alterations in membrane permeability, and presumably cytotoxicity. These effects were minimized when conjugated bile salts were added to the unconjugated bile salts in sufficiently high concentration. Bile acids such as deoxycholic acid and chenodeoxycholic acid also increase absorption of 1,2-dimethylhydrazine and 7,12-dimethylbenzanthracene in the colon of the rat and guinea pig.[68] Therefore, it is difficult to determine whether the effects of intrarectally instilled unconjugated bile salts that demonstrated classic tumor promotional activity were due to increased carcinogen absorption or resulted from nonspecific damage and repair activity in conjunction with greater cellular proliferation of the colonic mucosa caused by the high intraluminal concentration of the bile salts.

Nonspecific effects of tissue injury may be an important factor in the enhancement of tumorigenesis observed at high concentrations of bile acids. Increased cellular proliferation, which accompanies inflammation and repair, may be important in the tumor-enhancing effects of tissue injury.

Animal Experiments

The initial observation that dietary fat influences tumorigenesis was made in 1930 by Watson and Mellanby[69], who showed that by increasing dietary fat, total intake of calories increased. In the experiments of Watson and Mellanby addition of 12.5 to 25% butter to a basal (3% fat) diet given to coal-tar-treated mice increased the incidence of skin tumors from 34 to 57%. In another early experiment, 3-methylcholanthrene was applied topically to mice fed a basal diet.[70] When their diet was supplemented with 15% fat (shortening), the yield of skin tumors was increased from 12 to 83%. Fat was especially effective when fed 6 to 12 weeks after treatment with a carcinogen. These investigators also observed a minor effect of unsaturation: tumor incidence at 5 months was 33% for control diets, 66% for coconut oil diets, and 76% for added corn oil diets.

Mammary Tumors

Effects of Caloric Restriction, Obesity, and Carcinogen Level. Tannenbaum demonstrated that dietary fat enhanced the development of either spontaneously or chemically induced mammary tumors in mice.[71] If the high-fat diets were instituted at 24 weeks of age instead of 38 weeks, the incidence of spontaneous tumors was greater. Tannenbaum and Silverstone observed that tumor incidence was greater in obese mice than in normal mice and that caloric restriction inhibited mammary tumorigenesis in normal mice.[72] However, effects of caloric restriction on reducing the incidence of chemically induced tumors can be negated by increasing the dose of carcinogen. Waxler *et al.* induced obesity in mice with gold thioglucose and observed that spontaneous mammary carcinomas developed more quickly in obese mice than in controls.[73] When the weight of the obese mice was reduced below that of the controls, a decrease in mammary tumors was observed. By feeding mice isocaloric high- and low-fat diets, Tannenbaum provided evidence that calories *per se* were responsible for tumorigenesis.[71] This finding differed from that of Lavik and Baumann, who found that the caloric content of the diet had a greater effect than the level of fat on the induction of skin tumors in mice by 3-methylcholanthrene.[70]

Carroll and Khor pointed out that the level of dietary fat was just as important as the amount of 7,12-dimethylbenzanthracene (DMBA) administered to induce breast cancer.[74] These workers studied the effect of both high and low doses of DMBA fed to rats in corn oil. At low dose (1 mg), rats fed 20% corn oil had more tumors and a shorter latent period, but no difference in the number of tumors per tumor-bearing rat, compared with rats fed 0.5% corn oil diet. The high-fat diet increased tumor incidence and the number of tumors, but did not alter the latent period, when the dose of DMBA was increased to 2.5 mg.

Effect of the Quality and Type of Lipid. The quality or type of lipid was also shown to be important in the induction of breast cancer by DMBA.[75] The incidence of mammary tumors was uniformly high with all dietary fats tested at a level of 20% in the diet, but in the rats fed unsaturated fats the number of tumors per group and the number of tumors per tumor-bearing rat was greater in the rats fed unsaturated fats. It became apparent that the tumor yield per group was influenced by the levels of the essential fatty acid, i.e., linoleic acid, present in the fat. When the groups of rats were fed tallow or coconut oil, which have low linoleate levels, they had significantly fewer tumors than did groups fed polyunsaturated fats, which have adequate sources of linoleate. Since the enhancement of breast tumorigenesis by high-fat diets was demonstrated when the diets were fed after tumor initiation by DMBA, Carroll concluded that dietary fat exerted its effect during the promotional phase.[76] The promotional effect of high-fat diets became stronger, as the dose of carcinogen was increased. There seemed to be a limit to the promotional effects of dietary fats. Diets containing fat at levels greater than 20% were no more effective than those containing 20%.

The enhancement of DMBA-induced mammary tumorigenesis in rodents by high-fat diets and also those containing polyunsaturated fats has been observed by a number of investigators. If only a small amount of polyunsaturated fat (3% sunflower seed oil) was added to the saturated fat (17% coconut oil), saturated fat was as effective as polyunsaturated fat in enhancing carcinogenesis. The polyunsaturated fat used must also provide sufficient amounts of essential fatty acids, and the diet must contain high levels of total fat to increase the yield of breast tumors. There is a possibility that these two requirements are interrelated.

McCay et al. also found that both the level and quality of dietary fat appear to influence the growth rate of DMBA-induced breast tumors.[77] Rats fed high levels of polyunsaturated fat (20% corn oil) had an average tumor growth rate considerably greater than that for rats fed high levels of saturated fat (18% coconut oil and 2% linoleic acid). Therefore, the total dietary fat and its unsaturated fat content appears at least in part to determine the average tumor growth rate. Apparently a certain dose of DMBA could produce a similar number of initiated cells in the mammary gland, independent of the dietary regimen used, and the number of tumors that are palpable within a fixed time probably depends on the growth rate of the initiated clones. As a consequence, if a higher level of total dietary fat or a greater amount of polyunsaturated fat accelerated clonal growth, the number of tumors reaching palpable size within a fixed time would be greater.

Additional support for an association between dietary fat and DMBA-induced breast cancer derives the results from studies in rats with the known breast carcinogen, NMU. A significant reduction in the latent period for the development of NMU-induced breast tumors has been observed in female Fischer 344 rats fed high-fat diets as compared with rats fed low-fat diets.[78] In contrast to studies using the DMBA model of breast carcinogenesis, high-fat diets increased only the incidence, but not the multiplicity of NMU-induced breast tumors.

In a study of the relationship of dietary fat levels to X-ray-induced and NMU-induced mammary carcinogenesis, Silverman et al. reported similar effects.[79] The incidence and multiplicity of breast tumors induced by 350 rads of total-body irradiation were increased in Sprague-Dawley rats fed a calorie-controlled, 20% lard diet, compared with rats fed a 5% lard diet. The high-fat diet increased the multiplicity of the NMU-induced tumors, but not the occurrence.

Newberne and Ziegler observed that effects of a high-fat diet on breast carcinogenesis could be modified if the diet were marginal in lipotrope (choline and methionine content).[80] In Sprague-Dawley rats given 2-acetylaminofluorene (AAF) or DMBA to induce breast tumors, the tumor incidence was lower, and death from the tumors occurred later in marginally lipotrope-deficient rats than in the controls.

Effect of Corn Oil on the Metabolism of Benzpyrene. Baker *et al.* fed ICR Swiss mice either a fat-free diet or a diet containing 10% corn oil.[81] After 3 weeks the rates of benzpyrene metabolite formation and metabolism to products that covalently bind with macromolecules were compared with the use of hepatic nuclei and microsomal preparations. The high-fat diet enhances the ability of hepatic cytochrome P450-containing enzymes to metabolize benzpyrene. Accompanying the increases in benzpyrene metabolism resulting from feeding the corn oil diet were increases in the covalent binding of benzpyrene to calf-thymus DNA and microsomal protein.

Effect of Fat on Transplantable Tumors/Dietary fats also influence the growth of transplantable tumors. Hopkins and West observed that a transplantable mammary adenocarcinoma developed more readily in host mice fed a high level of polyunsaturated fat than in mice fed an equivalent amount of saturated fat.[82] Abraham and Rao added as little as 1.0% corn oil to the diet and stimulated the growth of a transplantable mammary tumor in mice.[83] Inhibitors of prostaglandin synthesis were used. They concluded that this effect was related to the level of essential fatty acids rather than to the synthesis of prostaglandin. As little as 0.1% of pure linoleic acid in the diet was as effective as 15% corn oil in enhancing the growth of a transplantable mammary carcinoma. Santiago-Delpin *et al.* observed that a high-fat diet prolongs survival of skin and tumor allografts in mice.[84]

Wicha *et al.* demonstrated that polyunsaturated fat enhanced the growth of both normal and neoplastic mammary epithelial cells from rats.[85] Corwin *et al.* measured the tumorigenicity of Kirsten sarcoma virus-transformed murine cell line, AK3T3, which was grown in delipidized tissue culture media.[86] The incidence of tumors after implantation of a constant number of cells was compared with that in a conventional line of FK3T3 cells maintained in a complete tissue culture medium. As the level of dietary polysaturated fats was increased from 4 to 8%, an increase of tumorigenicity with AK3T3 cells was observed, whereas an opposite effect on tumorigenicity was noted with the FK3T3 cells. Apparently, the lipid supply *in vitro* was affected.

Stoddart *et al.* studied the growth-promoting effect of dietary vegetable fats on the growth of the transplantable Morris hepatoma #7800 hepatocellular carcinoma in rats.[87] The groups fed coconut oil had a lower percentage of palpable tumor than did control groups or the group fed palm oil. The expression of the transformed phenotype of a transplantable tumor may be affected. This alteration, in turn, may change the response of the tumor to dietary lipids in the host. A high-fat level has also enhanced tumor incidence induced by herpes simplex virus type 2-transformed cells (H238 cells).[88]

Liver Tumors/When administered to Fischer rats, which are resistant to breast cancer, 2-acetylaminofluorene induced hepatic carcinomas.[80] A high-fat diet marginally deficient in lipotropes significantly increased the incidence of hepatic carcinomas, compared with the incidence in rats fed a high-fat diet with adequate lipotropes. Apparently the effect of marginal lipotrope deficiency on the relationship between dietary fat and carcinogen-induced tumorigenesis appears to differ from one target organ to another.

An increase in dietary fat increased the incidence of AAF-induced hepatomas in male rats.[89] Chronic feeding of AAF resulted in the cloning of hepatic cells with resistance to AAF toxicity. These hyperplastic nodules resulting from the regenerative activity of such clones eventually progress to form hepatomas. The influence of dietary fat in the early stages of hyperplastic nodule formation and during the later stages of hepatoma development has been studied by McCay *et al.*[77] Hyperplastic nodules formed from AAF more frequently, and the latent period was shorter in rats fed a low-fat diet (2% linoleic acid) than in rats fed diets high-saturated fat (18% coconut oil and 2% linoleic acid) or fed a high-polyunsaturated fat content (20% corn oil). However, there was a 100% incidence of hepatomas in the rats fed the high-polyunsaturated fat diet and a 20% increase in rats fed the low-fat diet. There was also a high mortality among those fed the high-saturated fat diet because of the excessive toxicity of AAF under these conditions.

Dietary lipids are also able to modify aflatoxin-B-1-induced liver tumors in rats.[90] When beef fat was fed to rats, the number of animals with tumors was about the same regardless of whether the beef fat was fed only after induction or both before and after induction. In contrast, feeding polyunsaturated fat (corn oil) before and after induction resulted in a 100% tumor yield, but when the oil was fed only after tumor induction, the yield was 66%. Apparently the unsaturated fats increase the tumor yield more effectively than do saturated fats, but this effect may occur during the initiation or early promotional phase of hepatic carcinogenesis.

Pancreatic Tumors/The incidence of pancreatic adenocarcinoma induced in rats by azaserine may be modified by dietary fat.[91] In Lewis rats fed diets containing either 20% corn oil or 20% safflower oil, the number of pancreatic neoplasms were greater than in animals fed the same percentage of saturated fat. The animals fed the control diet (5% corn oil) and treated with azaserine had the same incidence and number of pancreatic neoplasms as did animals fed an 18%

saturated fat diet. Compared with the controls, there was a marked increase in hepatocellular carcinomas in rats given azaserine, but maintained on a lipotrope-deficient diet. Birt *et al.* observed that Syrian golden hamsters fed a high-fat level of corn oil had a greater incidence of ductal adenocarcinomas induced by *N*-nitroso-bis(2-oxopropyl)amine.[92]

Intestinal Cancer/The effect of dietary fat on the carcinogenicity of a variety of bowel carcinogens has been studied in a number of animal models. More intestinal tumors and more metastatic lesions were observed in azoxymethane-treated Sprague-Dawley rats fed a diet containing 35% beef fat than when fed regular chow.[93] Because the caloric density of the beef-fat diet was significantly greater than that of the laboratory chow, it is difficult to separate the effect of calories from that of fat on tumorigenesis. Nonetheless, this tumor model is useful for studying diet-responsive intestinal tumorigenesis.

Dimethylhydrazine (DMH) has been used to induce tumors of the colon and to a lesser extent the small intestine in rats fed 5% or 20% lard or corn oil diets.[94] When the rats were fed the 5% corn oil diets, they had a greater tumor incidence and a higher average number of tumors per animal than those fed the 5% lard diet. Tumor incidence and the number of tumors increased with the higher levels of dietary fat. However, when the level of fat in the diet reached 20%, there were essentially the same incidence and multiplicity of tumors whether the fat was polyunsaturated or saturated. Animals maintained on these diets for two generations before tumor induction with DMH had about the same tumor incidence and numbers of tumors. There were essentially no differences in the quantity of daily diet among the groups. In these experiments the caloric density of the high- and low-fat diets differed; rats eating the high-fat diets consumed, in addition to more fat, about 20% more calories.

Broitman *et al.* fed atherogenic diets containing 5% or 20% coconut oil to Sprague-Dawley rats given DMH to induce tumors of the bowel. The rats fed the 20% saturated-fat diet had a greater incidence and multiplicity of tumors than did rats fed the 5% saturated fat diet.[95] However, the rats fed the low-fat diet consumed fewer calories, gained much less weight, and thus received less carcinogen than did the rats fed high-fat diets. The effects of serum cholesterol levels on DMH-induced tumorigenesis in the bowel was also studied in these experiments. Rats were fed isocaloric cholesterol-containing diets supplemented with either 20% coconut oil to promote hypercholesterolemia and vascular lipidosis or 20% safflower oil to maintain lower serum cholesterol levels and presumably to shunt cholesterol through the gut. The rats fed the 20% polyunsaturated-fat diet had less vascular lipidosis, but developed more bowel tumors than did rats fed the saturated-fat diet. These studies did not determine whether the enhanced bowel carcinogenesis was due to the polyunsaturated fat *per se* or whether the effects were related to its hypercholesterolemic action. However, Reddy and Watanabe observed that when cholesterol-5,6-epoxide, or cholestane-3,5,6-triol were administered intrarectally to rats, there was no increased tumor-promoting activity in rats given MNNG to induce bowel tumors.[96] However, Cruse et al. have suggested that dietary cholesterol may be cocarcinogenic.[97] Rats given DMH and fed a diet containing amino acid hydrolysate and added cholesterol had shorter life spans, decreased time to tumor appearance, and more colonic tumors than did rats fed the amino acid hydrolysate alone. Because these dietary regimens are markedly different from those consumed by humans, the applicability to human health is unclear.

In general, studies with a number of strains of rats and various carcinogens have demonstrated that intestinal tumorigenesis is enhanced as the quantity of dietary fat is increased. Using Wistar-Furth rats, Bansal et al. observed that rats fed a 30% lard diet developed more DMH-induced large bowel tumors than did those fed a low-fat standard diet.[98] Using Fischer 344 rats, Reddy et al. administered DMH or methylazoxymethanol acetate systemically on a weight basis or gave the animals constant intrarectal doses of 2,3-dimethyl-4-aminobiphenyl or nitrosomethylurea.[61] The tumor incidence in rats fed 20% beef fat was greater than that in the rats fed 5% beef fat, regardless of the carcinogen used to induce the intestinal tumors. It is known that the routes of metabolic activation for some of these carcinogens differ, and it is likely that the effects of increased levels of dietary fat were manifested after the carcinogen was activated, rather than during the various steps leading to activation.

Dietary fat was also suggested to have promoting effects by studies in which high-fat diets increased the frequency of small and large bowel tumors when fed to rats after administration of azoxymethane but not before or during carcinogen administration.[99] In these experiments the high-fat diet (30% beef fat) had a caloric density about 34% greater than did the low-fat diet (5% beef fat) and may have been responsible for the differences in weight gains between groups.

DMH-induced intestinal tumors were increased in rats fed diets marginally deficient in the lipotropes choline and methionine than in rats fed high-fat diets with adequate amounts of lipotropes.

PROTEIN

Dietary protein has often been associated with cancer of the breast, endometrium, prostate, colorectum, pancreas, and kidney. However, the major dietary sources of protein such as meat contain many other nutrients as well as nonnutritive components. The association of protein with cancer at these sites might not be a direct effect, but could be related to the action of another constituent such as fat, which may also be present in protein-rich foods.

Epidemiological Evidence

After examining incidence rates for 27 cancers in 23 countries as well as mortality rates for 14 cancers in 32 countries, Armstrong and Doll correlated the data with the per-capita intake of a wide range of dietary constituents and other environmental factors.[9] Several relationships were observed between many variables. The correlations of total protein and animal protein with total fat were 0.70 and 0.93, respectively. In comparison, correlations with the gross national product were 0.32 and 0.65, respectively. Kolonel *et al.* analyzed the diet histories of more than 4000 subjects. They calculated that the correlation between total protein and total fat consumption was 0.7.[20]

Breast Cancer

Per-capita intakes of total protein and animal protein were significantly correlated with the incidence of and mortality from breast cancer in the study of Armstrong and Doll.[9] There was a stronger association for animal protein than for total protein, and in this study the correlations of breast cancer with per-capita total fat intake were generally as good as or better than those for animal protein. Hems conducted a similar study in which the per-capita intakes of individual foods and nutrients were compared with the chief causes of mortality in 20 different countries including Canada, Japan, the United States, and 17 European countries.[100] The results also indicated a strong correlation between the per-capita intake of animal protein and mortality from breast cancer. Time-trend data for breast cancer and per-capita food intakes in England and Wales indicated that the association with fat was stronger than the association with protein. After controlling for weight, height, and age of menarche, Gray *et al.* found a direct correlation between the international incidence and mortality rates for breast cancer in relationship to the per-capita intake of animal protein.[101]

In a study based on diet histories obtained by interview, Kolonel *et al.* found a direct correlation between consumption of animal protein and incidence of breast cancer in five different ethnic groups in Hawaii.[4] Gaskill *et al.* correlated the age-adjusted breast cancer mortality with the per-capita protein intake by state within the United States.[2] There was a direct correlation, but this finding was not significant after controlling for age at first marriage, as an indicator of age at first pregnancy.

Large Bowel Cancer

Food Intake Studies. Gregor *et al.* first reported a direct correlation between per-capita of animal protein and mortality from intestinal cancer.[102] This study was confirmed by Armstrong and Doll, who observed a strong correlation between the per-capita intake of total protein, animal protein, as well as the total fat and the incidence and mortality from colon and rectal cancer for both sexes.[9] Their observations for cancer at these sites were similar to those observed for breast cancer in that there were stronger correlations for total fat and for animal protein than for total protein. A strong association between the intake of eggs and cancer of the colon and rectum was also reported by these investigators. This latter association was greater than that for total protein. However, Bingham *et al.* were unable to find any significant association for intakes of animal protein in a study that correlated average intakes of foods, nutrients, and fiber in different regions of Great Britain with the regional pattern of mortality from colon and rectal cancers.[103]

Case-Controlled Study. The only case-controlled study of large bowel cancer in which bowel cancer was specifically examined was reported by Jain *et al.*[27] Although these workers found a direct association between consumption of high levels of protein and risk of both colon and rectal cancer, they found an even stronger correlation for saturated fat.

Meat Intake. In most studies of the relationship of meat intake to the risk of colorectal cancer protein intake *per se* was not estimated. These findings may reflect associations with protein because meat is a major source of protein in the Western diet. However, fat is an important component of meat and may be responsible for these observations. After correlating international mortality rates for colon cancer with per capita intake data, Howell found the strongest correlations with meat.[28] In another study, by Armstrong and Doll, correlations were stronger for meat than for total protein and animal protein.[9] Knox reported the strongest correlations for eggs, followed by beef, sugar, beer, and pork.[20] However, Enstrom studied the time-trend data for per capita beef intake and colorectal cancer incidence and mortality in the United States and showed no clear association.[30]

After studying cases, of large bowel cancer and hospital controls among Japanese in Hawaii, Haenszel *et al.* found an association between cancer of the large bowel and consumption of legumes, starches, and meats.[29] The correlations were the strongest for beef. In a similar study among Japanese in Japan,[104] these findings were not reproduced, nor did they parallel case-controlled studies conducted in Norway and Minnesota[105] or in a study done at Roswell Park Memorial Institute.[106] These controlled studies depended solely on the frequency of consumption data for their assessments of dietary intake. In a large-scale group study in Japan, Hirayama observed a decrease in overall risk for cancer, including intestinal cancer, in association with daily meat intake.[107]

Pancreatic Cancer

In a study that examined the relationship between per-capita intake of foods and nutrients and cancer mortality resulting from up to 22 different types of neoplasms in 33 countries, Lea found a strong direct correlation between the intake of animal protein and pancreatic cancer.[108] Similar results were reproduced by Armstrong and Doll.[9]

Association has not directly been confirmed by any case-controlled or cohort studies. However, a study based on responses to a mailed questionnaire completed mostly by relatives of decreased patients showed an association of the disease with consumption of high-meat diets in men.[31] In a group of 265,118 Japanese subjects followed prospectively, Hirayama reported a relative risk of 2.5 for daily meat intake and pancreatic cancer incidence in Japan.[12] Because meat is a major source of dietary protein, these findings offer support for the results of the earlier correlation studies.

Other Cancers

A strong correlation coefficient (0.8) was found between animal protein intake and the incidence of renal cancer.[9] In a later study, Armstrong *et al.* found no clear association between renal cancer and consumption frequencies for several foods containing animal protein, such as meat, poultry, seafood, eggs, milk, and cheese.[109]

In a study by Kolonel *et al.* incidence of prostate cancer was significantly correlated with consumption of total and animal protein.[4] Mortality from, but not the incidence of, prostate cancer was similarly correlated.[9] Hirayama reported a sharp increase in intake of animal protein in Japan since 1950, and during this period the incidence of prostate cancer in that country increased correspondingly.[12] Mortality from prostate cancer has been correlated with the intake of meat, especially beef.[9]

The intake of total protein has been significantly correlated with the incidence of endometrial cancer.[4,9] These results may reflect the high correlation observed between the occurrence of endometrial cancer and breast cancer, with the latter also having been associated with protein intake. No controlled studies have been conducted to examine this association.

Experimental Evidence

Far fewer reports have been published on the results of laboratory studies to determine the relationship between cancer and dietary protein than for certain other nutrients such as fat. In general, animals fed minimum amounts of protein required for optimum growth developed fewer tumors than did similar groups fed two to three times the minimum requirements. However, a number of these earlier reports in animals are difficult to interpret for numerous reasons: (1) several factors were being varied at the same time in some experiments; (2) dietary levels of the carcinogen were different in the high- and low-dietary protein groups; (3) the total intake of food was less for animals fed very high levels of protein, and tumor growth is known to be inhibited at lower food (and lower calorie) intake; and (4) a higher dietary level of fat, which probably has a tumor-enhancing effect, was present in the experimental diet. Nevertheless, several earlier studies provided useful information either because they were well controlled or because they were confirmed by other studies.

The effect of dietary protein on tumor incidence has been observed both with and without pretreatment with chemical carcinogens. That is, both spontaneous and chemically induced tumor responses may not be distinct, since certain so-called spontaneous tumors may be related to the previous ingestion of, or other exposure to, some unknown initiator of carcinogenicity. There is a possibility that the high incidence of liver tumors observed in earlier reports may have been caused by aflatoxin contamination or peanut meal or corn meal fed to animals.

Effect on Benzpyrene-Induced Tumors

Dietary protein seems to have a mixed effect on chemical carcinogenesis. In some cases increased dietary protein enhances carcinogenesis, but in other cases it seems to have an inhibitory effect on carcinogenesis. Studies conducted by Tannenbaum, in which the percentage of casein in the diets was varied from 9 to 45%, demonstrated the difficulty of generalizing about the effects of protein.[110] In general, the formation of benzpyrene-induced skin tumors and sarcomas was not significantly influenced. However, with protein levels below or above 18% there was an increase in incidence, but a slight decrease in latency of spontaneous mammary tumors with protein levels below or above 18%. Even when rats were fed 9% protein, some growth was observed. Silverstone observed that dimethylaminoazobenzene-induced liver cancers were decreased when dietary protein was increased, while spontaneous tumors were decreased.[111]

Effect on 3-Methylcholanthrene-Induced Tumors

The effects of protein and cancer are often difficult to interpret in some studies. In several experiments, even though diets varied in protein, numerous natural ingredients were fed and dietary components other than protein were also varied. In a number of studies, protein concentrations were inadequate for normal growth. The development of 3-methylcholanthrene-induced leukemias in DBA mice was inhibited by a 4% protein diet.[112] When this diet was supplemented with sulfur amino acids, the growth of the mice was increased and the number of tumors increased as well. A similar pattern was observed in C3H mice for spontaneous mammary tumors.

Experiments by Shay *et al.* indicated that there were no significant differences in 3-methylcholanthrene-induced mammary tumors in rats fed various percentages of casein diets at usual dietary percentages.[113] These investigators concluded that the significant increase in tumors in the rats fed 64% casein compared with those fed laboratory chow containing 27% protein. The difference in source between the semipurified 64% protein diets and the commercially prepared diet as well as the large difference in percentages are too great to permit definite conclusions. Another possible reason for the difference in tumorigenicity of the two protein diets is that aryl hydrocarbon hydroxylase (AHH), an enzyme that specifically metabolizes polycyclic aromatic hydrocarbons (PAH's) such as 3-methylcholanthrene, is induced in rats fed commercial laboratory chow.[114] The induction of AHH protects against the carcinogenic action of PAH's. In an earlier experiment White *et al.* reported that a high-protein diet enhanced 3-methylcholanthrene induced leukemia in mice.[115]

Effect on 2-Acetylaminofluorene-Induced Tumors

Partially purified diets containing 2-AAF and varying amounts of protein containing 9 to 60% were fed to rats in a study by Engel and Copeland.[116] Feed intakes were about equal, and the number of tumors at various sites was inversely proportional to the ratio of dietary protein. The group of rats fed the partially purified diets containing 9–27% casein from the time of weaning had a 86% incidence of mammary tumors. In contrast, rats fed diets containing 40 to 60% casein had only a 12% tumor incidence. However, the number of animals in these experiments was small. It is possible that the highly reactive 2-AAF was reacting directly with the protein either *in vivo* or *in vitro,* thereby being unavailable for reaction with DNA or other important cellular components.

Morris *et al.* found more tumors of a greater variety appeared in rats treated with 2-AAF and fed synthetic diets containing 18% and 24% casein than in similarly treated animals fed diets containing 12% casein.[117] Harris found that dietary protein had a modest reducing effect on carcinogenesis induced by either 2-AAF or aminofluorene (AF), which was applied to the skin.[118] In the 2-AAF-treated rats, a modest reduction in dietary casein from 20 to 13% resulted in a decrease in the total incidence of skin tumors from 65 to 45% in males and from 80 to 70% in females. In the rats receiving the low-protein diet, the incidence of liver tumors was decreased from 50 to 30% in males and from 20 to 0% in females.

Effect on Aflatoxin-Induced Tumors

The carcinogenesis of aflatoxin was compared in rats fed 5% and 20% casein.[119] There was a 50% incidence of hepatic tumors, with the other half of the animals showing precancerous lesions in rats fed a 20% casein diet, whereas the rats fed the 5% casein diet had no tumors or precancerous lesions. Wells *et al.* found similar results. The severity of the liver involvement increased progressively with increased protein levels in the diet.[120] Cystine was also added to the casein diet of some other groups of rats fed similar levels of protein, since sulfur-containing amino acids are the most limiting amino acids in casein. When cysteine was included in the diet, tumors were also observed in the animals fed the low-protein diet. Furthermore, the livers of animal on "normal" and high-protein diets were much more severely involved than were the livers of animals on non-cystine-supplemented diets.

There may be a problem in comparing the carcinogenicity of these two dietary levels of casein because short-term toxicity studies have indicated that low-protein intake increases animal susceptibility to large doses of aflatoxins. However, monkeys receiving small daily doses of aflatoxin for extended periods were more resistant to aflatoxins when they were consuming low-protein diets. In addition, other studies have suggested that components of the dietary protein source may also act or interact with other dietary components to modify the severity of the response to aflatoxin.

Numerous studies have been undertaken to determine the mechanism by which dietary protein alters aflatoxin B-1 (AFB1)-induced carcinogenesis. The mixed-function oxygenases are depressed when the protein intake is low. The mixed-function oxygenase system is responsible for AFB1 metabolism as well as the *in vivo* formation of AFB1–DNA covalent adducts.[121,122] Although Campbell suggested that modification of AFB1 metabolism was responsible for the effect of dietary protein of AFB1 carcinogenesis, more recent studies indicate that the effect of dietary protein on postinitiation events may be more important.[123]

For example, the development of γ-glutamyltranspeptidase hepatocellular foci, thought to be an excellent early indicator of hepatocarcinogenesis,[124] is depressed more in rats fed a 5% casein diet more than in rats fed a 20% casein diet, both given after the administration of AFB1 is completed.[124] The low-protein diet postinitiation effect was even able to overcome the potential carcinogenic effects of a higher AFB1–DNA adduct level, which had already been established by feeding high levels of protein during AFB1 administration.[125]

Effect on Dimethylnitrosamine-Induced Tumors

Studies show that dietary proteins affect dimethylnitrosamine (DMN)-induced carcinogenesis. At the time of administration protein deficiency has reduced the acute toxic effects of DMN in rats, but later increased carcinogenesis in the kidney.[126] These results were obtained with protein-free diets or stock pellets fed for 1 week before DMN administration. From these results it is apparent that protein-free diets have a different influence on the metabolism of DMN in different tissues. DMN metabolism in the liver, which is essential for producing the active toxin or carcinogen, was decreased almost 50%, thus allowing a greater amount of unmetabolized DMN to circulate to other tissues. DMN is then metabolized to the active carcinogen in the kidney, and the greater amount of unmetabolized DMN in the circulation is believed to enhance carcinogenesis in the kidney. In these experiments feed intake was not controlled, and therefore the relative contribution of dietary protein to the observed results is difficult to evaluate.

Effect on Spontaneous Tumor Development

Ross and Bras have studied the influence of protein undernutrition and overnutrition on spontaneous tumor development.[127] With *ad libitum* and restricted feeding, the effects of dietary casein varied and a differential response depended on the tissue and type of tumor. In the case of *ad libitum* feeding, a slight protein deficiency increased the incidence of lymphoreticular and hematopoietic tumors. Urinary bladder papillomas were increased in the rats given a high-protein diet. The highest incidence of other tumors, such as of the pituitary, thyroid, and pancreas, occurred when protein was fed at intermediate levels. When rats were fed restricted diets, malignant epithelial tumors increased inversely to protein content. Rate of tumor formation was reduced with restricted food intake in a number of tissues. These data indicate that caution must be exercised in regard to generalizations about the role of protein in tumor formation in light of our present knowledge.

Tannenbaum and Silverstone described a study in which diets containing 9 to 45% protein were fed *ad libitum* to an inbred strain of mice.[110] In the mice fed 9% casein diets, the incidence of spontaneous hepatomas was 11/44; in the mice fed 18% casein diets, it was 28/46. However, no significant effect was observed on either the incidence or the average time of appearance for the spontaneous mammary tumors.

A 4% protein diet also inhibits spontaneous mammary tumors in C3H mice. Although food intake per unit body weight was similar, mice on low-protein low-cystine diets had no weight gain and showed aberrations in estrous cycles, which may have influenced mammary gland tumor development. When synthetic estrogens were implanted in mice deficient in protein, the development of tumors was increased and approximated the number observed with adequate protein. In the same strain of mice lysine-deficient diets were also studied and the development of spontaneous mammary tumors was greatly reduced.[128] In both the experiments with low cysteine and the lysine-deficient diets, the development of spontaneous mammary tumors were much reduced. In both instances, the reduction was similar to that expected from calorie restriction to similar body weights. Pair-feeding experiments showed no difference in spontaneous mammary tumors between deficient and amino acid-supplemented mice.

Effect on Azo Dye-Induced Tumors

McSheehy observed that a high-protein diet resulted in an earlier appearance of mammary adenocarcinoma in rats.[129] In contrast, malignant hepatic tumor induced by azo dyes tended to be inhibited by increasing the amount of dietary casein. Possibly, dietary protein may increase the resistance of the liver to carcinogenic hydrocarbons.

The type and composition of protein may also play an important role in hepatoma formation. Rats fed unpolished rice mixed with a carcinogenic hydrocarbon developed hepatomas. Other investigators were unable to repeat these results with wheat as the source of the protein.

Effect on Dimethylhydrazine-Induced Tumors

Visek *et al.* studied the possible role of dietary protein in dimethylhydrazine (DMH)-induced colon carcinogenesis in Sprague-Dawley rats.[130] The source of protein as a possible modifying factor on colon carcinogenesis was studied. Semipurified diets containing 20% protein as freeze-dried raw beef, charcoal-broiled beef, or soybean protein were fed to the rats along with 20% beef fat. Visek *et al.* concluded that the source of the protein was not a factor in the DMH-induced colon carcinogenesis in rats. However, in another study, rats fed 15 and 22.5% protein had a greater number of DMH-induced intestinal tumors exceeding 200 mm^3 than did those fed 7.5% protein.[131] Even though the total number of tumors was greater, the percentage of animals with colon tumors was not significantly different between various dietary groups. The number of rats with tumors was greater at the higher protein levels; however, this increase was not significant. Ear tumors were also greater in number and appeared earlier with the 22.5% protein compared with the other groups fed lower percentages of protein.

About 4% of the diet is the usual estimated protein requirement of mature rats, so that even 7.5% protein exceeded the requirements for most of the experiments. As the remainder of the diets was about the same, the difference in tumors between the treatment groups could not be ascribed to any other significant differences in the consumption of calories or other nutrients. DMN was given to the rats on a body weight basis and, even though the 7.5%-protein group weighed less, they received 85% of the carcinogen dosage given to the other groups. The differences in tumor yield cannot likely be explained on this basis alone. There is a possibility, however, that the decreased number of tumors in rats fed the 7.5% protein diet was due to suboptimal protein intake during the period of rapid body growth. However, the evidence suggests that the time of appearance of tumors and their size and number were influenced by protein intake.

Also in this experiment 2.5% urea was added to the three protein concentrations to enhance ammonia concentrations in the bowel lumen. No evidence was found that ammonia derived from urea in the diet affected tumor yield. Even though portal blood ammonia concentrations were significantly higher in the urea-supplemented rats, the colon and cecal ammonia concentrations were unaffected. However, as dietary protein increased there was an increase in ammonia concentrations of the cecum.

Effect on 7,12-Dimethylbenzanthracene-Induced Tumors

Effect of Dietary Level of Protein. In a study by Walters and Roe newborn pups of mice were fed diets containing either 15 or 25% casein and were then given a single dose of the polycyclic aromatic hydrocarbon 7,12-dimethyl-benzanthracene.[132] After they were weaned, they were fed the same diet as their mothers. Even though the difference in the proportion of mice was not significantly different, the group fed a 25% casein diet developed fewer tumors per mouse.

Clinton *et al.* examined the effects of dietary protein on the initiation of DMBA-induced mammary cancer.[133] They fed rats 7.5, 15, and 45% protein for 4 weeks before the rats were given a single dose of DMBA. There were no significant differences in caloric intake for this period. After DMBA administration, all rats were fed the 15% protein diet. As the percentage of dietary protein increased, the tumors developed more rapidly and in greater number (Fig. 2-5). In addition, the latent period of tumor induction was increased and the percentage of rats with multiple tumors and the number of cancers per animal were decreased. The latent period of tumor induction was increased from 84 days in the rats fed 7.5% protein to 126 days in the rats fed the 45% protein diet. The percentage of the rats with multiple tumor incidence and the number of tumors per tumor-bearing rat was 81% and 2.5% for the rats fed the 7.5% protein diet and 0% and 1.0% for the rats fed the 45% protein diet.

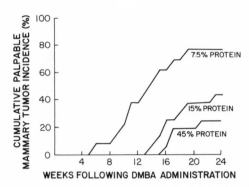

Figure 2-5. Cumulative palpable mammary tumors in female Sprague-Dawley rats maintained on diets containing 7.5%, 15%, and 45% protein prior to DMBA administration. All rats were maintained on the 15% protein diet following DMBA administration. (By permission of Clinton 1977, *J. Nutr. 109:* 55–62.)

Effect on Aryl Hydrocarbon Hydroxylase. Rats killed at the time of carcinogen administration but not given DMBA showed increasing AHH activity as the percentage of dietary protein was increased. AHH is known specifically to metabolize DMBA as well as several other PAH's to more soluble and therefore more rapidly excretable derivatives. This evidence seems to support the concept that increasing dietary protein decreases the carcinogenic response to DMBA by stimulating the production of its detoxification products. There is also the possibility that DMBA is binding to protein and is unable to bind to other macromolecules such as DNA.

Effect of Dietary Protein on Prolactin. Clinton *et al.* observed an increased prolactin level in DMBA-treated rats fed higher protein levels.[134] There is a possibility that the increased prolactin level may be responsible for the increased tumorigenesis in the rats fed higher protein levels. Increasing the fat concentration, however, had no effect on prolactin levels.

The results of the several experiments with carcinogens and the various levels of dietary protein indicate that influence of protein varies with species and strain, tissue origin of the tumor, malignancy, feeding conditions, and whether tumors are spontaneously or chemically induced. It is certainly clear that the influence of dietary protein on carcinogenesis is not resolved and, since each experimental model seems to differ, the problem will not be resolved by a single experimental model.

Effect on Tumor Transplantation

The general inhibition of the growth of transplanted tumors has been associated with low-protein diets. Haley and Williamson fed a no-protein diet and a diet containing 20% casein to rats implanted with HAD-1 tumors.[135] These workers observed that the resultant tumors were smaller in the no-protein diet group. Babson found that increasing dietary casein from 0 to 18% increased tumor growth rates in rats implanted either with the sarcoma R-1 tumor or the Flexner-Jobling carcinosarcoma.[136] In another experiment, there was a prolonged inflammatory reaction to the implantation of the Walker carcinosarcoma 256 as well as incomplete connective tissue encapsulation in animals fed 5% casein diets, compared with animals fed 20% diets.[137]

The effect of low-protein diets on the "take" of implanted mammary carcinoma 15091 has been studied by White and Belin.[138] Even though the number of takes was higher (16/31) in the low-protein group than in the adequate dietary protein group (10/31), the growth rate at 3 weeks was only 74% the rate for the higher protein diet.

A low incidence of herpes 2-transformed cell-induced tumors was found in mice fed low protein from a milk or fish source.[88] In addition, mice fed the low amounts of milk protein had fewer transplantable colon tumors than did mice fed low amounts of protein from other sources.[139]

The mechanism for the inhibition of tumor growth by low-protein diets is unknown. The cellular immune response may be involved; it is believed to be enhanced through a deficiency of blocking serum antibody production at low levels of protein intake. Or the low-protein intake may cause a restricted amount of amino acid to enter the tumor, and other body functions may compete for the amino acid pool. Thus, the evidence from both epidemiological and laboratory studies suggests that protein intake may be associated with an increased amount of risk at certain sites. The limited data on protein as compared with fat and the strong correlation between fat and protein intake in the Western diet mitigate against a definite conclusion about an independent protein effect.

AMINO ACIDS

Deficiencies

Certain amino acid deficiencies appear to have tumor-suppressing action. It was postulated that if a minimal amount of an essential amino acid was fed to a tumor-bearing animal, the normal tissues would use this nutrient to maintain biochemical integrity. It was believed that if normal tissues were able to retain functional capacity they might compete successfully with the tumor for the limited amount of the essential nutrient. The tumor would have to survive with a reduced intake of essential amino acid(s) and would have to compete with healthy cells for the limited supply of a metabolite. The growth of the tumor would be decreased without damaging normal tissue or metabolic wasting.

Greenstein and co-workers demonstrated that tube-fed synthetic diets, each totally deficient in a single essential amino acid, could inhibit Walker carcinoma in rats in short-term experiments.[140] These experiments represented the first use of synthetic mixtures of precisely determined compositions. As with previous experiments designed to control tumor growth with amino acid deficiency, significant inhibition—in some cases as great as 90% with some diets—could be achieved. Unfortunately, since the host animals suffered severe body weight loss, clinical applications of these diets to human patients may thus be severely limited.

Low dietary cystine has been reported to inhibit the induction of leukemia in DBA mice. Cystine added to low-protein casein diets enhanced the liver tumorigenicity of aflatoxin in rats.[121] Spontaneous mammary carcinoma in C3H female mice was inhibited by lysine-deficient or cystine-deficient diets.

Experiments using phenylalanine-tyrosine-limited diets against transplanted mouse hepatoma BW 7756 and mouse mammary adenocarcinoma C3HBA showed significant tumor inhibition over 2–4 weeks of feeding. During the experiments there was only a moderate weight loss with no downward changes in hemoglobin or serum proteins.[141]

These results encouraged application of the diet to patients who had far-advanced malignancies no longer responsive to conventional therapy. Early experiments on a variety of tumors (melanoma, Hodgkin's disease, cervical, endometrial, and ovarian carcinomas) showed pronounced regression of some cancers, reduced ascites, less pain, and even occasional weight gain.

The inhibition of mouse melanomas and regression of human melanomas have been observed with an aromatic amino acid-restricted diet.[142] In addition, chronic myelogenous leukemia in mice and human subjects benefited from a low-phenylalanine diet.[143] Using phenylalanine-tyrosine-restricted diets Lorincz et al. found that the growth of BW 7756 hepatomas, CaD2 and H2712 mammary adenocarcinoma, as well as S180 pleomorphic sarcomas was inhibited in the mouse.[141]

On the same type of restricted phenylalanine-tyrosine diet, a 54-year-old woman with differentiated bilateral papillary serous cystadenocarcinoma of the ovary with extensive abdominal metastases showed improvement with some regression of her abdominal tumors.[15] Previous treatment with endocrine agents including stilbestrol and testosterone had had no effect. This case illustrates the benefits of essential amino acid restriction even with tumors not controlled by hormonal substances. It suggests that diet therapy does not exert an effect by producing an endocrine balance secondary to caloric restriction. This seems to agree with the findings in the mouse hepatoma experiments, since such tumors are not ordinarily dependent on hormones for their growth.

Chan et al. studied the effect of dietary leucine restriction on the tumor growth of Lewis's lung carcinoma. Severely restricted leucine diets brought about a reduction in tumor growth.[144]

Effect on Immunity

The tumor-suppressing action of amino acids may be explained by the split effect on humoral and cellular immunity.[18] Cellular immunity is believed to be a major immunological defense against cancer. Humoral response, i.e., antibody formation, may enhance tumor development by protecting the tumor from cell-mediated immune responses.[145] It is believed that certain amino acid deficiencies can maintain cell-mediated immunity in its entirety, while simultaneously depressing antibody production. The inhibitory effect of low-protein intake on certain types of neoplasms could be explained by this mechanism. Severe protein deficiency could, in addition, alter tumor incidence or site by changing the metabolism of the carcinogenic agent.

Ross and Bras have studied the widely varying effects of protein on different tumors by analyzing the impact of protein nutrition on the endocrine system and on the cell-mediated immune system.[107] These two systems apparently represent opposite forces with respect to their role in the cancer process. It is possible that the net effect of protein metabolism on the endocrinological and immunological systems determines the type and the numbers of tumors.

CARBOHYDRATE

In contrast to lipids and proteins (the other two main macronutrients in the diet), little attention has been directed toward the study of carbohydrate intake and the occurrence of cancer. Sugars, starches, and cellulose are the principal carbohydrates in foods. Evidence related to sugars and starches are evaluated in this section. However, data on cellulose are discussed under dietary fiber in Chapter 3.

Epidemiological Evidence

Sugar and Cancer

There is little epidemiological evidence to support a role for carbohydrates *per se* in the etiology of cancer. The per-capita intake of foods and specific nutrients has been correlated with cancer incidence and mortality in 23 and 32 countries, respectively.[9] A significant direct correlation between sugar intake and pancreatic cancer mortality, but not incidence, was found in women only, in addition to a weak association between liver cancer incidence and the intake of potatoes, which are a starch-rich vegetable. No support for either of these observations has been reported in any case-control studies.

In a study of diet and breast cancer among 41 women in 41 countries, a high intake of refined sugar was one of the dietary components associated with increased incidence of breast cancer.[99] Drasar and Irving observed a direct correlation between breast cancer and the intake of simple sugars in a study of per-capita food intake and cancer risk in 37 countries.[146] These results are consistent with findings in laboratory experiments. However, in an earlier study an inverse relationship was reported between breast cancer incidence and another dietary carbohydrate—starch.[147]

Flour, Cereal, and Cancer

The age- and sex-adjusted mortality rates for stomach cancer in 16 countries were studied by Hakama and Saxen.[148] They found a strong correlation ($r = 0.75$) with the per-capita intake of cereal used as flour from 1934 to 1938.

Starches and Gastric Cancers

Several studies have suggested that the incidence of gastric cancer is influenced by environmental factors. These observations are based on both descriptive and analytical studies. The descriptive data include the wide variation in incidence rates among ethnic, socioeconomic, or racial groups that occurred with migration, as well as the marked decline of incidence rates with time. In analytical studies gastric cancer has been associated with certain food items.

In a controlled study, Modan et al. found more frequent consumption of starches among patients with gastric cancer.[149] This was not merely attributable to a higher frequency of only a few items. For each high-starch food item eaten less frequently by gastric cancer patients, approximately three starchy foods were eaten more frequently. The three foods consumed significantly more frequently among gastric cancer patients were noodles, root beer, and cholent, an Eastern European Jewish dish composed of potatoes, dried beans, barley, beef, and fat cooked together at low heat for 24 hr. High consumption of cereal and potatoes was previously suggested to be related to gastric cancer.[149]

However, in view of the higher incidence of gastric cancer and higher consumption of starches in the lower socioeconomic group, doubts have been raised as to the validity of this association. The greater consumption of starches may merely reflect the fact that gastric cancer patients belong to a lower socioeconomic group. In the study of Modan et al., controls were matched on factors strongly associated with socioeconomic status, i.e., ethnic groups, age, residence, and period of immigration.[149] When these factors were controlled, results still indicated a true increase in starch consumption in gastric cancer cases.

Modan *et al.* proposed that an association between starch consumption and gastric cancer may be related to the physiological effect of food on the stomach. The relationship between hypochlorhydria and gastric cancer is well established. The acid-producing portion of the stomach is highly resistant to carcinogenic agents. Animal studies have shown carbohydrates to have much less of a stimulating effect on gastric acid secretion than do proteins.[150] Possibly long-term habits of frequent consumption of starchy food affect the mechanism of secretion of gastric acid, thereby rendering the gastric mucosa more susceptible to exogenous carcinogens.

An alternate hypothesis may be that higher consumption frequency of carbohydrates associated with some specific eating habits could in turn lead to a greater risk of gastric cancer. A general excess of food consumption may be a possible mechanism leading to a mechanical effect on the gastric mucosa. Although Modan *et al.* found no significant differences between gastric cancer cases and controls for food groups, it is possible that overeaters consume more starches; consequently, starch is the only food group that showed significant differences.

Findings in the study by Modan *et al.* may be spurious, however, if participants in the study did not give accurate reports of foods consumed, which might confound differences between gastric patients and controls. In addition, dietary factors common to both gastric and intestinal cancers might have been overlooked.

De Jong *et al.* studied cases of esophageal cancer and hospital controls in Singapore.[151] These workers reported a direct association between consumption of bread and potatoes—major sources of carbohydrate—and risk of esophageal cancer. However, observations by other investigators have not supported such associations.

Other Dietary Factors and Stomach Cancer

Although consumption of starches may have an important role in the gastric cancer process, other factors may be important in the gastric cancer process.

Incidence. Gastric cancer mortality patterns show widely varying cross-national incidence.[61] Areas of high incidence include Japan, Latin America west of the Andes, parts of the Caribbean, Iceland, and Northern and Eastern Europe.

The high incidence of stomach cancer observed in Japan might be related to the consumption of large amounts of starch in the form of rice. In contrast, low incidences have been observed in Western Europe, the United States, Canada, Australia, New Zealand, and other Anglo-Saxon countries. Even though gastric cancer was the most common cancer in the United States 40 years ago, the age-adjusted death rates in the United States are among the lowest of all countries, with a rate of 8:100,000 in White males and 17:100,000 in Black males.

In addition to the marked international variation in risk, variation within countries has been observed with the northern or colder regions having greater risk. The rate of cancer of the stomach is higher in the mountainous region of Croatia, Yugoslavia, in contrast to the lower risk observed on the Adriatic coast. Mortality from gastric cancer in the Japanese prefectures of southern Kyushu is extremely low. An especially high mortality has been observed in the north-western part of Iceland and in certain cities in the tropical zone of Latin America, including Bogota and Cali, Colombia, Guatemala City, and Lima, and the population in the mountainous central Andean region. In contrast to this latter incidence, the residents of the tropical coastal zones in Latin America are at low risk.

The incidence of stomach cancer in males is greater than in females within cell populations, with the overall female rate one-half to two-thirds the male rate. Cancer of the glandular stomach with its antecedent intestinalization has a different etiology; it can be distinguished from diffuse stomach cancer, which is associated with blood group A, and possibly pernicious anemia. A marked inverse socioeconomic gradient in risk is a prominent characteristic of this disease with the risk for the lower class about 2.5 times that of the higher.

Migratory Studies. Several important clues to the etiology of stomach cancer have come from the study of the epidemiological data of human migration. Immigrants to the United States from countries with a high risk of stomach cancer continued to experience a risk characteristic of that seen in their nation of origin. In general, similar gastric cancer mortality did not appear until the succeeding generation. Studies of Australian immigrants yielded similar results. In Cali, Colombia, a marked excess of stomach cancer was observed among migrants born in the mountainous region bordering Ecuador.

In a controlled study of Hawaiian Japanese, Haenszel *et al.* found that migrants from Japanese areas of high stomach cancer risk continued to experience an excess risk in Hawaii, but this effect did not persist among their nisei (second-generation) offspring.[152] Lower risks were observed for the niesei, but not issei (first-generation), who probably still had not adopted Western-style diets. These results seem to reinforce earlier influences from migrant study data on the critical nature of early life exposures.[153] The decrease in stomach cancer mortality among second-generation Hawaiian Japanese is not likely due to the result of improved diagnostic or treatment methods, but may be explained by the decreased consumption of traditional Japanese foods.

Food Consumption and Gastric Cancer

Per-Capita Food Consumption Studies/Numerous investigators have correlated the national per-capita average amounts of selected food items and available nutrients with stomach cancer mortality. In general, negative correlations
have been found between age-standardized international mortality from stomach
cancer and the consumption of fats, oils, animal protein, and sugar. Another
study has shown a negative correlation between incidence and mortality rates of
stomach cancer with total fat consumption and a positive association between
incidence rates and fish consumption. This latter positive association for fish
consumption is entirely dependent on the extreme values for Japan and Iceland.
Although the fish-consumption factor is highly relevant to Iceland and Japan, it
probably does not contribute significantly with the stomach cancer in other
countries.

In other countries high stomach cancer incidence in certain areas has been
related to high intake of salted foods and certain smoked foods and has been
associated with widespread use of sodium intake as a fertilizer and high levels of
nitrate in the drinking water. Where sweet potatoes are a staple food in some
areas of Japan, stomach cancer is particularly low. Sweet potatoes and vegetables are relatively abundant in the southernmost district of Kagoshima, which has
the lowest mortality from stomach cancer. Higher intakes of vitamin C due to
higher consumption of potatoes and rutabagas have been observed in the low-
mortality areas of Iceland. The prevalent availability of fruits and vegetables in
Yugoslavian areas along the Adriatic coast may be responsible for the low gastric
cancer mortality.

Dietary Surveys/Surveys of dietary habits of the people of Chokai village in
a rural Akita district, Japan, which has high death rates for stomach cancer, as
well as comparisons with dietary habits of Hawaiian Japanese and Hawaiian
Caucasians indicate that the specific food items are extremely different among
the three groups. The Hawaiian Japanese have a higher intake of uncooked
vegetables such as celery, lettuce, and tomato and of fresh fruit juices. However,
the most prominent dietary item in the district of Akita is a large intake of dried
fish and miso soup, both of which have a high salt content.

Controlled Studies/Controlled studies of diet and stomach cancer have been
complicated by problems with accuracy of histories and informant control. Some
studies have not been rewarding, but diet inquiries have steadily improved.

Haenszel *et al.* associated elevated gastric cancer risk with consumption of
pickled vegetables and dried salted fish as well as greater risk with increased
consumption of these food items.[152] However, the companion controlled study
in Hiroshima and the Miyagi districts of Japan did not reproduce the associations
with pickled vegetables and salted dried fish, which were reported for the Hawai-

ian Japanese. Low risks were identified for Hawaiian Japanese for several Western-type vegetables, such as lettuce, celery, tomatoes, and corn; and the latter effects appeared to be independent of the associations with Japanese foods.

In Norway and Minnesota, USA controlled studies of stomach cancer have been conducted for people of Scandinavian descent.[154] In Norway there was greater use of cooked cereal (high starch) and consumption of salted fish was greater among the stomach cancer patients than among the controls. The greatest differences from the controls were observed for total vegetable intake and for vitamin C intake with the greatest differences observable among young patients and women.

Recent use of cooked cereals, smoked fish, and canned fruits was greater and intake of lettuce and tomatoes lower among Minnesota stomach cancer patients than among controls. In addition, whereas total intake of cereal products and or fish was only slightly greater than among the control groups, the index for total vegetables was considerably lower among the gastric cancer patients. In both the Norway and Minnesota studies, lower vegetable and vitamin C intake among the gastric cancer patients which had persisted for a long time was more pronounced among women, and the type of gastric carcinoma was mainly the diffuse type in both sexes. In another study the diet of gastric cancer patients in the United States has been found to include fewer vegetables.[155]

Nitrates/Hartman observed a correlation coefficient of 0.88 between the gastric cancer death rate and the nitrate intake per person per day in 12 countries (Fig. 2-6).[156] An association was reported between the consumption of salted fish and the incidence of gastric cancer in Japan, which had the highest death rate due to gastric cancer. Crude salt for fish preservation may contain nitrate, which can be reduced to nitrite. High rates of gastric cancer are reported in South America, Chile, and some regions of Colombia and Costa Rica, which have large nitrate deposits and correspondingly elevated levels of nitrate in the food and drinking water. Hill *et al.* observed a positive correlation between nitrate levels in drinking water and the incidence of gastric cancer in Worksop, England.[157] In Worksop, the high nitrate content of the drinking water resulted in a weekly nitrate intake more than double that of people living in Paddington, England, which is a low-risk area for gastric cancer. Measurements of daily excretion of nitrate in the urine of Worksop people showed levels three times higher than in Paddington. Similar results were also observed in another study in Colombia.

Tannenbaum *et al.* investigated human gastric juice samples from high- and low-risk areas (Colombia and Boston) for factors that influence the stability of nitrite and its potential for nitrosamine formation.[158] Samples from individuals with chronic atrophic gastritis and intestinal metaplasia were not reactive to nitrite and supported a rate of nitrosation largely compatible with the nitrite and thiocyanate concentration. Samples from normal individuals contained factors

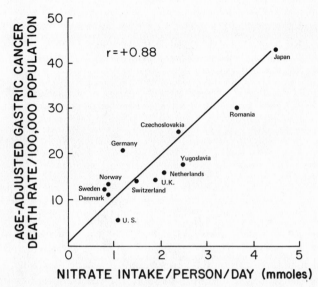

Figure 2-6. Relationship of age-adjusted gastric cancer mortality rates and nitrate ingestion in 12 countries. (By permission of Hartman 1983, *Envir. Mutagen. 5:* 111–121.)

that destroyed nitrite and inhibited nitrosation. Some samples from both groups had an elevated rate of nitrosation catalyzed by unknown factors. There is possibility that continued hypochlorhydria might deplete gastric juice of its natural protective factors and lead to an elevated risk of gastric cancer. The etiology of gastric cancer seems to be complex, and apparently the nitrate factor is insufficient to explain the occurrence of this disease.

Summary of Factors/The above studies indicate that a population with risk consumes a diet high in carbohydrates and low in fat with limited protein intake, limited micronutrients on an annual basis, and perhaps of greater relevance, low levels of select micronutrients, especially vitamin C, on a seasonal basis. People prone to gastric cancer consume limited amounts of fresh fruits and vegetables. Other risk factors include increased consumption of pickled, highly salted, and smoked foods or foods grown in soils high in nitrate content. Studies on migrants from high- to low-risk regions have indicated that people with lowered risk include lettuce and other fresh greens as part of their daily diet.

Experimental Evidence

The relationship between carbohydrates and cancer has been studied only in a few laboratory experiments. In general, these studies have been conducted by varying the concentration of the test substance such as starch, sucrose, dextrin or glucose, in a basal diet. In many experiments little attention has been given to the differences in the caloric content of the control and the experimental diets. The variation in carbohydrate content, resulting from attempts to "balance" diets on a weight basis, has generally been overlooked. There have been several studies that have focused on the effects of long-term carbohydrate feeding on tumorigenesis.

Sucrose

The results of long-term (more than 1 year) feeding or systemic administration of sucrose on spontaneously occurring tumors have been studied in both mice and rats. In one experiment sucrose was fed to mice at 10% by weight of the diet (15 gm/kg body weight), and in the other, rats were fed sucrose at 77% by weight of the diet (40 gm/kg body weight).[159,160] There were no increases in the incidence of tumors in either study. In several other experiments neither intraperitoneal or subcutaneous injections of sucrose given over various lengths of time nor systemic administration of 20% sucrose given twice weekly for 2 years produced any evidence of carcinogenesis in either rats or mice.

A higher incidence of hepatocellular tumors was observed in females, but not the male CFLP mice fed 20% sucrose for 2 years.[161] The same investigators also conducted parallel feeding studies in which 20% sucrose diets were fed to male and female Sprague-Dawley rats for up to 1 year and to male and female beagle dogs for up to 2 years. There was no evidence that sucrose contributed to tumorigenesis.

The effect of dietary carbohydrates has been evaluated on chemically induced tumors in rats.[162] After breast tumors were induced with DMBA, rats were fed diets containing either refined sugars or complex starches. Significantly more breast tumors were observed in the rats fed refined sugar than in those fed starch. Obviously much more experimental work is required before a conclusion can be reached in regard to a possible relationship between sucrose and carcinogenesis.

Lactose

The interaction of dietary lactose (49%) or sucrose (43–55% total weight) with vitamin A deficiency in the production of primary urinary bladder calculi in male Charles River rats has been studied by Gershoff and McGandy.[163] There was a small percentage of the rats fed lactose in a diet with sufficient vitamin A that developed vesicle stones. In contrast, about 60% of the rats fed lactose in vitamin A-deficient diets developed bladder calculi. The bladder walls in most of the affected rats were grossly hypertrophic and also had focal areas of transitional cell hyperplasia. Histologic changes consistent with grade I to II transitional cell carcinomas were observed in about 30% of the stone-containing bladders. In these experiments it was not possible to determine whether the deficiency of vitamin A contributed directly to bladder tumors or indirectly via stone formation and subsequent physical irritation of the bladder. The rats fed sucrose with or without superimposed vitamin A deficiency did not exhibit calculi or histological changes of the bladder. Apparently this was one of the first studies to demonstrate the production of tumors without an exogenous source of a carcinogen in animals that were not genetically predisposed to tumor formation.

Glucose

Dietary glucose has been implicated in the development of carcinogen-induced tumors in the large bowel in a preliminary report by Ingram and Castleden.[164] Male Wistar rats were fed Milne's Standard Laboratory Diet and were given drinking water *ad libitum* either with or without 1.6% glucose. Both groups were injected subcutaneously with 1,2-dimethylhydrazine to induce bowel tumors. There were no significant differences in the number of small bowel tumors per rat in the two groups; however, the rats given the glucose solution developed almost twice the number of small bowel tumors in rats given the drinking water alone. There are some problems in interpreting this experiment because about 35% of the Milne Standard Laboratory Diet is composed of carbohydrates, and this diet was fed to both groups of animals. Therefore, the contribution of this diet to blood glucose levels is much greater than the carbohydrates supplied by the 1.6% glucose in water solution. There is a possibility that the observed results were an indirect effect of the glucose in water solution rather than a direct effect of glucose.

Xylitol

Xylitol is present in many natural foods and its sweetness is approximately equal to that of sucrose. In a 2-year feeding study, Hunter *et al.* fed CFLP male and female mice either 0, 2%, 10%, or 20% xylitol in the diet for as long as 106 weeks.[165] In the groups fed the 10% or 20% xylitol diets, there was a reduction in spontaneous hepatocellular tumors in the males, but not in the females. In the male mice fed the 10% or 20% xylitol diets, there was a reduction in the spontaneous hepatocellular tumors. This effect was not observed in the females. In general, the males in these dietary groups had more crystalline bladder calculi as well as an associated increase in hyperplasia, metaplasia, and neoplasia of the transitional epithelium of the bladder than did the females fed similar diets, the control mice, or the mice fed 2% xylitol.

In another experiment Sprague-Dawley CD rats were fed 2%, 5%, 10%, or

20% xylitol for 26 weeks without evidence of increased renal calculi or hepato-cellular abnormalities at autopsy.[165] However, in the rats fed 5%, 10%, or 20% xylitol, the incidence of adrenal medullary hyperplasia was greater than in the controls. When male and female beagle dogs were fed 10% or 20% mannitol for 52 weeks, the only different pathological change was an increased liver weight at autopsy. Along with this slight hepatomegaly there was a hepatocyte enlarge-ment as well as an altered hepatocyte appearance in the periportal areas of the dogs.

The amount of xylitol in the 20% diet approaches the LD_{50} for xylitol in mice. In rats, ingestion of a 20% xylitol diet may exceed the maximum metabolic turnover rate as calculated from rates observed in humans.

The evidence concerning the role of carbohydrates in the development of cancer in humans is extremely limited. The data from the few laboratory experi-ments designed to study the role of carbohydrates in carcinogenesis are difficult to interpret because of generally poor experimental design and there is also uncertainty about the actual carbohydrate content of the foods used in the experi-mental test diets. Thus, the evidence from both epidemiological and laboratory studies is too sparse to suggest a direct role for carbohydrates (excluding fiber) in carcinogenesis. However, excessive carbohydrate consumption contributes to caloric excess, which has in turn been implicated as a modifier of carcinogenesis. Caloric restriction has also been shown to be important in modifying carcino-genesis.

Raw Soya Flour and Azaserine Carcinogenesis

Animals. A diet of raw soya flour is known to stimulate pancreatic prolifera-tion, with the production of pancreatic hyperplasia and subsequently neo-plasia.[166] Tissues in a state of cellular proliferation are known to be abnormally sensitive to the action of carcinogens. For this reason McGuinness et al. de-signed a study to determine whether a diet of raw or cooked soya flour would sensitize the pancreas of rats to the action of a weak pancreatic carcinogen (azaserine). The rats fed a diet of raw soya flour and given weekly injections of azaserine developed benign and malignant neoplasms of the pancreas earlier in life and much more frequently than rats given raw soya flour alone. However, azaserine alone in the dose used in this study did not produce pancreatic cancer. Apparently the raw soya flour sensitizes the pancreas to the action of azaserine. Cooked soya flour had no cancer-enhancing effect.

It is not known which component(s) of soya flour is/are responsible for the pancreatic carcinogenic and sensitizing effects. It is likely that the soybean trypsin inhibitor is responsible, at least in part (as shown by the beneficial effects of heat treatment on the soya flour) responsible for the production of experimen-tal pancreatic cancer. Because of the probable effect of soybean trypsin inhibitor, the effect of other protease inhibitors in legumes, cereals, tubers, and so forth should also be assessed in the production of experimental pancreatic cancer.

These results also indicate that in the studies of experimental pancreatic carcinogenesis, it would be important to control dietary conditions, because some of the commercial rat chows contain much soya flour.

Humans. It is not known whether the human pancreas is affected by soya flour. However, soya products are used widely in human nutrition. In many cases soya products are sometimes the sole source of nutrition, as in some infant foods, and are sometimes recommended in the treatment of other diseases, such as in the treatment of hyperlipoproteinemia. These observations illustrate the great complexity of the interaction of nutrition and carcinogens, because it has been shown that dietary protease inhibitors actually protect against the promotion of experimental cancer, i.e., skin and mammary gland. From the results of these studies, it is apparent that a complex balance exists between the deleterious and beneficial effects of nutrients.

Caloric Intake

A number of factors complicate the interpretation of the effect of caloric intake on cancer incidence. Even though this discussion is placed in the carbohydrate section of this chapter, certainly caloric density can be modified either by changing the ratio of fat (9.5 kcal/gm) to carbohydrate (4.0 kcal/gm) or by varying the concentration of nonnutritive bulk (fiber). However, since dietary fat and fiber may also affect carcinogenesis, it is difficult to measure any independent effect of calories.

In general, it is not possible to identify the effect of caloric intake on cancer incidence in human studies. Although total caloric intake by two populations can be compared, the interpretation of the data is limited. It is also difficult to interpret studies in which the prevalence of obesity is compared with cancer incidence. Obesity is known to be related to the balance between caloric intake and caloric expenditure, but the relative contributions of caloric intake and caloric expenditure to cancer risk is not known. There is also evidence that obesity is related to the consumption of diets with increased caloric density. Thus, the concentrations of fat, fiber, and carbohydrate cannot be easily assessed independently.

Epidemiological Evidence. Few epidemiological studies have been done correlating total caloric intake to cancer risk, partly because most dietary studies have been based on preselected food lists, which do not permit the quantification of total dietary intake. International distribution of hormone-dependent cancers has generated suspicion that these cancers may be related to a high standard of living.[167] It is possible that diets typical of affluent populations, when ingested since childhood, could overstimulate the endocrine system, leading to aberrations in the metabolic processes that could result in cancer.

Gastrointestinal Cancer/Gregor et al. compared data on caloric intake and the incidence of gastric and intestinal cancers.[102] They found that as per-capita food intake (or gross national product) increases, gastric cancer mortality decreases, but those for intestinal cancer increase. In a study of mortality from colorectal cancer in three socioeconomic groups in Hong Kong, Hill *et al.* found that the most affluent group has more than twice the mortality of the least affluent group (i.e., 26.7 in 100,000 vs. 11.7 in 100,000.[54] The relative proportions of nutrients in their diets were similar, but in the lowest socioeconomic group the estimated daily caloric intake was 2700 and 3900 in the highest.

Armstrong and Doll correlated the per-capita total caloric intake to the cancer incidence in 23 countries and to cancer mortality in 32 countries.[9] Significant correlations were observed for total calories and rectal cancer incidence in males, leukemia in males, and mortality from breast cancer in females. The per-capita intake of calories was highly correlated with intake of total fat, total protein, and animal protein. Gaskill *et al.* reproduced the findings for breast cancer.[2] Mortality from breast cancer was directly correlated to the per-capita intake for foods by state within the United States. However, they found no correlation when they controlled for age at first marriage. This latter factor reflects age at first pregnancy.

In a controlled study, a number of dietary variables, including total caloric and fat intake, were estimated for individuals with cancer of the colon and rectum as well as for matched controls.[11] Jain *et al.* found a direct association with caloric intake and both colon and rectal cancer, but the associations were not as strong as they were for intake of saturated fat. Jain *et al.* concluded that the relevant variable in each study was more likely to be dietary fat than caloric intake.[27]

Breast Cancer/In another case-control study, a number of dietary variables including total caloric and fat intake were estimated for subjects with breast cancer as well as for matched controls.[6] Miller *et al.* found no association between caloric intake and breast cancer and a weak association between total dietary fat and caloric intakes.[38] In a cohort of postmenopausal women in the Netherlands, associations were made in two studies between breast cancer and body weight and height. Associations of weight and cases have been reported in Taiwan and in Sao Paulo, Brazil. The concept that susceptibility to breast cancer could be related to body mass, which in turn could be related to nutrition was suggested by deWaard,[168] but this hypothesis has not been accepted universally. In a subsequent study de Waard *et al.* examined the influence of height and weight on the age-specific incidence of breast cancer in the Netherlands and Japan, and computed age-specific incidence curves for the various height and weight groups.[169] The highest incidence of breast cancer was found in the postmenopausal women who were heavier and taller. However, there appeared to be little independent effect of weight if there was an adjustment for its correlation with height. In de Waard's earlier study lean body mass seemed to be an important variable. If height is important (and it is critical to the calculation of lean body mass, nutritional factors, if important, may begin to operate during adolescence or earlier. de Waard *et al.* suggested that approximately one half of the difference in the incidence of breast cancer between Holland and Japan may result from differences in body weight and height.[169]

Other Sites. Lew and Garfinkel studied the relationship between mortality from cancer and other diseases and variation in weight among 750,000 men and women selected from the general population.[170] This analysis was based on a long-term propective study conducted by the American Cancer Society from 1959 to 1972. Total cancer mortality was significantly elevated in both sexes who had other diseases, but only among those who were 40% or more overweight. In the case of males, most of the excess mortality resulted from cancer of the colon and rectum; for women, cancer of the gallbladder and biliary passages, breast, cervix, endometrium, and ovary were the major sites. It was not possible to evaluate the relative importance of overweight in comparison to the total caloric intake or intake of other nutrients. Therefore, assumptions that obesity is the major risk factor may not be correct. However, since most studies confirm a relationship between obesity and caloric intake, and in the absence of definite information from studies that separated the effects of caloric intake and fat intakes,[6,27] it seems reasonable to assume that high total caloric intake is a risk factor for some sites.

Experiments in Animals

Caloric Restriction and Benzpyrene-Induced Tumors/The effects of caloric restriction on the development of spontaneous and chemically induced tumors in several strains of mice have been examined by Tannenbaum.[171] Caloric restriction inhibited the growth of benzpyrene-induced tumors to different extents in ABC, Swiss, or DBA mice. The growth of skin tumors or spontaneous and chemically induced breast tumors was affected by the level of dietary fat, but the growth of sarcomas and lung tumors were not affected. Caloric intake was restricted by controlling the amount of starch added to a diet containing commercial ration and skim milk powder. In the groups of mice whose daily dietary intake was 11.7 calories, there were 25% more spontaneous mammary tumors than the mice whose intake was limited to 9.6 tumors. The incidence of benzpyrene-induced tumors was similar in the groups of mice ingesting 11.7 and 9.6 cal/day, but when the caloric intake dropped to 8.1 cal/day, tumor incidence fell by 38%. Among the mice receiving 11.7 cal/day, those receiving 18% of their calories from fat developed 70% more spontaneous mammary tumors than those whose diets contained only 2% fat (about 4% of calories). Tannenbaum concluded that dietary fat intake exerted a specific influence over and above its caloric contribution.

Caloric Restriction and 3-Methylcholanthrene-Induced Tumors/The influence of caloric restriction was also tested in a study of 3-methylcholanthrene-induced skin tumors in mice fed *ad libitum* and in a control group placed on a restricted diet. After the carcinogen was painted on the skin for 10 weeks, the mice were then observed for 1 year. From this and earlier studies, Tannenbaum concluded that the carcinogen-induced changes occur regardless of diet, but that *ad libitum* ingestion of diet promotes development of tumors.[42]

The promoting action of different levels of dietary fat on 3-methylcholanthrene-induced skin tumors in mice were studied by Lavik and Baumann.[70] The fewest tumors resulted from a low fat, low-calorie diet. Similar results were found when either lard with high (saturated) and low (unsaturated) melting points. The addition of riboflavin to the diet had a slight promoting effect, but the major effect on carcinogenesis was produced by high caloric intake.

Other Carcinogens

Some studies show that caloric restriction has not caused tumor reduction. Tumorigenesis of the liver by azo dyes appeared to be enhanced by low caloric intake.[172] However, the carcinogen was so highly concentrated in the diet of the calorie-restricted animals that most died, making it difficult to evaluate the effects of energy intake. In another experiment castrated C3H mice showed an equal incidence of adrenal adenomas whether fed *ad libitum* or a calorie-restricted diet.[173]

Ross and Bas studied the influence of caloric restriction during the early postweaning period on tumors later in life.[174] Rats were fed *ad libitum* throughout life or restricted for 7 weeks immediately after weaning followed by *ad libitum* feeding for the remainder of their life. If there was a limited period of restricted food intake, even if followed by *ad libitum* feeding, the number of animals with tumors was reduced. The amount of reduction varied from 14% to 83%, depending on the tissue. Rats feed on a restricted intake regimen for 7 weeks after weaning consistently ate less even if subsequently allowed to eat *ad libitum*. This may have contributed to the lower body weights and fewer tumors in this treatment group. The lighter half of each population consistently showed fewer tumors than the heavier subgroup. These results are consistent with the epidemiological studies in man that show that cancer mortality increases with the degree of overweight. It is likely that undernutrition reduces cell division and may permantly influence cell populations in various organs.

Thus neither the epidemiological nor the experimental studies show a clear pattern of the specific effect of caloric intake on the risk of cancer. However, animal studies show that a reduction in total food intake decreases the age-specific incidence of cancer. The evidence for humans is much less clear.

REFERENCES

1. Carroll, K. K., and Khor, H. T. 1975. Experimental evidence of dietary factors and hormone-dependent cancers. *Cancer Res. 35:*3374–3383.
2. Gaskill, S. P., McGuire, W. L., Osborne, C. K., and Stern, M. P. 1979. Breast cancer mortality and diet in the United States. *Cancer Res. 39:*3628–3637.
3. Hems, G. 1980. Associations between breast-cancer mortality rates, child-bearing and diet in the United Kingdom. *Br. J. Cancer 41:*429–437.
4. Kolonel, L. N., Hankin, J. H., Lee, J., Chu, S. Y., Nomura, A. M. Y., and Hinds, M. W. 1981. Nutrient intakes in relation to cancer incidence in Hawaii. *Br. J. Cancer 44:*332–339.
5. Phillips, R. L. 1975. Role of life-style and dietary habits in risk of cancer among seventh-Day Adventists. *Cancer Res. 35:*3513–3522.
6. Miller, A. B., Kelly, A., Choi, N. W., Matthews, V., Morgan, R. W., Munan, L., Burch, J. D., Feather, J., Howe, G. R., and Jain, M. 1978. A study of diet and breast cancer. *Am. J. Epidemiol. 107:*499–509.
7. Lubin, J. H., Burns, P. E., Blot, W. J., Ziegler, R. G., Lees, A. W., and Fraumeni, J. F. 1981. Dietary factors and breast cancer risk. *Int. J. Cancer 28:*865–869.
8. Nomura, A., Henderson, B. E., and Lee, J. 1978. Breast cancer and diet among the Japanese in Hawaii. *Am. J. Clin. Nutr. 31:*2020–2025.
9. Armstrong, B., and Doll, R. 1975. Environmental factors and cancer incidence and mortality in different countries, with special reference to dietary practices. *Int. J. Cancer 15:*617–631.
10. Howell, M. A. 1974. Factor analysis of international cancer mortality data and *per capita* food consumption. *Br. J. Cancer 29:*328–336.
11. Blair, A., and Fraumeni, J. F. 1978. Geographic patterns of prostate cancer in the United States. *J. Natl. Cancer Inst. 61:*1379–13844.
12. Hirayama, T. 1977. Changing patterns of cancer in Japan with special reference to the decrease in stomach cancer mortality. in H. H. Hiatt, J. D. Watson, and J. A. Winsten (eds.) *Origins of human cancer*, Book A: *Incidence of cancer in humans.* pp. 55–75. Cold Spring Harbor, New York: Cold Spring Harbor Laboratory.
13. Rotkin, I. D. 1977. Studies in the epidemiology of prostatic cancer: Expanded sampling. *Cancer Treatm. Rep. 61:*173–180.
14. Schuman, L. M., Mandell, J. S., Radke, A., Seal, U., and Halberg, F. 1982. Some selected features of the epidemiology of prostatic cancer: Minneapolis-St. Paul, Minnesota case-control study, 1976–1979. in K. Magnus (ed.) *Trends in cancer incidence. Causes and practical implications.* pp. 345–354. New York: Hemisphere.
15. Lingeman, C. M. 1974. Etiology of cancer of the human ovary: A review. *J. Natl. Cancer Inst. 53:*1603–1618.
16. Carroll, K. K., and Khor, H. T. 1975. Dietary fat in relation to tumorigenesis. *Prog. Biochem. Pharmacol. 10:*308–353.

17. Higginson, J. 1966. Etiological factors in gastrointestinal cancer in man. *J. Natl. Cancer Inst.* *37*:527–545.
18. Graham, S., Schotz, W., and Martino, P. 1972. Alimentary factors in the epidemiology of gastric cancer. *Cancer 30*:927–938.
19. Lea, A. J. 1967. Neoplasma and environmental factors. *Ann. R. Coll. Surg. Engl. 41*:432–438.
20. Knox, E. G. 1977. Foods and diseases. *Br. J. Prev. Soc. Med. 31*:71–80.
21. Enig, M. G., Munn, R. J., and Keeney, M. 1979. (Response to letters.) *Fed. Proc. 38*:37–39.
22. Lyon, J. L., and Sorenson, A. W. 1978. Colon cancer in a low-risk population. *Am. J. Clin. Nutr. 31*:5227–5230.
23. MacLennan, R., Jensen, O. M., Mosbech, J., and Vuori, H. 1978. Diet, transit time, stool weight, and colon cancer in two Scandinavian populations. *Am. J. Clin. Nutr. 31*:5239–5242.
24. Reddy, B. S., Hedges, A. R., Laakso, K., and Wynder, E. L. 1978. Metabolic epidemiology of large bowel cancer: Fecal bulk and constituents of high-risk North American and low-risk Finnish populations. *Cancer 42*:2832–2838.
25. Dales, L. G., Friedman, G. D., Ury, H. K., Grossman, S., and Williams, S. R. 1978. A case-control study of relationships of diets and other traits to colorectal cancer in American blacks. *Am. J. Epidemiol. 109*:132–144.
26. Martinez, L., Torres, R., Frias, Z., Colon, J. R., and Fernandez, M. 1979. Factors associated with adenocarcinomas of the large bowel in Puerto Rico. in J. M. Birch (ed.) *Advances in medical oncology, research and education.* Vol. 3: *Epidemiology.* pp. 45–52. New York: Pergamon Press.
27. Jain, M., Cook, G. M., Davis, F. G., Grace, M. G., Howe, G. R., and Miller, A. B. 1980. A case-control study of diet and colo-rectal cancer. *Int. J. Cancer 26*:757–768.
28. Howell, M. A. 1975. Diet as an etiological factor in the development of cancers of the colon and rectum. *J. Chronic Dis. 28*:67–80.
29. Haenszel, W., Berg, J. W., Segi, M., Kwihara, M., and Locke, F. B. 1973. Large-bowel cancer in Hawaiian Japanese. *J. Natl. Cancer Inst. 51*:1765–1779.
30. Enstrom, J. E. 1975. Colorectal cancer and consumption of beef and fat. *Br. J. Cancer 32*:432–439.
31. Ishii, K., Nakamura, K., Ozaki, H., Yamada, N., and Takeuchi, T. 1968. Epidemiological problems of pancreas cancer. *Jpn. J. Clin. Med. 26*:1839–1842.
32. Liu, K., Stampler, J., Moss, D., Garside, D., Persky, V., and Soltero, I. 1979. Dietary cholesterol, fat and fibre, and colon-cancer mortality. *Lancet 2*:782–785.
33. Pearce, M. L., and Dayton, S. 1971. Incidence of cancer in men on a diet high in polyunsaturated fat. *Lancet 1*:464–467.
34. Miettinen, M., Turpeinen, O., Karronen, J., Elosuo, R., and Paavilainen, E. 1972. Effect of cholesterol-lowering diet on mortality from coronary heart—causes and other causes: A twelve-year clinical trial in men and women. *Lancet 2*:835–838.
35. Ederer, F., Leven, P., Turpeinen, O., and Frantz, D. 1971. Cancer among men on cholesterol-lowering diets: Experience from five clinical trials. *Lancet 2*:203–206.
36. Rose, G., Blackburn, H., Keys, A., Taylor, H. L., Kannel, W. B., Paul, O., Reid, D. D., and Stamler, J. 1974. Colon cancer and blood-cholesterol. *Lancet 1*:181–183
37. Bjelke, E. 1974. Colon cancer and blood-cholesterol. *Lancet 1*:1116–1117.
38. Nydegger, U. E., and Butler, R. E. 1972. Serum lipoprotein levels in patients with cancer. *Cancer Res. 32*:1756–1760.
39. Committee on Principal Investigators. 1978. A cooperative trial in the primary prevention of ischaemic heart disease using clofibrate. *Br. Heart J. 40*:1069–1118.
40. Beaglehole, R., Faulkes, M. A., Prior, A. M., and Eyles, E. F. 1980. Cholesterol and mortality in New Zealand Maoris. *Br. Med. J. 280*:285–287.

41. Rose, G., and Shipley, M. J. 1980. Plasma lipids and mortality: A source of error. *Lancet* *1*:523–526.
42. International Collaborative Group. 1982. Circulating cholesterol level and risk of death from cancer in man aged 40 to 69 years. *JAMA 248*:2853–2859.
43. Williams, R. R., Sorlie, P. D., Feinleib, M., McNamara, P. M., Kannel, W. R., and Dawber, T. R. 1981. Cancer incidence by levels of cholesterol. *JAMA 245*:247–252.
44. Kark, J. D., Smith, A. H., and Hames, C. G. 1980. The relationship of serum cholesterol to the incidence of cancer in Evans County, Georgia. *J. Chronic Dis. 33*:311–322.
45. Stamler, J., Berkson, D. M., Linber, H. A., Miller, W. A., Soyugene, C. R., Tokish, T., and Whipple, T. 1968. Does hypercholesterolemia increase risk of lung cancer in cigarette smokers? *Circulation* 6 (*Suppl.*) 188.
46. Kagan, A., McGee, D. L., Yano, K., Rhoads, G. G., and Nomura, A. 1981. Serum cholesterol and mortality in a Japanese-American population. *Am. J. Epidemiol. 114*:11–20.
47. Kozarevic, D., McGee, D., Vojvodic, N., Gordon, T., Racic, Z., Zukel, W., and Dawber, T. 1981. Serum.cholesterol and mortality. The Yugoslavia cardiovascular disease study. *Am. J. Epidemiol. 114*:21–28.
48. Garcia-Palmieri, M. R., Sorlie, P. D., Costas, R., and Havlik, R. J. 1981. An apparent inverse relationship between serum cholesterol and cancer mortality in Puerto Rico. *Am. J. Epidemiol. 114*:29–40.
49. Peterson, B., Trell, E., and Sternby, N. H. 1981. Low cholesterol level as risk factor for noncoronary death in middle-aged men. *JAMA 245*:2056–2057.
50. Lilienfeld, A. M. 1981. The humean fog: Cancer and cholesterol. *Am. J. Epidemiol. 114*:1–4.
51. Westlund, K., and Nicolaysen, R. 1972. Ten-year mortality and morbidity related to serum cholesterol. *Scand. J. Clin. Invest. Suppl. 127*:1–24.
52. Dyer, A. R., Stamler, J., Paul, O., Shekelle, R. B., Schoenberger, J. A., Berkson, D. M., Lepper, M., Collette, P., Shekelle, S., and Lindberg, H. A. 1981. Serum cholesterol and risk of death from cancer and other causes in three Chicago epidemiological studies. *J. Chronic Dis. 34*:249–260.
53. Miller, S. R., Tartter, P. I., Papatestas, A. E., Slater, G., and Aufses, A. H. 1981. Serum cholesterol and human colon cancer. *J. Natl. Cancer Inst. 67*:297–300.
54. Hill, M., MacLennan, R., and Newcomb, K. 1979. Diet and large bowel cancer in three socioeconomic groups in Hong Kong. *Lancet 1*:436.
55. Reddy, B. S. 1979. Nutrition and colon cancer. *Adv. Nutr. Res. 2*:199–218.
56. Nomura, A. M. Y., Wilkins, T. D., Kamiyami, S., Heilbrun, L. K., Shimada, A., Stemmermann, G. N., and Mower, H. F. 1983. Fecal neutral steroids in two Japanese populations with different colon cancer risks. *Cancer Res. 43*:1910–1913.
57. Reddy, B. S., and Wynder, E. L. 1973. Large bowel carcinogenesis: Fecal constituents of populations with diverse incidence rates of colon cancer. *J. Natl. Cancer Inst. 50*:1437–1442.
58. Hill, M. J., Drasar, B. S., Aries, V., Crowther, J. S., Hawksworth, G., and Williams, R. E. O. 1971. Bacteria and aetiology of cancer of the large bowel. *Lancet 1*:95–100.
59. Reddy, B. S., Mangat, S., Sheinfil, A., Weisburger, J. H., and Wynder, E. L. 1977. Effect of type and amount of dietary fat and 1,2-dimethylhydrazine on biliary bile acids, fecal bile acids, and neutral sterols in rats. *Cancer Res. 37*:2132–2137.
60. Marisawa, T., Magadia, N. E., Weisburger, J. H., and Wynder, E. L. 1974. Promoting effect of bile acids on colon carcinogenesis after intrarectal instillation of N-methyl-N-nitro-N-nitrosoguanidine in rats. *J. Natl. Cancer Inst. 53*:1093–1097.
61. Reddy, B. S., Cohen, L. A., McCoy, G. D., Hill, P., Weisburger, J. H., and Wynder, E. L. 1980. Nutrition and its relationship to cancer. *Adv. Cancer Res. 32*:237–345.
62. Cohen, B. I., Raicht, R. F., Deschner, E. E., Fazzini, E., Takahashi, M., and Sarwal, A.

1978. Effects of bile acids on induced colon cancer in rats. *Proc. Am. Assoc. Cancer Res. Am. Soc. Clin. Oncol. 19*:48.

63. Broitman, S. A. 1981. Cholesterol excretion and colon cancer. *Cancer Res. 41*:3738–3740.

64. Nigro, N. D., Campbell, R. L., Gantt, J. S., Lim, Y. N., and Singh, D. V. 1977. A comparison of the effect of the hypocholesteremic agents, cholestyramine and candicidin on the induction of intestinal tumors by azoxymethane. *Cancer Res. 37*:3198–3203.

65. Chomchai, C., Bhadrachari, N., and Nigro, N. D. 1974. The effect of bile on the induction of experimental intestinal tumors in rats. *Dis. Colon Rectum 17*:310–312.

66. Williamson, R. C. N., Sorlie, P. D., Feinleib, M., McNamara, P. M., Kannel, W. B., and Dawber, T. R. 1981. Cancer incidence by levels of cholesterol. *JAMA 245*:247–252.

67. Vahouny, G. V., Cassidy, M. M., Lightfoot, F., Grau, L., and Kritchevsky, D. 1981. Ultrastructural modifications of intestinal and colonic mucosa induced by free or bound bile acids. *Cancer Res. 41*:3764–3765.

68. Rose, R. C., and Nahrwold, D. L. 1982. Bile acids: Effects on absorption of 1,2-dimethylhydrazine and 7,12-dimethylbenzanthracene in the colon of the rat and guinea pig. *J. Natl. Cancer Inst. 68*:619–622.

69. Watson, A. F., and Mellanby, E. 1930. Tar cancer in mice; condition of skin when modified by external treatment or diet, as factors in influencing cancerous reaction. *Br. J. Exp. Pathol. 11*:311–322.

70. Lavik, P. S., and Baumann, C. A. 1943. Further studes on tumor-promoting action of fat. *Cancer Res. 3*:749–756.

71. Tannenbaum, A. 1942. The genesis and growth of tumors. III. Effects of a high-fat diet. *Cancer Res. 2*:468–475.

72. Tannenbaum, A., and Silverstone, H. 1957. Nutrition and the genesis of tumours. in R. W. Raven (Ed.) *Cancer*. Vol. 1. pp. 306–334. London: Butterworth.

73. Waxler, S. H., Tabar, P., and Melcher, L. R. 1953. Obesity and the time of appearance of spontaneous mammary carcinoma in C3H mice. *Cancer Res. 13*:276–278.

74. Carroll, K. K., and Khor, H. T. 1970. Effects of dietary fat and dose level of 7,12-dimethylbenzanthracene on mammary tumor incidence in rats. *Cancer Res. 30*:2260–2264.

76. Carroll, K. K., and Khor, H. T. 1971. Effects of level and type of dietary fat on incidence of mammary tumors induced in female Sprague-Dawley rats by 7,12-dimethylbenzanthracene. *Lipids 6*:415–420.

77. McCay, P. B., King, M., Rikans, L. E., and Pitha, J. V. 1980. Interactions between dietary fats and antioxidants on DMBA-induced mammary carconomas and on AAF-induced hyperplastic nodules and hepatomas. *J. Environ. Pathol. Toxicol. 3*:451–465.

78. Chan, P. C., Head, J. F., Cohen, L. A., and Wynder, E. L. 1977. Influence of dietary fat on the induction of mammary tumors by N-nitrosomethylurea: Associated hormone changes and differences between Sprague-Dawley and F344 rats. *J. Natl. Cancer Inst. 59*:1279–1283.

79. Silverman, J., Shellabargar, C. J., Holtzman, S., Stone, J. P., and Weisburger, J. H. 1980. Effect of dietary fat on x-ray-induced mammary cancer in Sprague-Dawley rats. *J. Natl. Cancer Inst. 64*:631–634.

80. Newberne, P. M., and Ziegler, E. 1978. Nutrition, carcinogenesis, and mutagenesis. in W. G. Flamm and M. A. Mehlman (Eds.) *Advances in modern toxicology*. Vol. 5: *Mutagenesis*. pp. 53–84. New York: Wiley.

81. Baker, M. T., Karr, S. W., and Wade, A. E. 1983. The effects of dietary corn oil on the metabolism and activation of benzopyrene by the benzopyrene metabolizing enzymes of the mouse. *Carcinogenesis 4*:9–15.

82. Hopkins, G. J., and West, C. E. 1977. Effect of dietary polyunsaturated fat on the growth of a transplantable adenocarcinoma in C_3HAvyf B mice. *J. Natl. Cancer Inst. 58*:753–756.

83. Abraham, S., and Roe, G. A. 1976. Lipids and lipogenesis in a murine mammary neoplastic

system. in W. E. Criss, T. Ono, and J. A. Sabine (Eds.) *Progress in cancer research and therapy.* Vol. 1, Control Mechanisms in Cancer. Raven Press, New York, pp. 363–378.

84. Santiago-Delpin, E. A., and Szepsenwol, J. 1977. Prolonged survival of skin and tumor allografts in mice on high-fat diets. *J. Nat. Cancer Inst. 59:*459–461.

85. Wicha, M. S., Liotta, L. A., and Kidwell, W. R. 1973. Effects of free fatty acids on the growth of normal and neoplastic rat mammary epithelial cells. *Cancer Res. 39:*426–435.

86. Corwin, L. M., Varshavsky-Rose, F., and Broitman, S. A. 1979. Effect of dietary fats on tumorigenicity of two sarcoma cell lines. *Cancer Res. 39:*4350–4355.

87. Stoddart, A., Knight, E., Criss, W., and Adkins, J. 1983. The effect of dietary fats on growth of transplantable hepatocellular carcinoma in rats. *Fed. Proc. 42:*802.

88. Gridley, D. S., Kettering, J. D., Garaza, C. D., Andres, M. L., Slater, J. M., and Nutter, R. L. 1982. Modification of herpes 2-transformed cell-induced tumors in mice fed different sources of protein, fat and carbohydrate. *Cancer Lett. 17:*161–173.

89. Sugai, M., Witting, L. A., Tsuchiyama, H., and Kummerow, F. A. 1972. The effect of heated fat on the carcinogenic activity of 2-acetylaminofluorene. *Cancer Res. 22:*510–519.

90. Newberne, P. M., Weigert, J., and Kula, N. 1979. Effects of dietary fat on hepatic mixed function oxidases and hepatocellular carcinoma induced by aflatoxin B-1 in rats. *Cancer Res. 39:*3986–3991.

91. Longnecker, D. S., Roebuck, D. E., Yager, J. D., Lilja, H. S., and Siegmund, B. 1981. Pancreatic carcinoma in azaserine-treated rats: Induction, classification and dietary modulation of incidence. *Cancer 47:*1562–1572.

92. Birt, D. F., Salmasi, S., and Pour, P. M. 1981. Enhancement of experimental pancreatic cancer in Syrian golden hamsters by dietary fat. *J. Natl. Cancer Inst. 67:*1327–1332.

93. Nigro, N. D., Singh, D. V., Campbell, R. L., and Pak, M. S. 1975. Effect of dietary beef fat on intestinal tumor formation by azoxymethane in rats. *J. Natl. Cancer Inst. 54:*439–442.

94. Reddy, B. S., Weisburger, J. H., and Wynder, E. L. 1974. Effects of dietary fat level and dimethylhydrazine on fecal acid and neutral sterol excretion and colon carcinogenesis in the rats. *J. Natl. Cancer Inst. 52:*507–511.

95. Broitman, S. A., Vitale, J. J., Vavrousek-Jakuba, E., and Gottlieb, L. S. 1977. Polyunsaturated fat, cholesterol and large bowel tumorigenesis. *Cancer 40:*2455–2463.

96. Reddy, B. S., and Watanabe, K. 1979. Effect of cholesterol metabolites and promoting effect of lithocholic acid in colon carcinogenesis in germ-free and conventional F-344 rats. *Cancer Res. 39:*1521–1524.

97. Cruse, J. P., Lewis, M. R., Ferulano, P., and Clark, C. G. 1978. Cocarcinogenic effects of dietary cholesterol in experimental colon cancer. *Nature 276:*822–825.

98. Bansal, B. R., Rhoads, J. E., and Bansal, S. C. 1978. Effects of diet on colon carcinogenesis and the immune system in rats treated with 1,2-dimethylhydrazine. *Cancer Res. 38:*3293–3303.

99. Bull, A. W., Schullier, B. K., Wilson, P. S., Hayden, M. T., and Nigro, N. D. 1979. Promotion of azoxymethane-induced intestinal cancer by high-fat diet in rats. *Cancer Res. 39:*4956–4959.

100. Hems, G. 1978. The contributions of diet and childbearing to breast cancer rates. *Br. J. Cancer 37:*974–982.

101. Gray, G. E., Pike, M. C., and Henderson, B. E. 1979. Breast-cancer incidence and mortality rates in different countries in relation to risk factors and dietary practices. *Br. J. Cancer 39:*1–7.

102. Gregor, O., Toman, R., and Prusova, F. 1969. Gastrointestinal cancer and nutrition. *Gut 10:*1031–1034.

103. Bingham, S., Williams, D. R. R., Cole, T. J., and James, W. P. T. 1979. Dietary fibre and regional large-bowel cancer mortality in Britain. *Br. J. Cancer 40:*456–463.

104. Haenszel, W., Locke, F. B., and Segi, M. 1980. A case-control study of large bowel cancer in Japan. *J. Natl. Cancer Inst. 64:*17–22.

105. Bjelka, E. 1978. Dietary factors and epidemiology of cancer of the stomach and large bowel. Aktuel Ernaehrungsmed. *Klin. Prax. Suppl. 2:*10–17.

106. Graham, S., Dayal, H., Swanson, M., Mittelman, A., and Wilkinson, G. 1978. Diet in the epidemiology of cancer of the colon and rectum. *J. Natl. Cancer Inst. 61:*709–714.

107. Hirayama, T. 1981. A large-scale cohort study on the relationship between diet and selected cancer of the digestive organs. in W. R. Bruce, P. Correa, M. Lipkin, S. R. Tannenbaum, and T. D. Wilkins (Eds.) *Gastrointestinal cancer, endogenous factors:* Banbury Report 7. pp. 409–429. Cold Spring Harbor, New York: Cold Spring Harbor Laboratory.

108. Lea, A. J. 1977. Neoplasms and environmental factors. *Ann. R. Coll. Surg. Engl. 41:*432–438.

109. Armstrong, B., Garrod, A., and Doll, R. 1976. A retrospective study of renal cancer with special reference to coffee and animal protein consumption. *Br. J. Cancer 33:*127–136.

110. Tannenbaum, A., and Silverstone, H. 1949. The genesis and growth of tumors. IV. Effects of varying the proportion of protein (casein) in the diet. *Cancer Res. 9:*162–173.

111. Silverstone, H. 1948. The levels of carcinogenic azo dyes in the livers of rats fed various diets containing p-dimethylaminoazobenzene. *Cancer Res. 8:*301–308.

112. White, J., and Mider, G. B. 1941. The effect of dietary cystine on the reaction of dilute brown mice to methylcholanthrene. *J. Natl. Cancer Inst. 2:*95–97.

113. Shay, H., Gruenstein, M., and Shimkin, M. B. 1964. Effect of casein, lactalbumin and ovalbumin on 3-methylcholanthrene induced mammary carcinoma in rats. *J. Natl. Cancer Inst. 33:*243–253.

114. Wattenberg, L. W. 1975. Effects of dietary constituents on the metabolism of chemical carcinogens. *Cancer Res. 35:*3326–3331.

115. White, J., White, F. R., and Mider, G. B. 1947. Effects of diets deficient in certain amino acids on the induction of leukemia in dba mice. *J. Natl. Cancer Inst. 7:*199–202.

116. Engel, R. W., and Copeland, D. H. 1952. The influence of dietary casein level on tumor induction with 2-acetylaminofluorene. *Cancer Res. 12:*905–912.

117. Morris, H. P., Westfall, B. B., Dubnik, C. S., and Dunn, T. B. 1948. Some observations on carcinogenicity, distribution and metabolism of N-acetyl-2-aminofluorene in the rat. *Cancer Res. 8:*390.

118. Harris, P. N. 1947. Production of tumors in rats by 2-aminofluorene and 2-acetylaminofluorene: Failure of liver extract and of dietary protein level to influence liver tumor production. *Cancer Res. 7:*88–94.

119. Mgbodile, M. U. K., and Campbell, T. C. 1972. Effect of protein deprivation of male weaning rats on the kinetics of hepatic microsomal enzyme activity. *J. Nutr. 102:*53–60.

120. Wells, P., Aftergood, L., and Alfin-Slater, R. B. 1976. Effect of varying levels of dietary protein on tumor development and lipid metabolism in rats exposed to aflatoxin. *J. Am. Oil Chem. Soc. 53:*559–562.

121. Madhaven, T. V., and Gopalan, C. 1968. The effect of dietary protein on carcinogenesis of aflatoxin. *Arch Pathol. Lab. Med. 80:*123–126.

122. Preston, R. S., Hayes, J. R., and Campbell, T. C. 1976. The effect of protein deficiency on the in vivo binding of aflatoxin B_1 to rat liver macromolecules. *Life Sci. 19:*1191–1197.

123. Campbell, T. C. 1979. Influence of nutrition on metabolism of carcinogens. *Adv. Nutr. Res. 2:*29–55.

124. Tsuda, H., Lee, G., and Farber, E. 1980. Induction of resistant hepatocytes as a new principle for a possible short-term in vivo test for carcinogens. *Cancer Res. 40:*1157–1164.

125. Appleton, B. S., and Campbell, T. C. 1981. Effects of dietary protein levels and phenobarbital

on aflatoxin (AFBI)-induced hepatic γ-glutamyl transpeptidase (GGT) in the rat. *Fed. Proc. 40:*842.

126. McLean, A. E. M., and Magee, P. N. 1970. Increased renal carcinogenesis by dimethyl-nitrosamine in protein deficient rats. *Br. J. Exp. Pathol. 51:*587–590.

127. Ross, M. H., and Bras, G. 1973. Influence of protein under and overnutrition on spontaneous tumor prevalence in the rat. *J. Nutr. 103:*944–964.

128. White, F. R., and White, J. 1944. Effect of diethylstilbesterol on mammary tumor formation in strain C3H mice fed a low cystine diet. *J. Natl. Cancer Inst. 4:*413–415.

129. McSheey, T. W. 1974. The onset of mammary adenocarcinoma in mice: A possible correlation with nutrition. *Ecol. Food Nutr. 3:*147–150.

130. Visek, W. J., Clinton, S. K., and Truex, C. R. 1978. Nutrition and experimental carcinogenesis. *Cornell Vet. 68:*3–39.

131. Topping, D. C., and Visek, W. J. 1976. Nitrogen intake and tumorigenesis in rats injected with 1,2-dimethylhydrazine. *J. Nutr. 106:*1583–1590.

132. Walters, M. A., and Roe, F. J. C. 1964. The effect of dietary casein on the induction of lung tumors by the injection of 9,10-dimethyl 1,2-benzanthracene (DMBA) into newborn mice. *Br. J. Cancer 18:*312–316.

133. Clinton, S. K., Truex, C. R., and Visek, W. J. 1977. Dietary protein, aryl hydrocarbon hydroxylase, and chemical carcinogenesis. *J. Nutr. 109:*55–62.

134. Clinton, S. K., Li, P. S., Mulloy, A. L., Palmer, S. S., and Visek, W. J. 1983. Dietary-protein-fat interactions on prolactin homeostasis in female rats. *Fed. Proc. 42:*1314.

135. Haley, H. B., and Williamson, M. B. 1960. Growth of tumors in experimental wounds. *Proc. Am. Assoc. Cancer Res. 3:*116.

136. Babson, A. L. 1954. Some host-tumor relationships with respect to nitrogen. *Cancer Res. 14:*89–93.

137. Devik, F., Elson, L. A., Koller, P. C., and Lamerton, L. F. 1950. Influence of diet on Walker rat carcinoma 256, and its response to X-radiation—cytological and histological investigations. *Br. J. Cancer 4:*298–314.

138. White, F. R., and Belkin, M. 1945. Source of tumor proteins. I. Effect of low-nitrogen diet on the establishment and growth of a transplanted tumor. *J. Natl. Cancer Inst. 5:*261–263.

139. Nutter, R. L., Gridley, D. S., Kettering, J. D., Andres, M. L., Aprecio, R. M., and Slater, J. M. 1983. Modification of a transplantable colon tumor and immune responses in mice fed different sources of protein, fat and carbohydrate. *Cancer Lett. 18:*49–62.

140. Sugimura, T., Bernbaum, S. M., Winitz, M., and Greenstein, J. P. 1959. Quantitative nutritional studies with water-soluble chemically defined diets. 8. The forced feeding of diets each lacking one essential amino acid. *Arch. Biochem. 81:*448–455.

141. Lorincz, A. B., Kuttner, R. E., and Brandt, M. B. 1969. Tumor response to phenylalanine-tyrosine limited diets. *J. Am. Dietet. Assoc. 54:*198–205.

142. Demopoulos, H. R. 1966. Effects of reducing the phenylalanine-tyrosine intake of patients with advanced malignant melanoma. *Cancer 19:*657–664.

143. Yuki, K., Tachikawa, T., Hirata, M., Ando, R., Nakashima, N., Sata, T., and Nomura, H. 1966. Low-phenylalanine diet therapy for chronic myelogenic leukemia. *Eiyogaku Zasshi 24:*195–201.

144. Chan, W., McElhanon, S., Shu, G., and Banks, W. L. 1983. Effect of dietary leucine restriction on its utilization by tumor and host tissues. *Fed. Proc. 42:*670.

145. Worthington, B. S. 1974. Effect of nutritional status on immune phenomena. *J. Am. Diet Assoc. 65:*123–129.

146. Dresar, B., and Irving, D. 1973. Environmental factors and cancer of the colon and breast. *Br. J. Cancer 27:*167–172.

147. Hems, G., and Stuart, A. 1975. Breast cancer rates in populations of single women. *Br. J. Cancer 31:*118–123.
148. Hakama, M., and Saxen, E. A. 1967. Cereal consumption and gastric cancer. *Int. J. Cancer 2:*265–268.
149. Modan, B., Lubin, F., Barell, V., Greenberg, R. A., Modan, M., and Graham, S. 1974. The role of starches in the etiology of gastric cancer. *Cancer 34:*2087–2092.
150. Saint-Hilarie, S., Lavers, M. K., Kennedy, J., and Code, C. F. 1960. Gastric acid secretory value of different foods. *Gastroenterology 39:*1–11.
151. De Jong, U. W., Breslow, N., Hong, J. G. E. Sridharan, M., and Shanmugaratnam, K. 1974. Aetiological factors in oesophageal cancer in Singapore, Chinese. *Int. J. Cancer 13:*291–303.
152. Haenszel, W., Kurihara, M., Segi, M., and Lee, R. K. C. 1972. Stomach cancer among Japanese in Hawaii. *J. Natl. Cancer Inst. 49:*969–988.
153. Haenszel, W. Correa, P., and Cuello, C. 1975. Social class differences among patients with large-bowel cancer in Cali, Columbia. *J. Natl. Cancer Inst. 54:*1031–1035.
154. Bjelke, E. 1974. Epidemiologic studies of cancer of the stomach, colon and rectum. *Scand. J. Gastroenterol 9*(Suppl. 31):1–235.
155. Graham, S. 1975. Future inquiries into the epidemiology of gastric cancer. *Cancer Res. 35:*3464–3468.
156. Hartman, P. E. 1983. Review: Putative mutagens and carcinogens in foods. I. Nitrate/nitrite ingestion and gastric cancer mortality. *Envir. Mutagen. 5:*111–121.
157. Hill, M. J., Hawksworth, G., and Tattersall, G. 1973. Bacteria, nitrosamines and cancer of the stomach. *Br. J. Cancer 28:*562–567.
158. Tannenbaum, S. R., Moran, D., Falchuk, K. R., Correa, P., and Cuello, C. 1981. Nitrite stability and nitrosation potential in human gastric juice. *Cancer Lett. 14:*131–136.
159. Roe, F. J. C., Levy, L. S., and Carter, R. L. 1970. Feeding studies on sodium cyclamate, saccharin and sucrose for carcinogenic and tumour-promoting activity. *Food Cosmet. Toxicol. 8:*135–145.
160. Friedman, L., Richardson, H. L., Richardson, M. E., Lethco, E. J., Wallace, W. C., and Sauro, F. M. 1972. Toxic response of rats to cyclamates in chow and semisynthetic diets. *J. Natl. Cancer Inst. 49:*751–764.
161. Hunter, B., Graham, C., Heywood, R., Prentice, D. E., and Roe, F. J. C., and Noakes, D. N. 1978. Tumorigenicity and Carcinogenicity Study with Xylitol in Long-Term Administration to Mice (final report). Huntington Research Centre, Huntingdon, Cambridgeshire, England. Volumes 20–23 of Xylitol. F. Hoffman La Roche Company, Ltd., Basel, Switzerland. 1500 pp.
162. Hoehn, S. K., and Carroll, K. K. 1978. Effects of dietary carbohydrate on the incidence of mammary tumors induced in rats by 7,12-dimethylbenzanthracene. *Nutr. Cancer 1:*27–30.
163. Gershoff, S. N., and McGandy, R. B. 1981. The effects of vitamin A-deficient diets containing lactose in producing bladder calculi and tumors in rats. *Am. J. Clin. Nutr. 34:*483–489.
164. Ingram, D. M., and Castleden, W. M. 1981. Glucose increases experimentally induced colorectal cancer: A preliminary report. *Nutr. Cancer 2:*150–152.
165. Hunter, B., Colley, J., Street, A. E., Heywood, R., Prentice, D. E., and Magnusson, G. 1978. Xylitol tumorigenicity and toxicity study in long-term dietary administration to rats (final report). Huntingdon, Research Centre, Huntingdon, Cambridgeshire, England. Volumes 11–14 of Xylitol. F. Hoffman La Roche Company, Ltd., Basel, Switzerland. 2225 pp.
166. McGuinness, E. E., Morgan, R. G. H., Levison, D. A., Hopwood, D., and Wormsley, K. G. 1981. Interaction of azaserine and raw soya flour on the rat pancreas. *Scand. J. Gastroenterol. 16:*49–56.
167. Berg, J. W. 1975. Can nutrition explain the pattern of international epidemiology of hormone-dependent cancers? *Cancer Res. 35:*3345–3350.

168. de Waard, F. 1975. Breast cancer incidence and nutritional status with particular reference to body weight and height. *Cancer Res.* *35:*3351–3356.
169. de Waard, F., Cornelis, J. P., Aoki, K., and Yoshida, M. 1977. Breast cancer incidence according to weight and height in two cities of the Netherlands and in Aichi prefecture, Japan. *Cancer 40:*1269–1275.
170. Lew, E. A., and Garfinkel, L. 1979. Variations in mortality by weight among 750,000 men and women. *J. Chronic Dis. 32:*563–576.
171. Tannenbaum, A. 1945. The dependence of tumor formation on the composition of the calorie-restricted diet as well as on the degree of restriction. *Cancer Res. 5:*616–625.
172. Clayton, C. C., and Bauman, C. A. 1949. Diet and azo dye tumors: Effect of diet during a period when the azo dye is not fed. *Cancer Res. 9:*575–582.
173. King, J. T., Casas, C. B., and Visscher, M. B. 1949. The influence of estrogen on cancer incidence and adrenal change in ovariectomized mice on caloric restriction. *Cancer Res. 9:*436–437.
174. Ross, M. H., and Bras, G. 1971. Lasting influence of early caloric restriction on prevalence of neoplasms in the rat. *J. Natl. Cancer Inst. 47:*1095–1113.

Chapter 3

Dietary Fiber and Cancer

Some interest has been directed toward the physiological significance of dietary fiber, which generally includes indigestible carbohydrates and carbohydrate and carbohydrate-like components of food, such as cellulose, lignin, hemicellulose, pentosans, gums, and pectins. The major characteristic of these indigestible substances is that they provide bulk in the diet. The major types of foods that provide dietary fiber are vegetables, fruits, and whole grain cereals.

Because of the complex makeup of dietary fiber, the physiological functions, and metabolic activity of its individual components have not been studied adequately. Early reports may have underestimated the fiber content, since crude fiber assays only measure cellulose and lignin. Consequently, these early reports provided only incomplete data on the amount and type of fiber consumed.

During the past few decades, the consumption of dietary fiber has decreased in many parts of the Western world. On the basis of observations about the relationship of diet and the incidence of disease, Burkitt and Trowell have hypothesized that many chronic diseases including cancer are associated with a low intake of dietary fiber.[1] Some of the types of disease that may be related to dietary fiber deficiency are summarized in Table 3-1.

The McGovern Report on Dietary Goals for the United States suggested seven changes in food selection and preparation. Heading the list was advice to increase consumption of fruit and vegetables and whole grains. This advice aimed at achieving an intake of carbohydrate corresponding to 55–60% of energy intake. This increase in the consumption of starch implies an increased intake of nonstarch polysaccharides or, in other words, dietary fiber. Dietary guidelines also published in Australia, Norway, and Sweden have similarly encouraged increased fiber in the diet, and in the United Kingdom the Centre for Agricultural Strategy suggests that health may benefit by increased fiber consumption, especially in the form of cereals.

Some of the types of fiber, their physiological action, and their physical and chemical problems are listed in Table 3-2. The practical sources of fiber types are listed in Table 3-3.

Table 3-1. Dietary Fiber and Disease

Primary bowel conditions
Spastic bowel disease
Appendicitis
Benign tumors of the colon
Malignant tumors of the colon
Constipation
Hemorrhoids
Hiatus hernia
Extrabowel diseases
Hyperlipidemia
Coronary heart disease
Cholelithiasis
Obesity
Diabetes
Varicose veins
Gallstones

The carbohydrate composition of the plant cell wall varies widely between various plant types: cellulose, 40–96%, hemicellulose 5–45%; and pectins 1–45%. In ruminants, a large and variable portion of the cell wall is digestible, but there is much less in man where the cellulose is least digested.

The most plentiful organic compound on earth is cellulose, which creates the fibrous character of many plants by the formation of long chains 1–48 linked D-glucose molecules. In plants the celluloses are combined with lignin and hemicellulose thus changing the physical characteristics of pure cellulose as seen in cotton. Cellulose can be degraded only by microbial cellulose.

The hemicelluloses are known to be complexed polymers. In the hemicellulose A there are branched and linear polysaccharides comprised mostly of xylose units with additional salts, such as galactose, glucose, mannose, arabinose, and other sugars. Hemicellulose B are acidic substances which include uronic acids, hexoses and pentoses.

The pectins contain galacturonic acid, arabinose, and galactose and are amorphous rather than fibrous substances.

Lignin is the major noncarbohydrate fraction in the plant cell wall and is relatively resistant to microbial breakdown. Lignin reduces the digestibility of the carbohydrates with which it is associated with in the cell wall. Cell wall digestibility is more closely related to the lignin cellulose ratio than to any other measurement. In addition, the lignin content increases with increasing age of the plant and with increasing age there is a decreasing digestibility of the plant material.

Table 3-2. Data on the Type of Fiber Including the Physiological Action, Major Monomers, Degree of Polymerization, and the Molecular Weight

Type	Physiological action	Monomers	Degree of polymerization	Molecular weight
Cellulose	Holds water May reduce colonic intraluminal pressure May affect trace mineral excretion Reduces transit time	Glucose	1,400–12,000	250,000–2,000,000
Hemicellulose A and B	Holds water; increases stool bulk May bind bile acids Reduces elevated colonic intraluminal pressure Reduces transit time	Xylose Arabinose Mannose Glucuronic acid	70–150	11,000–24,000
Pectins, cutins, gums, and mucilages	Slow gastric emptying May bind bile acids May affect trace mineral excretion Possible antioxidant	Galacturonic acid Galactose Arabinose	350–550	60,000–90,000
Lignin[a]	Holds water May bind trace minerals Affects fecal steroids	Phenylpropanes	—	Several thousand

[a]Noncarbohydrate.

Table 3-3. Practical Sources of Fiber Types[a]

Celluloses	Natural sources
	Soy bran (soybean hulls)
	Fruit juice sacs (e.g., from citrus fruits)
	Legumes (e.g., beans, peas)
	Carrots
	"Artificial" sources
	Solkafloc powdered cellulose, from wood, highly purified and standardized
	Avicel microcrystalline cellulose, from wood highly purified and standardized
	Methylcellulose, a polymer derived from cellulose by alkali and other treatments
	Carboxymethylcellulose (CMC), a synthetic water-soluble polymer derived from cellulose
Hemicelluloses	Natural sources
	Corn hulls (maize)
	Barley hulls
	Oat hulls
	Corn brans
	Wheat brans
	Brewer's grains, residues from malting, mainly barley; mixture usually contains rice and sometimes other grains as well
	Soy fiber concentrate, residue after soy protein has been extracted
	"Artificial" sources
	Masonex extract of wood fibers by acid hydrolysis
	Xylan, the polysaccharide polymer of D-xylose units extracted from various plant sources
Lignins	Wheat straw
	Cottonseed hulls
	Alfalfa stems
	Bagasse, the sugarcane residue after sugar has been extracted
	Tannins, e.g., $C_{76}H_{52}O_{46}$ or penta(m-digalloyl)glucose; gallic acid derivatives found widely in plants

(*continued*)

EPIDEMIOLOGICAL EVIDENCE

Most of the epidemiological data on fiber are related mainly to its possible role in protection against large bowel cancer.

Mechanisms of Protection

Several different mechanisms have been proposed for this protective effect: Fiber can dilute carcinogens present in the large bowel; fiber can decrease transit

Table 3-3. (*Continued*)

Pectins	Citrus pulp
	Apple pulp
	Cabbages and other brassicas
	Sugarbeet pulp
	Legumes (e.g., peas and beans)
	Alfalfa leaves
	Sunflower heads
Cutins	Apple peels
	Tomato peels
	Berries (seeds of)
	Peanut skins
	Almond skins
	Onion skins
Gums	Guar gum from ground endosperms of the legume, *Cyamopsis tetragonolobus* L. Taub.
	Gum arabic, from locust beans
	Oat gums, from oat flour
	Agar, a phyllocolloid polysaccharide mixture of agarose and agaropectin derived from red algae
	Gum tragacanth, a mixture of polysaccharides of galactose, fructose, xylose, arabinose, and glucuronic acid from *Astragalus* spp., legumes
	Alginate, from kelp (seaweed), mixtures of hydrophilic colloids
	Xanthan, a polysaccharide from prickly ash trees
	Psyllium or fleaseed, from plantains (*Plantago* spp.)
	Konjac nannan, a polysaccharide from a Japanese source unspecified by the workshop
	Glycan, from yeast

[a]Reprinted from L. Crosby 1978, *Nutrition and Cancer* 1 (1)*16*, and the Franklin Institute Press, Philadelphia. Copyright 1968.

time, thereby decreasing contact time between the carcinogen and tissue; fiber may affect the production of putative carcinogens or procarcinogens in the stool such as the bile acids; or, by influencing the composition and metabolic activity of the fecal flora, it can alter the spectrum of fecal bile acids and their derivatives that are present in the stool. Because they pertain only to crude fiber, most data on the fiber content of foods are incomplete. Since certain selected components of the fiber may be responsible for the fiber effect, epidemiological studies of dietary fiber will have limited value until detailed information on each of its components becomes available.

Correlations

Inverse

Correlations of the fiber content of diets with colorectal cancer risk have yielded mixed results.[2] The differences in colon cancer incidence among northern and southern populations in India may be explained by the high levels of roughage, cellulose, and vegetable fiber in the northern Indian diet and the very low levels in the southern Indian diet. In the Punjabis in the north there was a virtual absence of the disease and vegetable fibers were more abundant in the stools of Indians from the north, but completely absent in the stools from inhabitants of the southern regions.

In another study similar differences were observed when the diets of adult men from Copenhagen, Denmark (high risk) were compared to the diets from Kuopio, Finland (low risk group). The Danes consumed less fiber and their stools weighed less than those of the Finns. These latter two studies lend support to the hypothesis that dietary fiber plays a protective role in carcinogenesis. In contrast, Bingham et al. calculated the average fiber intake by populations in different regions of Great Britain.[3] No significant correlations were found between total fiber intake and the corresponding mortality rates for colon and rectal cancers. However, the mean intakes of the pentosan fraction of total dietary fiber and of vegetables other than potatoes were inversely correlated with mortality from colon cancer. Their report suggested the importance of looking at the specific components of the fiber rather than at crude or total fiber in studies of large bowel cancer.

Correlation

Other correlation analyses have not supported the hypothesis that fiber intake is inversely related to the risk of colon cancer. Mortality from colon cancer in 20 industrialized countries between 1967 and 1973 has been compared with the rates of per-capita food intake for these same areas from 1954 to 1965.[4] Even though fiber intake was inversely correlated with colon cancer mortality, this relationship was no longer significant in a partial correlation analysis controlling for cholesterol intake. This study suggests that cholesterol, not fiber, was an important risk factor for colon cancer. In other studies, there was not correlation found between colon cancer incidence in 37 countries and the per-capita intake of various fiber-containing foods.[5] There was also little difference found in fiber intake between the population of Utah (low risk) and the population of the United States as a whole.[6]

Case-Control Studies

Investigators have attempted to relate the intake of dietary fiber and the risk of large bowel cancer in a number of case-control studies, again with inconsistent results. The frequency with which certain food items were consumed by colon and rectal cancer cases and both hospital and neighborhood controls has been assessed.[7] The consumption of high-fiber foods by colon cancer cases has been found to be significantly lower than that of both groups of controls, but no such difference was found between rectal cancer cases and controls. Using a similar approach, the consumption of dietary fiber was observed to be lower in colorectal cancer cases than that of controls in parallel studies conducted in Minnesota and Norway.[8]

Another case-control study of colorectal cancer was done on American Blacks. Controls were chosen from two hospitals and a multiphasic health checkup clinic.[9] By measuring the frequency of consumption of selected food items, it was found that the cases consumed fewer fiber-containing foods than did the controls and that there was a consistent dose–response relationship as well. There were significantly more cases than controls which reported the consumption of a diet high in saturated fat but low in fiber.

Another case-control study of diet and colorectal cancer in Canada[10] attempted to compute consumption of dietary fiber on the basis of the actual fiber content of food rather than on a simple grouping of food items as other investigators had done. An elevated risk associated with increased consumption of calories, total fat, total protein, saturated fat, oleic acid, and cholesterol was found, but there was no association found with the consumption of crude fiber, vitamin C, or linoleic acid. However, data on the specific components of fiber were not available for their analysis.

In a case-control study in Puerto Rico, an inverse association between fiber consumption and large bowel cancer was reported. Higher consumption of fiber and total residue was found in the cases than in controls when frequency-of-consumption dietary histories were compared. There was no explanation given for this unusual finding, which, however, is consistent with the observation of Hill *et al.* who reported that the highest socioeconomic group studied in Hong Kong has the greatest incidence of colon cancer and a high intake of fiber and calories, whereas the middle and lowest socioeconomic groups had correspondingly lower incidence rates and intakes.[12]

Fiber and Transit Time

Comparisons have been made of bowel transit times in men from three different populations: Japanese in Japan (low risk for colon cancer), Japanese in Hawaii (high risk for colon cancer), and Caucasians in Hawaii (also high risk for colon cancer).[13] Bowel transit times were similar in both Japanese populations and were shorter than in the Caucasians. However, the mean stool weight was similar in the two high-risk populations and was notably less than that for the Japanese in Japan. Stool weight and transit time were measured in four groups of 30 men, aged 50–59 years, randomly selected from populations in urban Copenhagen, rural Them, Denmark, urban Helsinki, and rural Parikkala, Finland.[14] These populations exhibited a three- fourfold difference in risk for large bowel cancer, but the mean transit time was not significantly different among populations. The average stool weights were different and had a significant inverse relationship to total large bowel cancer incidence, with larger stool weights being found in the low-risk population. These results do not support the hypothesis that dietary fiber protects against colon cancer by decreasing transit time in the bowel, thereby decreasing the contact time between carcinogens and tissues.

Fiber and Bile Acid Excretion

The amounts of bile acids that can be excreted into the lumen of the intestine can also be affected by dietary fiber. Fiber, when fed to animals or man will usually cause increased excretion of bile acids. The bile acid level of bile salt excretion appears to be a function of the fiber structure. Fiber binds bile acids and bile salts *in vitro*. The degree of binding is characteristic for each fiber type and each substrate. Bile acid binding may be one mechanism of the physiological action of fiber. In addition, fecal steroid concentration is inversely related to fecal bulk.[15] However, dietary fat also influences bile acid excretion as well, the relative effects of both of these dietary components need additional study. Studies of the composition of bile acids in the feces of humans are summarized in Chapter 2.

EXPERIMENTAL EVIDENCE

A number of chemical carcinogens cause colon cancer in rats. Among these colon carcinogens are 1,2-dimethylhydrazine (DMH), azoxymethane (AOM), methylazoxymethanol (MAM) acetate, 2,3-dimethyl-4-aminobiphenyl (DAB), and nitrosomethylurea (NMU). Colon cancer can be induced in these laboratory animals in several ways: by parenteral administration of DMH, AOM, MAM, and DAB; by feeding DMH; and by intrarectal instillation of NMU.

DMH-induced colon cancer is protected against in rats by bran, regardless of whether the carcinogen is administered orally or subcutaneously.[16] However, bran has no effect on the incidence or number of tumors in the duodenum or cecum. Cellulose has been found to protect rats against DMH-induced tumors,[17] but pectin does not protect against DMH-induced tumors.[17] However, cellulose does not appear to protect against DMH-induced tumors.[17] However, cellulose does not appear to protect against tumors induced by AOM or NMU.[18,19]

The effects of different levels of fiber on DMH-induced colon cancer in rats have been studied by Fleiszer *et al.*[20] Four diets were tested: very high fiber (28%) supplied as bran cereal; high fiber (15%) supplied as a special rat chow; low fiber (5%) supplied as standard rat chow; and a fiber-free semipurified diet.

Rats fed the very-high-fiber and high-fiber diets had fewer cancers than did those fed the low-fiber diet. However, the basal diet for the fiber-free group was considerably different, and the response of these animals cannot be reasonably compared with those of other animals.

Even though components of dietary fiber generally appear to have a protective effect against DMH-induced carcinogenesis, Glauert *et al.* have reported that dietary agar (a fiber-rich component of the diet) enhanced DMH-induced colon cancer in mice.[21]

Rats treated with AOM or NMU have also been fed several types of dietary fiber.[22] The substances tested were alfalfa, pectin, and wheat bran fed as 15% of a diet that also contained 5% cellulose. Pectin exerted a protective effect, but alfalfa and bran were ineffective when the carcinogen was given parenterally. But when the carcinogen was given by intrarectal instillation, alfalfa increased carcinogenesis, but pectin and bran were not protective. Alfalfa is known to have a relatively strong ability to bind bile acids. Substances with this binding capacity disrupt the topography of the colonic mucosa. The denuded epithelium may then be more susceptible to the action of a locally administered carcinogen.

Although some data suggest that certain types of fiber (e.g., bran and cellulose) can protect rats from the action of certain chemical carcinogens, the data from different experiments are difficult to compare or interpret, mainly because of a lack of uniform experimental plans. The experiments differed in the strains of rats, their diets, age, the carcinogens used, and the routes of administration. Reddy *et al.*[23] have studied the effect of a low lignin containing corn bran diet and autohydrolyzed lignin on 3,2'-dimethyl-4-aminobiphenyl-induced intestinal carcinogenesis in male inbred F344 rats. The incidence and multiplicity of small intestinal tumors as well as the number of colon adenocarcinomas per tumor-bearing animal were lower in animals fed the lignin diet than those fed the control diet. The daily output of total bile acids was increased in animals fed the lignin diet. Perhaps the varied effect of fiber on carcinogenesis in other experiments is related to the lignin content of the fiber.

REFERENCES

1. Burkitt, D. P., and Trowell, H. C. 1975. *Refined carbohydrate foods and disease. Some implications of dietary fiber.* pp. 1–356. New York: Academic Press.
2. Malhotra, S. L. 1977. Dietary factors in a study of cancer colon from cancer registry with special reference to the role of saliva, milk and fermented milk products and vegetable fibre. *Med. Hypotheses 3*:122–126.
3. Bingham, S., Williams, D. R. R., Cole, T. J., and James, W. P. T. 1979. Dietary fibre and regional large-bowel cancer mortality in Britain. *Br. J. Cancer 40*:456–463.
4. Liu, K., Stamler, J., Moss, D., Garside, D., Persky, V., and Soltero, I. 1979. Dietary cholesterol, fat, and fibre, and colon-cancer mortality. *Lancet 2*:782–785.

5. Drasar, B. S., and Irving, D. 1973. Environmental factors and cancer of the colon and breast. *Br. J. Cancer 27:*167–172.

6. Lyon, J. L., and Sorenson, A. W. 1978. Colon cancer in a low-risk population. *Am. J. Clin. Nutr. 31:*S227–S230.

7. Modan, B., Barell, V., Lubin, F., Modan, M., Greenberg, R. A., and Graham, S. 1975. Low-fiber intake as an etiologic factor in cancer of the colon. *J. Natl. Cancer Inst. 55:*15–18.

8. Bjelke, E. 1978. Dietary factors and the epidemiology of cancer of the stomach and large bowel. *Aktuel. Ernaehungsmed. Klin. Prax. Suppl. 2:*10–17.

9. Dales, L. G., Friedman, G. D., Ury, H. K., Grossman, S., and Williams, S. R. 1978. A case-control study of relationships of diet and other traits to colorectal cancer in American blacks. *Am. J. Epidemiol. 109:*132–144.

10. Jain, M., Cook, G. M., Davis, F. G., Grace, M. G., Howe, G. R., and Miller, A. B. 1980. A case-control study of diet and colo-rectal cancer. *Int. J. Cancer 26:*757–768.

11. Martinez, I., Torres, R., Frias, Z., Colon, J. R., and Fernandez, M. 1979. Factors associated with adenocarcinomas of the large bowel in Puerto Rico. in J. M. Birch (Ed.) *Advances in medical oncology, research and education.* Vol. 3: *Epidemiology.* pp. 45–52. New York: Pergamon Press.

12. Hill, M., MacLennan, R., and Newcombe, K. 1979. Diet and large-bowel cancer in three socioeconomic groups in Hong Kong. *Lancet 1:*436.

13. Glober, G. A., Nomura, A., Kamiyama, S., Shimada, A. and Abba, B. C. 1977. Bowel transit-time and stool weight in populations with different colon-cancer risks. *Lancet 2:*110–111.

14. Cummings, J. H., Branch, W. J., Bjerrum, L., Paerregaard, A., Hels, P., and Burton, R. 1982. Colon cancer and large bowel function in Denmark and Finland. 1982. *Nutr. Cancer 4:*61–66.

15. Zafar, M., Nomani, A., Lim, J. K., Watne, A. L., and Rodriguez, N. R. 1983. Relationship of fecal steroid concentration with the fecal steroid output and bulk. *Fed. Proc. 42:*801.

16. Barbolt, T. A., and Abraham, R. 1978. The effect of bran on dimethylhydrazine-induced colon carcinogenesis in the rat. *Proc. Soc. Exp. Biol. Med. 157:*656–659.

17. Freeman, H. J., Spiller, G. A., and Kim, Y. S. 1980. A double-blind study on the effects of differing purified cellulose and pectin fiber diets on 1,2-dimethylhydrazine-induced rat colonic neoplasia. *Cancer Res. 40:*2661–2665.

18. Ward, J. M., Yamamoto, R. S., and Weisburger, J. H. 1973. Cellulose dietary bulk and azoxymethane-induced intestinal cancer. *J. Natl. Cancer Inst. 51:*713–715.

19. Watanabe, K., Reddy, B. S., Wong, C. Q., and Weisburger, J. H. 1978. Effect of dietary undegraded carrageenin on colon carcinogenesis in F344 treated rats treated with azoxymethane or methylnitrosourea. *Cancer Res. 38:*4427–4430.

20. Fleiszer, D. M., Murray, D., Richards, G. K., and Brown, R. A. 1980. Effects of diet on chemically induced bowel cancer. *Can. J. Surg. 23:*67–73.

21. Glauert, H. P., Bennink, M. R., and Sander, C. H. 1981. Enhancement of 1,2-dimethyl-hydrazine-induced colon carcinogenesis in mice by dietary agar. *Food Cosmet. Toxicol. 19:*281–286.

22. Watanabe, K., Reddy, B. S., Weisburger, J. H., and Kritchevsky, D. 1979. Effect of dietary alfalfa, pectin and wheat bran on azoxymethane- or methylnitrosourea-induced colon carcinogenesis in F344 rats. *J. Natl. Cancer Inst. 63:*141–145.

23. Reddy, B. S., Maeura, Y., and Wayman, M. 1983. Effect of dietary corn bran and autoanalyzed lignin on 3,2'-dimethyl-4-aminobiphenyl-induced intestinal carcinogenesis in male F344 rats. *J. Nat. Cancer Inst. 71:*419–423.

Vitamins and Cancer

VITAMIN A

Of the entire collection of chemically diverse substances classified as vitamins, vitamin A is of greatest current interest in terms of its possible role in the process of carcinogenesis. In this discussion the term *vitamin A* is used to describe vitamin A itself as well as its synthetic analogues of vitamin, called retinoids. The only well-understood function of vitamin A is its role in the visual cycle.

Ingested vitamin A is absorbed in the bloodstream and stored in the liver; if large amounts are consumed, vitamin A can reach toxic levels. The recommended daily requirement of vitamin A by the Food and Nutrition Board of the National Academy of Sciences—National Research Council is 1000 retinol equivalents for males and 800 retinol equivalents for females, with a retinol equivalent equal to 1 microgram (μg) retinol or 6 μg β-carotene. Blood levels are regulated by a feedback mechanism, but do not immediately reflect the amounts consumed or stored in the liver. The involvement of this vitamin in cell differentiation, although not well documented, provides important insight into its relationship to cancer.

Vitamin A plays an important role in the control of growth, differentiation, and function of epithelial tissues. Vitamin A deficiency results in hyperkeratosis of the skin, and vitamin A deficiency causes metablastic changes in the epithelium of the gastrointestinal, respiratory, and urogenital tracts. Squamous epithelium lines the external part of the body and its orifices (mouth, pharynx, anus, and vagina). The gut, lower respiratory passages, gallbladder, and endocervix are lined by glandular epithelium. In vitamin A deficiency, it is known that the bronchial mucus-producing, ciliated columnar epithelium undergoes metaplastic change into a cornified, stratified squamous epithelium. Of relevance to the relationship between vitamin A and cancer is the occurrence of metaplasia early in the evolution of many neoplasms. Some investigators believe that metaplasia is the first step in the transformation from normal to neoplastic tissue. In the tissue undergoing malignant transformation, the normal differentiation pattern is lost and a new form of epithelium appears.

Effects of Vitamin A on Metaplasia and Carcinogenesis in Animals

Vitamin A deficiency is often related to keratinizing disorders and squamous metaplasia of the skin. Deficiency of vitamin A causes phrynoderma, a skin disease characterized by dryness, roughness, and follicular hyperkeratosis. Upon microscopic examination, hyperkeratosis, distended follicular openings with keratinous plugging, and atrophy of sweat and sebaceous glands are observed. Later keratinizing metaplasia develops in these glands. The histological picture cannot be clearly distinguished from ichthyosis or keratosis pilaris. Squamous metaplasia associated with a marked keratinization is also especially common in bronchi and the uterine cervix; this hyperplasia can be inhibited by adequate intake of vitamin A.

Organ Culture

Because the appearance of metaplasia is common to both vitamin A deficiency and early neoplasia as well, a deficiency of this vitamin might enhance the neoplastic response to chemical carcinogens. Experiments *in vitro* in organ cultures have supported this concept.

Lasnitzki demonstrated that the extensive hyperplasia and squamous metaplasia produced by carcinogenic polycyclic hydrocarbons in an organ culture of mouse prostate can be reversed or inhibited by naturally occurring vitamin A or by snythetic retinoids.[1,2] In organ cultures of hamster trachea, vitamin A inhibited the induction of squamous cell metaplasia as well as the proliferative epithelial lesions by benzpyrene.[3] The inhibition of hyperplasia seems to be mediated through a reduction of DNA synthesis.

Experiments in Animals

Many *in vivo* experiments have produced similar results. A number of experiments have suggested that vitamin A deficiency is related to cancer of the skin, stomach, nasopharynx, lower respiratory tract, and the endocervix, which are lined by glandular epithelium.

Skin Cancer. In Rhino mice fed a diet containing 100 IU vitamin A/g feed, fewer 7,12-dimethylbenzanthracene (DMBA)-induced papillomas were produced than in mice fed a diet deficient in vitamin A.[4] When vitamin A was given orally, the time of tumor induction was influenced as well as the growth of DMBA–croton oil induced papillomas of the skin.[5] When vitamin A was applied topically, the number of mouse skin papillomas induced by DMBA–croton oil was reduced.[5] The beneficial effect of vitamin A on the development of chemically induced papillomas may be due to its regulatory effect by controlling cellular differentiation of the epithelium.

Lung Cancer. Saffiotti *et al.* observed that oral administration of vitamin A palmitate after benzpyrene treatment markedly inhibits not only squamous metaplasia, but tracheal bronchigenic carcinomas in hamsters as well.[7] Cone and Nettesheim demonstrated that vitamin A protects against the development of respiratory squamous tumors in response to the carcinogen, 3-methylcholanthrene, administered by endotracheal instillation.[8] Nettesheim and Williams reported that the induction of neoplastic lesions of the lungs by 3-methycholanthrene was enhanced in rats deprived of vitamin A.[9] This conclusion was based on observations of squamous nodules in the lungs, which have been demonstrated to be precursors of squamous cell carcinomas. In contrast, Smith *et al.* observed that high levels of vitamin A intake increase the incidence of respiratory tract tumors in hamsters.[10]

Bladder Cancer. Vitamin A deficiency also affects the mucus of the urinary bladder, producing squamous cell metaplasia as well as a high incidence of cystitis, ureteritis, and pyelonephritis.

The effects of a vitamin A deficiency have been studied in rats given *N*-[4-(5-nitro-2-furyl)-2-thiazolyl]formamide (FANFT), a known bladder carcinogen. Sprague-Dawley rats maintained on a diet deficient in vitamin A exhibited an accelerated neoplastic response to FANFT, which resulted in an earlier appearance of urinary bladder tumors as well as the development of ureteral and pelvic carcinomas.[11] In addition, a high incidence of squamous cell papilloma of the urinary bladder was observed in rats fed a vitamin A-free diet and given *N*-methyl-*N*-nitrosoguanidine (MNNG).[12]

Intestinal Cancer. Even though squamous cell metaplasia in the mucosa of the large bowel does not occur with vitamin A deficiency, several studies have been conducted to determine what effect such a deficiency would have on the large bowel in the rat. Rogers *et al.* studied the effects of a low vitamin A dietary intake on the response of rats to intragastric administration of 1,2-dimethylhydrazine.[13] In these experiments a slight increase in the incidence of tumors of the large bowel in the animals fed the low vitamin A diet was observed. However, in the same experiments Rogers *et al.* reported that the induction of neoplasia in the large bowel of rats by 1,2-dimethylhydrazine was slightly enhanced by a high intake of the vitamin. Narisawa *et al.* administered the carcinogen MNNG intrarectally to rats and found that animals fed a diet free of vitamin A developed fewer neoplastic lesions of the large bowel than did those supplemented with vitamin A or those fed a commercial chow diet containing an adequate vitamin A content.[12]

In another experiment, rats were exposed to the carcinogen aflatoxin and were fed diets containing various amounts of vitamin A.[14] The animals that were deficient in vitamin A developed tumors of the large bowel, whereas rats fed a diet containing adequate levels of vitamin A did not develop tumors. In both groups of animals, neoplasms of the liver developed; however, there were fewer liver tumors in the group deficient in vitamin A. Therefore, the overall affect was a shift in the site of neoplasms rather than an overall change in tumor incidence.

Stomach. Chu and Malmgren observed that a high intake of vitamin A inhibits the formation of tumors of the forestomach and of the cervix in hamsters.[15]

Solid Tumors. Vitamin A has been used as a chemotherapeutic agent against several solid tumors. Vitamin A has reduced the tumor size of mice inoculated with a murine sarcoma virus of the Moloney strain.[16] Tumors induced by inoculation with C3HBA tumor cells have a decreased rate for the first 19 days.[17] Survival time has also been increased in vitamin A-treated mice. In addition, the growth of Shope rabbit papilloma has been inhibited by hypervitaminosis A.[18]

Synergistic Effect on Chemotherapy. Vitamin A enhances the antitumor effect of cyclophosphamide in mammary gland adenocarcinoma in rats and mice and also of 1,3-bis(2-chloro-ethyl-1-nitrosourea) BNCU in leukemic mice.[19,20] The combined effect of retinyl palmitate (RP) and 5-fluorouracil (5-FU) has been examined with the use of allostransplantable and syngeneic murine tumor systems.[21] The combined intraperitoneal administration of RP and 5-FU was shown to suppress the tumor growth in 1CR/JCL mice given subcutaneous inoculations of allotransplantable sarcoma 180 cells and to prolong the survival time of mice, as compared with the survival time of mice given a single administration of either RP or 5-FU. Similar results were observed with BALB/c mice were inoculated subcutaneously with a syngeneic BALB/c Meth A fibrosarcoma and treated with RP and 5-FU.

Prutkin also found a synergistic effect of vitamin A and fluorouracil used in combination on the skin tumor, kerotoacanthroma.[22] Tani *et al.* reported a synergistic effect of vitamin A and 5-FU as chemotherapeutic agents in glioma.[23] Synergistic combinations of 5-FU, vitamin A, and cobalt-60 have been reported effective on head and neck tumors.[24] In these experiments, vitamin A might be enhancing the regression of tumors by labilizing lysosomes. The labilization of lysosomes is a known property of vitamin A in normal tissues.

Effect of Retinoids on Cell Transformation. Merriman and Bertram used cultured C3H/10T-½ clone 8 cells to study the effects on 3-methylcholanthrene (MCA)-induced neoplastic transformation. At concentrations that did affect cell survival, retinyl acetate was found to inhibit MCA-induced transformation.[25] Complete inhibition of transformation was observed when MCA-treated cells were continuously treated with retinyl acetate starting 7 days after MCA exposure. A brief exposure to retinyl acetate on days 7–14 caused a 70% inhibition in transformation. If treatment was delayed with retinyl acetate up to 3 weeks after MCA exposure, transformation was still decreased by 80%. Nontoxic concentrations of retinol and retinal were found to be about equal in potency to retinyl acetate. The inhibition of neoplastic transformation by retinoids was found to be fully reversible on maintaining initiated cultures for 3–5 weeks in retinoid-free medium. It is likely that the retinoids are acting to delay the progression of preneoplastic cells to fully neoplastic cells. The mechanism by which retinoids inhibit the expression of neoplastic transformation in the 10T-½ system is unknown.

Murine sarcoma virus (MSV)-transformed cells are known to lack available receptors for epidermal growth factor (EGF).[25] This altered phenotype is the result of the endogenous production of growth factors by the MSV-transformed cells themselves. The major activity, isolated and purified from transformed cells, has been found in a 12,000-mw peak and competes with EGF in an EGF-receptor-binding assay. The growth factor, called sarcoma growth factor (SGF), stimulates cell division. This process causes normal cells to grow in soft agar and also produces rapid, reversible morphological transformation of cells in monolayer cultures. There is no evidence that SGF acts as a complete carcinogen, producing permanent cell transformation; its properties resemble the classical chemical promotors of carcinogenesis, like 12-O-tetradecanoylphorbol-13-acetate (TPA), the highly active component of croton oil. In the experiments of Todaro *et al.*, retinoids were found to block the transforming effect of the polypeptide hormone, SGF.[26] Only one concentration of each retinoid was used, and both the growth promoter and the antagonists were added to the cells at the same time.

Lotan and Nicolson studied the ability of vitamin A derivatives (retinoids) to inhibit the growth of 31 untransformed, transformed, or tumor cell lines *in vitro*.[27] Two retinoids, retinyl acetate and, to a greater extent, retinoic acid have inhibited the growth of a considerable number of transformed and tumor cells. The inhibition *in vitro* suggested that the previously observed antitumor activity of retinoids *in vivo* at least partly due to direct inhibition of cell proliferation. The availability of transplantable homogeneous tumor cell lines inhibited by retinoids may be useful for screening vitamin A derivatives for antitumor activity.

Effect on Mutagenesis

Mammalian Cells/Retinol by itself failed to induce an increase of sister–chromatid exchanges (SCE) or a cycle delay in Chinese hamster V79 cells with or without the metabolic activation of S-9 mix.[28] However, retinol inhibited SCE frequencies and cell cycle delay in V79 cells induced by the indirect mutagen cyclophosphamide or aflatoxin B-1. The inhibitor was found to be both dose and time dependent. The results of Huang *et al.* suggest that retinol itself may have no direct effect on the genetic materials, but rather may possibly act by inhibiting the metabolic activation of an indirect mutagen or carcinogen.[28] These workers suggest that the antitumor activities of retinoids might not be limited to the widely accepted role of preventing the promotion step, but could affect the initiation step of carcinogenesis as well.

Bacterial Cells/Vitamin A (retinol) has been shown to inhibit the mitogenic activity of aflatoxin B-1 when added to the Ames *Salmonella*/mammalian microsome assay.[29] The inhibition was found to be dose dependent and not caused by a direct toxic effect on the test bacteria. The same inhibitory effect was observed on the mutagenicity of an aminoazo dye, *o*-aminoazotoluene. Furthermore, the inhibitory effect was exerted by retinol esters such as retinol acetate and retinol palmitate, the later being the physiological storage form of vitamin A. The inhibition was interpreted by the investigators as an effect on the mixed-function oxidases that convert *o*-aminoazotoluene to its ultimate mutagenic form.

Vitamin A has also been shown to modify the mutagenic activity of the aromatic amines 2-aminofluorene (2-AF) and 2-acetylaminofluorene (2-AAF) when added to the Ames *Salmonella*/mammalian microsome assay. Low amounts of retinol were found to increase the mutagenicity of both 2-AF and 2-AAF. At higher doses, the mutagenicity of 2-AAF remained unchanged, while the mutagenicity of 2-AF was gradually decreased. The data from this latter experiment do not support the hypothesis that retinol generally acts as an inhibitor of *in vitro* metabolic activation of procarcinogens.

Retinoids

Toxicity

The toxic effects of vitamin A certainly limit its effective use on cancer prevention. The toxicity problem has led to searches for more effective vitamin A derivatives that have high vitamin A activity but low toxicity. These investigations have led to the discovery of retinoids (Fig. 4-1). The effectiveness of retinoids has been summarized by Sporn *et al.*[3] One of the more effective retinoids is retinyl methyl ether, which is 20–100 times less toxic than retinol or retinoid acid in comparative toxicity to tracheal cartilege in organ culture. More than 1000 retinoids have been tested with only partial success in regard to their toxicity and their vitamin A activity.

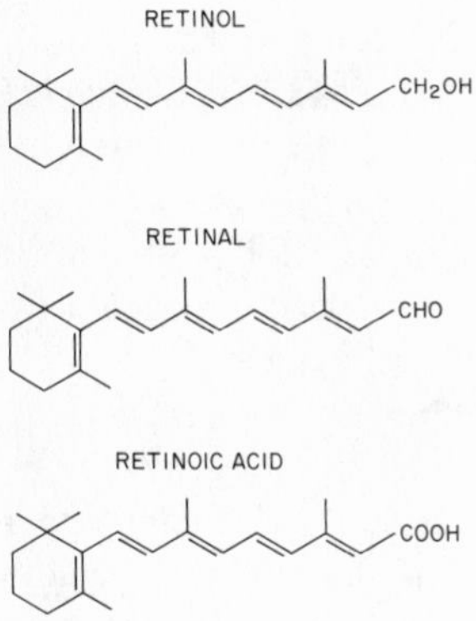

RETINOL

RETINAL

RETINOIC ACID

Figure 4-1. Structures of retinol, retinal, and retinoic acid.

Anticarcinogenic Effect

The major advantage of retinoids is that they have the same anticarcinogenic effects as vitamin A, but are not as toxic as vitamin A. Several synthetic retinoids have been observed to prevent the development of skin cancer,[31] cancer of the respiratory tract,[33] cancer of the mammary gland,[33] and cancer of the urinary bladder.[30] Todaro *et al.* reported that the retinoids may work by inhibiting the mitogenic action of a growth factor produced in cells transformed by a mouse sarcoma virus.[35] This factor seems to be a polypeptide that stimulates cell proliferation by binding to a receptor on the plasma membrane. Apparently retinoids abrogate the cell proliferation signal that results from interaction between the receptor and the tumor-derived growth factor.

Sporn *et al.* concluded that in some circumstances retinoids could prevent the development of epithelial cancer, but were of limited use as agents for chemoprevention because of their inadequate tissue distribution, excessive toxicity, or both.[35] One might speculate whether a clinical trial with retinoids would be useful. However, because high doses of retinoids are also known to produce hypervitaminosis A, which is characterized by changes in the skin and mucous membranes as well as liver dysfunction and headache, the systemic use in a clinical trial or a clinical practice seems to be limited.

Carotenoids

Plants contain a group of compounds, the carotenoids, which can be converted into vitamin A *in vivo*. Carotenoids can also be absorbed unchanged from the gastrointestinal tract and may also exist in tissues in their original form. In a review of epidemiological data on vitamin A and related compounds, Peto *et al.*

postulated that β-carotene itself, rather than its derivative vitamin A, may have the capacity to inhibit carcinogenesis in epithelial cells.[37] Because one form can be converted to the other, it is difficult to determine which of the two forms is more important in the cancer inhibitory process.

Mathews-Roth *et al.* observed that β-carotene, canthaxanthin (4-4'-di-keto-β-carotene), and phytoene can produce a significant protective effect against the development of ultraviolet (UV)-induced skin tumors in hairless mice.[38] Because canthaxanthin and phytoene are carotenoids that do not exhibit vitamin A activity, the protective effect appears to be an inherent part of the carotenoid structure *per se.* In contrast, Shamberger reported earlier experiments in which β-carotene applied to the skin of mice at the same time that croton oil greatly increased the formation of epidermal tumors previously initiated by DMBA.[39] There is a possibility that the great degree of unsaturation of the carotene molecule and its exposure to air on the skin increased carcinogenesis through a greater peroxidative effect. It is likely that increased peroxidation and tissue damage and free radical damage enhance carcinogenesis. On the other hand, dietary carotene would not be exposed to air and would be available to be metabolized to vitamin A in the tissues. Certainly further research is necessary to evaluate the effects of carotenoids on carcinogenesis in laboratory animals.

Decreased tumor frequency, increased latent period, and an increased tumor regression rate were observed in male inbred CBA/J mice fed supplemental β-carotene before and/or after they were inoculated with Moloney sarcoma virus.[40] β-carotene feeding begun after tumors were already present markedly increased the rate of tumor regression.

Retinol-Binding Protein

Although retinoic acid is known to be involved in epithelial differentiation and in the control of tumorigenesis, the biochemical mechanism displayed by retinoic acid at the genetic level is unknown. The binding affinity of various retinoic acid analogues for retinoic acid binding protein (RABP) has been correlated with their ability to reverse the metaplasia of hamster trachea and their ability to reverse the keratinization of chick embryo skin in organ culture.[41,42] RABP has been detected in the nuclei of chick embryo skin, and some experimental colon tumors as well as the transmigration of retinoic acid–RABP complex into the nuclei in retinoblastoma cells have suggested that retinoic acid may be functioning as steroid hormones do through the mediation of receptor proteins.[43–45]

Like most of the steroid hormone receptors, RABP is primarily detected in the cytosol, followed by nuclei, and then by mitochondria. Ligand specificity studies have indicated that the nuclear-binding component shares similar properties with cytoplasmic RABP. RABP has been detected in the nuclei of chick embryo skin and Lewis lung tumor.[45] In this study, the nuclear binding component showed the same ligand specificity and sedimentation valve as the cytosol RABP. The nonspecific uptake of retinoic acid by Lewis lung nuclei and chick embryo skin nuclei was inhibited up to 50% by cytosol RABP. Demonstration of the localization of RABP in the nuclei of chick embryo skin may be the first step in delineating the molecular mechanism of retinoic acid for gene activation in differentiation.

Huber *et al.* checked 75 specimens of human breast tissue for the presence of cellular retinoic acid-binding protein (CRABP). Fifty-two percent of the primary carcinomas and 43% of the dysplastic breast lesions (stage MII) were found to contain detectable amounts of CRABP, whereas no CRABP was found in normal tissue.[47] Basu *et al.* measured serum vitamin A and retinol-binding protein (RBP) in 53 myeloma and 28 epithelial cell cancer cases.[48] In these patients, vitamin A levels were found to be more marked in the patients with cancer of epithelial origin. RBP serum concentrations fell in parallel with vitamin A in the epithelial cancer patients, while the RBP levels remained unaffected in the patients with myeloma, suggesting that an underlying factor for resulting low vitamin A levels may be different in these two groups of patients.

Mechanisms of Action

There are several possible mechanisms for the anticancer effect of vitamin A.

Mixed-Function Oxidase

Several vitamin A compounds and analogues have been observed to inhibit the *in vitro* microsomal mixed function oxidases that metabolize carcinogenic polycyclic aromatic hydrocarbons (PAH's).[49] This could be an important mechanism in the protection of vitamin A-induced squamous metaplasia. In addition, Carruthers observed that intraperitoneally administered 3,4-benzpyrene and MCA results in a marked reduction in hepatic vitamin A in rats.[50] These results suggest that the depletion of vitamin A by PAH's may be an important process in the development of carcinogenesis.

DNA Binding

The binding of carcinogens to DNA has been indicated as a critical step in the carcinogenic process. For phytohemaglutinin (PHA), the binding to DNA may be a measure of the carcinogenic potential toward a given tissue. Vitamin A deficiency has been observed to enhance the binding of benzopyrene to the DNA of hamster tracheal cells.[51]

Effect on Metabolic Activation

Huang et al. found that retinol affects neither the frequency of SCEs nor cell delay in Chinese hamster V79 cell with or without metabolic activation of S-9 mix, but inhibits the SCE frequencies and cell cycle delay in V79 cells induced by the indirect mutagen cyclophosphamide or aflatoxin B-1.[28] The results suggest that retinol itself may have no direct effect on the genetic materials, but rather exerts its effect by possibly inhibiting the metabolic activation of an indirect mutagen or carcinogen.

Inhibition of Ornithine Decarboxylase

Application of the potent tumor promoter 12-otetradecanoyl-phorbol-13-acetate (TBA) to mouse skin leads to a more than a 200-fold increase in epidermal ornithine decarboxylase activity.[51] This phenotypic change may be essential for skin tumor promotion. Verma et al. found that vitamin A and its analogues applied to the skin inhibit both the TPA-induced ornithine decarboxylase activity and the formation of skin papillomas. Systemic administration of retinoic acid also inhibited ornithine decarboxylase activity. In another type of experiment, nude mice were irradiated once daily with ultraviolet light.[52] In the experimental group, topical retinoic acid was applied immediately after each irradiation. After 52 weeks, the groups treated with retinoic acid tended to have fewer mice with tumors, fewer tumors per mouse, smaller tumor diameters, and slower-growing tumors than did the appropriately irradiated control groups. Retinoic acid also reduced the activity of UV-light-induced epidermal ornithine decarboxylase activity. Similar inhibitions of UV-light-induced carcinogenesis were reported by Conner et al.[54]

Effect on Lysosomal Membranes

One of the known properties of vitamin A and the polyene antibiotics is their ability to labilize lysosomal membranes. Several investigators have proposed that retinoids labilize lysosomal membranes, which are able to act on preneoplastic and neoplastic cells alike. In the experiments of Lotan and Nicolson, who incubated retinoids with tumors cells in vitro, the viability of the treated cells were not affected.[27] Direct determinations of free lysosomal enzymes in the cytoplasms of the melanoma cell lines S91 and B16, which are known to be sensitive to inhibition of growth by retinoic acid, did not show any increased release or change in the ratio of free to bound acid phosphatase or arylsulfatase. Therefore, labilization of lysosomal membranes may not be an important mechanism in the chemopreventative action of vitamin A on tumors.

Effect on Immune Functions

As a consequence of their presence in certain organs, tissues, and body fluids other than blood plasma, such as lymph, vitamin A, and β-carotene may influence the growth and maturation of cells that regulate various immune functions, such as thymus function, thereby moderating tumor growth. Stimulation of the immune response by vitamin A compounds is adequately documented and reviewed by Hill and Grubbs.[57] Vitamin A administration can cause increased humoral responses to foreign proteins and to heterologous red blood cells, accelerated graft rejection, increased cellularity of lymph nodes draining injection depots, and enhanced resistance to infection with variety of bacterial pathogens.

Evidence for Involvement of Retinoids in the Immune Response. Various retinoids stimulate the induction of cytotoxic thymus-derived lymphocytes both *in vivo* and *in vitro*. Increased lymphocyte blastogenesis and immunostimulation occur in response to PHA, and an increased lymphocyte blastogenesis was observed in lung cancer patients dosed with retinyl palmitate or 13-*cis*-retinoic acid. Several studies of retinoids and experimental animal tumors support involvement of the immune response. The results of these studies are as follows:

1. The dose of radiation needed to achieve eradication of immunogenic tumors was lowered by retinyl palmitate.
2. Prophylactic treatment of animals with retinyl palmitate did not reduce the "take" of nonimmunogenic tumors.
3. The inhibition by retinyl palmitate on the growth of an immunogenic tumor was reversed by the administration of antilymphocyte serum (ALS), and the retinoid reversed stimulation of tumor growth by ALS.
4. For a transplantable syngeneic sarcoma, retinyl palmitate potentiated the reduction in tumor incidence mediated by *Mycobacterium bovis,* strain bacille Calmette-Guérin (BCG).
5. The growth of several experimental tumors was restricted by retinoic-treated animals, but only in immunocompetent animals. The growth restriction appeared to be the result of stimulation of thymus-dependent, immune-mediated factors that reduce growth of tumors. Furthermore, investigators studying rat chondrosarcoma have suggested that its inhibition by retinoids, which is one of the most dramatic examples of the inhibition of a transplantable tumor, was due to chondrocyte recognition and rejection by the immune system.

6. Established skin papillomas have undergone spontaneous regressions, implying that immunostimulation by retinoids plays a role in their regression during experiments. In addition, x-irradiation and thymectomy delayed, and a methanol extract of BCG accelerated, regression of papillomas.

Apparently by a different mechanism, retinoids also modify cells that change the neoplasia in such a way that progression is reversed, and the cells do not become malignant. Retinoids are able to block tumor induction, at least in some models, by inhibiting the promotion phase. However, the application of various retinoids to skin after carcinogen exposure, but 1 hr before application of promoting agents results in the inhibition of papillomas on mouse skin. Because of the time necessary to synthesize proteins, it is unlikely that the immune response could be so quickly involved as to overcome the action of the promoter. It is also unlikely that direct cytotoxicity or endocrine factors are involved. Rather, the inhibition seems to correlate with the ability of the drugs to impede stimulation of synthesis of epidermal ornithine decarboxylase by the promoter. Consistent with this concept is the idea that the retinoids are like steroids, binding to cytosolic receptors, which are able to translocate to the cell nucleus to alter messenger RNA and protein synthesis.

Evidence Supporting the Nonimmunologic Role of Retinoids. Additional evidence supports a nonimmunologic role of retinoids in the chemoprevention of cancer, which may be summarized as follows:

1. Investigations *in vitro* demonstrate that retinoids, present in the medium, inhibit the oncogenic transformation of 10T-½ cells exposed to γ-radiation or previously exposed to 3-MCA. Retinoids also block cell transformation caused by sarcoma growth factor in rat kidney fibroblasts.
2. Several natural and synthetic retinoids inhibit carcinogen-induced hyperplastic or anaplastic tissue changes *in vitro* as well as the growth of established cell lines *in vitro*.
3. Because retinoids are involved, especially for epithelial tissues, in the induction or enhancement of cellular differentiation, retinoids may be able to arrest or reverse the process of carcinogenesis through the same mechanism as in normal differentiation, a process that presumably does not involve the immune system. The mechanism whereby retinoic acid painted onto the skin is able to promote the carcinogenic effect of DMBA or of UV light in some cases is also unknown.

The antipromoting effect seems to be important in the prevention by retinoids of at least some types of cancer, but these compounds may also inhibit established, immunogenic tumors by enhancing the immunologic response of the host. There is a possibility that a common mechanism exists for both pre-neoplastic and neoplastic lesions. Formation of these lesions may be influenced by the antipromoting properties of retinoids. However, the host may also mount an immunologic response to both preneoplastic and neoplastic lesions, this latter response perhaps being enhanced by retinoids.

Epidemiological Evidence

The marked anticancer effect of vitamin A in animals has led to numerous epidemiological investigations, most of which are case-control studies. These studies have indicated an inverse relationship between vitamin A intake and a large variety of cancers. Most studies of vitamin A were based on the frequency of ingestion of a group of foods (e.g., green and yellow vegetables) known to be rich in β-carotene (a provitamin that may be enzymatically converted to vitamin A *in vivo*) as well as a few foods such as whole milk and liver containing preformed retinol (vitamin A). Therefore, to a large extent, these epidemiological studies have measured indirect indices of β-carotene intake. In this section the term vitamin A is also used to include β-carotene intake, since the effect of the two components is not separated in most reports cited.

Lung Cancer

Bjelke was one of the first investigators to report epidemiological data that suggested that vitamin A plays a protective role against cancer.[58] Using frequency of consumption data collected from a questionnaire mailed to a group of Norwegian men, Bjelke calculated a vitamin A index using limited sources of the vitamin. After controlling for cigarette smoking, lower values were observed for lung cancer cases than for controls. In another case-control study among Chinese women in Singapore, MacLennan *et al.* found an inverse association between consumption of green leafy vegetables rich in vitamin A and lung cancer.[59]

A case-control study conducted by Gregor *et al.*, included hospital outpatients, mostly from a rheumatology clinic, as controls.[60] Significantly less vitamin A was consumed by male lung cancer patients than by the controls. The male lung cancer patients had consumed fewer vitamin A supplements as well as less liver. This study included only a small number of female participants, however; in general, these cases had a different relative distribution of tumor cell type than was found in the males, but showed an opposite (direct) association with vitamin A intake, even though they consumed fewer vitamin A supplements than did the controls.

In another case-control study,[61] Smith and Jick noted an inverse association between the use of vitamin A supplements and the incidence of cancer, including lung cancer in men, but not women. After controlling for cigarette smoking, Mettlin *et al.* conducted a case-control study in which an index of vitamin A consumption, based on the frequency of consumption of a group of food items, was found to be inversely associated with lung cancer in males.[62] Plasma levels of vitamin A were lower in 28 patients with bronchial carcinoma than in a small group of controls.[63]

In a 19-year follow-up study of 1954 men in Chicago, lung cancer incidence showed an inverse correlation with carotene intake both with and without adjustment for cigarette smoking.[64] However, there was no significant association of lung cancer with the intake of preformed vitamin A.

Laryngeal Cancer

Laryngeal cancer in male patients has been studied by Graham *et al.*[65] After controlling for cigarette smoking and alcohol consumption, these investigators reported an inverse relationship, with a dose–response gradient, between cancer risk and the vitamin A and C intake, based on the frequency of consumption of selected foods. Similar results have been reported for vegetable consumption in general, but not for cruciferous vegetable in particular.

Bladder Cancer

In a case-control study designed along the lines of their investigation of lung cancer, Mettlin *et al.* reported a similar inverse association of their vitamin A consumption index with bladder cancer. This study controlled for coffee consumption, smoking, and occupational exposure.[62]

Esophageal Cancer

The frequency of milk consumption and of leafy green and yellow vegetables, both sources of vitamin A and β-carotene, has been reported to be lower among patients with esophageal cancer than in the diets of controls.[45] After controlling for cigarette smoking and alcohol consumption, Mettlin *et al.* reported a similar inverse association and a dose–response gradient for frequency of consumption of fruits and vegetables in a study of male cases and controls.[67] Although these workers also observed an inverse relationship for an index of vitamin A consumption based on selected foods, there was an even stronger inverse relationship for an index of vitamin C consumption. These findings were consistent for populations in the Caspian littoral of Iran, a region for which a particularly high esophageal cancer incidence has been reported.[68] These studies indicated that consumption of green vegetables and fresh fruit as well as the estimated vitamin A and C intake in high-risk areas were lower than in areas of low risk. In a subsequent case-control study in this area of Iran, investigators also found that cases had consumed smaller amounts of uncooked vegetables (as well as fruits) than had the controls.[69]

Stomach Cancer

Hirayama reported an inverse relationship between daily consumption of milk (a source of vitamin A) and stomach cancer in a case-control study conducted in Japan.[70] Hirayama also reported a similar protective effect of milk based on data from a prospective group involving 265,118 subjects.[71] In addition, there was a lower risk for stomach cancer among nonsmokers who consumed leafy green and yellow vegetables. In a case-control study of gastric cancer in New York state, Graham et al. reported a higher consumption of uncooked vegetables (likely sources of β-carotene) by controls than by gastric cancer cases.[72] In a case-control study in Hawaii, a similar inverse association with the consumption of raw vegetables was observed by Haenszel et al.[73]

Colon/Rectal Cancer

In studies of cancer cases and controls in Norway and Minnesota, Bjelke observed that milk and several vegetables have been consumed with less frequency by colorectal cancer cases than by controls.[74] In addition, an index of vitamin A intake (which was highly correlated with vegetable consumption) showed the same inverse relationship.

Prostate Cancer

Schuman et al. have related foods rich in vitamin A (e.g., liver) and β-carotene (e.g., carrots) to prostate cancer and observed that the vitamin A-rich foods were consumed less frequently by cases than by controls.[75]

Cervical Dysplasias

Women with abnormal cytology were matched with normal control subjects for age, parity, ethnicity, and socioeconomic class.[76] These women participated in a blind case-control study focused on a nutritional survey to study the role of nutrition in cervical dysplasia. In addition, sucrose-gradient ultracentrifugation studies were done to determine the presence and concentration of the binding proteins for retinol and retinoic acid from colposcopic biopsy specimens. The nutritional survey revealed statistically significant differences for vitamins A and C and β-carotene. Retinol-binding protein was absent or minimally detectable and inversely related to the severity of the dysplasia.

General

In three recent reports based on data from groups studied in the United States and England, Kark *et al.* observed an inverse relationship between serum levels of vitamin A and the subsequent risk of cancer in general.[80] The interrelationship between the dietary intake of vitamin A and its serum level (which appears to be under homeostatic control) is not clear in these populations, which are generally not deficient in this nutrient. There is also a known correlation between retinol and cholesterol concentrations and cancer mortality, which may reflect a relationship between their carrier proteins—retinol-binding protein and low-density lipoprotein. There is a possibility that the determinants of the blood concentrations of these carrier proteins have the same genetic origin. A study of serum cholesterol, serum retinol, and serum carotene concentrations in relation to the incidence of cancer may elucidate the cholesterol–cancer relationships previously described.

VITAMIN B

B vitamins are known to be essential components of any adequate diet and are necessary for the continued maintenance of cellular integrity as well as metabolic function. In general, several deficiencies of any of the B vitamins will clearly reduce the growth rate of tumor cells and also interfere with the normal functioning of the organism. However, only a few of the vitamins, such as thiamine, riboflavin, pyridoxine, vitamin B12, and folic acid, have been tested. Even though choline is not a vitamin by strict definition, it is generally included in the vitamin B complex. In order to consider the roles of choline and the B vitamins in carcinogenesis, one should recognize the complex interrelationships of these vitamins with one another and with other dietary components, such as protein and total calories. Certainly if there were secondary changes in protein, nucleic acid, carbohydrates, fat, and/or mineral metabolism, this could account for many of the effects observed with specific vitamins. Even though certain experimental models have defined the roles of several of the vitamins at the molecular level, their individual contribution to the overall carcinogenic effect is difficult to assess.

General Effect in Animals

There has been little or no control for intake of other dietary constituents, notably protein and calories, in much of the work demonstrating effects of specific B vitamins on carcinogenesis in model systems. An improved experimental design would make the results of these experiments more useful, because protein and caloric intake are two major components that have considerable effect on the overall outcome of carcinogenesis. A couple of the early experiments were exceptions and were designed appropriately. These studies showed that the intake of B vitamins has either no effect, or at most a minimal effect, on carcinogenesis.

Tannenbaum and Silverstone reported no significant differences in tumor incidence amoung groups of animals fed minimal, moderate, of high levels of B vitamins.[81] However, in three of four experiments, the rate of tumor development was faster in mice ingesting moderate amounts of vitamins than in mice ingesting either high or low amounts. In another experiment, no effects of specific components were detected, but when the intake of all B vitamins was low, the incidence of tumors in mice was decreased.[82]

Riboflavin

Requirements and Effect of Deficiency. The recommended daily intake of riboflavin for infants is 0.4–0.6 mg; for children aged 1–10 years, 0.8–1.4 mg; for women, 1.2–1.3 mg; and for men, 1.4–1.7 mg. The amount of riboflavin that might have an effect on cancer is unknown. Riboflavin deficiency manifests as a corneal vascularization. Angular stomatitis, glossitis, alopecia, ulceration, and seborrheic dermatitis also occur about the nose and scrotum. Erythrocyte glutathione reductase, which is a riboflavin-dependent enzyme, has been used to evaluate population groups.

Effect on Carcinogenesis in Animals. Enzymatic activation or deactivation of procarcinogens involves competing pathways. Many of these metabolic pathways can be altered by dietary constituents such as vitamins and other nutrients, which in turn may alter carcinogenesis. Kensler *et al.* demonstrated that riboflavin provided partial protection against hepatic cancer induced by orally administered dimethylaminoazobenzene by possibly enhancing the detoxification of that carcinogen through a flavin-dependent enzyme system.[83,84] It seems likely that the opposite effect, i.e., enhancement of carcinogenic potential, might be observed if vitamin B_2 (riboflavin) were necessary for activation to the ultimate carcinogen.

The growth and spread of spontaneous mammary cancers are markedly reduced in animals that have become deficient in riboflavin. Morris indicated that the size of spontaneous mammary tumors is smaller in the riboflavin-deficient animals than in the control animals.[85]

Riboflavin has been shown to enhance skin carcinogenesis by 7,12-dimethylbenzanthracene-croton oil and to enhance azo dye-carcinogenesis.[86] The activation of DMBA may be also due to an increase of activity of arylhydrocarbon hydroxylase, thereby forming active metabolites, which may lead to increased binding to DNA.

When placed in the drinking water, riboflavin was ineffective against UV-induced carcinogenesis.[87] However, riboflavin has reduced hepatoma incidence induced by a single dose of aflatoxin B-1.[88] Riboflavin deficiency has been observed to enhance hepatic carcinogenesis by azo dyes; riboflavin administration to deficient animals has also been shown to inhibit the development of hepatomas. Diminished activities of flavin-dependent enzymes may be responsible for this latter effect. In riboflavin deficiency, the hepatic concentration of flavin-adenine dinucleotide (FAD) is reduced to one-third of normal and its likely under these conditions there is decreased degradation of azo dyes by azo reductase. The activity of an enzyme that metabolizes 3,4-benzpyrene is also reduced in riboflavin deficiency. In the special case of azo compounds attached to benzidine, azo reduction leads to a more potent mutagenic compound, rather than an activated one. The major drug metabolizing hepatic enzymes, the mixed-function oxidase system, requires FAD. Therefore, potential changes in the riboflavin status could alter the rates of a large number of foreign chemicals and carcinogens in addition to the azo dyes and could therefore be a major factor in regulating carcinogenesis.

Chemotherapeutic Use of Riboflavin and Its Derivatives. Riboflavin deficiency has been shown to result in marked reduction in the size of transplanted lymphosarcomas in mice.[89] Diethyl riboflavin, a structural analogue of riboflavin that antagonizes the biological action of the vitamin, decreases the growth rate of Walker carcinoma in rats.[90] Lane combined riboflavin deficiency with galactoflavin in treating patients having polycythemia vera and lymphoma.[91] In this study, partial remissions were obtained in two of four patients with lymphosarcoma and in one of two patients with Hodgkin's disease. Prolonged remissions were observed in two patients with polycythemia vera.

Pantothenic Acid

Requirements and Effect of Deficiency. The recommended daily intake of pantothenic acid for infants up to 1 year of age is 2–3 mg; for children aged 1–11, 3–7 mg; and for adults, 4–7 mg. This vitamin is so widely distributed in foods that a deficiency of the vitamin is extremely rare. When foods are cooked, canned, frozen, or processed, significant amounts of pantothenic acid are lost. In malnutrition, multiple deficiencies often occur, and a pantothenic acid deficiency may not be apparent. Serum contains free pantothenic acid and no coenzyme A, while most of the vitamin is present in the erythrocytes as coenzyme A.

Symptoms have been observed in human volunteers on a pantothenic acid-deficient diet and on a pantothenic acid antagonist ω-methyl pantothenic acid. Subjects on the pantothenic acid-deficient diet experienced such initial symptoms as vomiting, malaise, abdominal distress, and burning cramps, followed by tenderness in the heels, as well as fatigue and insomnia. The amount of pantothenic acid that might be required in order to alter the cancer process in humans is unknown.

Effect on Carcinogenesis in Animals. Spontaneous mammary carcinoma in C3H mice was depressed by pantothenic acid deficiency.[92] The semicarbazone of pantothenic acid (3-ethoxy-2-oxobutyraldehyde) has been observed to be a potent antitumor against several transplanted tumors.[93] A decrease in liver thiamine and pantothenic acid results when animals are treated with this semicarbazone. In contrast, supplementation with excess amounts of thiamine and pantothenic acid in tumor-bearing rats will also increase the antitumor activity of the semicarbazone.

Choline

Requirements and Effect of Deficiency. The requirement for choline is dependent to some extent on methionine availability, as well as the folacin and vitamin B_{12} content in the diet. Because of the interaction of choline with these and other dietary components, the human requirement for choline is unknown. However, in animals, the most common deficiency signs are fatty infiltration of the liver and hemorrhagic kidney damage. Poultry suffer from perosis, a tendon defect resulting in permanently deformed legs. Choline participates in transmethylation reactions in which choline donates a labile methyl group of homocystine to form methionine, which in turn reacts with guanidoacetic acid to form creatinine. Transmethylation reactions permit replacement of choline with methionine or homocystine, betaine, and ethanolamine in diets without incurring a specific choline deficiency.

In humans the use of choline in the treatment of the fatty liver of alcoholism and kwashiorkor has proven to be ineffective. Administration of choline may help alleviate symptoms of tardive dyskinesia and Huntington diseases, but the effect appears to go far beyond specific dietary needs for choline for normal people. The amount of choline which may have an effect on human cancer is unknown.

Effects of Carcinogenesis in Animals. Liver tumors observed in rats fed choline-deficient diets were linked to the presence of aflatoxin in the diets.

Inhibition of tumor incidence was found when the diet was supplemented with choline.[94] In addition, Lombardi and Shinozuka found a choline-deficient diet to enhance the induction in rats of liver tumors induced by 2AAF.[95] In general, azaserine is a weak inducer of liver tumors, but Shinozuka *et al.* observed a 60–70% incidence of hepatocellular carcinomas after 4–5 months when azaserine was administered to choline-deficient rats. Liver tumor induction was also increased in a similar manner when ethionine was fed to rats maintained on a methionine choline-deficient diet. It appears that a choline-deficient diet acts as a strong promoter of further evolution to neoplasia of initiated liver cells.

Feeding a choline-deficient diet to rats strongly promotes the evolution of liver cells initiated by a liver carcinogen diethylnitrosamine to foci of γ-glutamyltranspeptidase (GGTP)-positive hepatocytes. Takahashi *et al.* investigated whether a choline-deficient diet might promote the evolution of GGTP-positive foci to hepatomas.[97] During the first 7 weeks after initiation, the number and size of the foci increased in both groups. At 12–16 weeks, the number and size of foci began to decline in rats fed a choline-supplemented diet. However, in the choline-deficient group, there was a progressive increase in the size with coalescence of the foci, as well as development of the neoplastic nodules.

The most conspicuous pathological lesion caused by a choline-deficient diet in rat liver is an accumulation of fat; this accumulation progresses, causing a rupture of the plasma membrane and formations of extracellular collections, termed fatty cysts. The fatty cysts apparently result from the fusion of several large droplets of fat contained originally within single hepatocytes, the remnants of which constitute the wall of the cysts. This accumulation of fat is accompanied by liver necrosis and an elevated glutamic oxaloacetic transaminase. Giambarresi *et al.* observed that feeding a choline-deficient diet to rats causes a loss of prelabeled DNA, and therefore of liver cells, accompanied by a stimulation of liver cell proliferation.[98] These workers conclude that feeding a choline-deficient diet causes a low grade of liver cell regeneration.

Effect on Mutagenesis in Bacteria. Reddy *et al.* used *Salmonella* mutagenesis assays to evaluate the mutagenicity of several chemical carcinogens using liver S-9 fractions from rats fed a choline-supplemented or choline-devoid (CD) diet.[99] The liver S-9 fraction from CD diet-fed rats was found to have a significantly decreased ability to activate 2AAF; 2-aminoanthracene, but not *N*-hydroxy-2-acetylaminofluorene (HO-N-2-AAF), and dimethylnitrosamine. The same CD liver S-9 fraction was less effective in deactivating *N*-methyl-*N*-nitro-*N*-nitrosoguanidine, but not methylnitrosourea. In addition, a 20% decrease was found in the cytochrome P450 content in liver microsomes of CD diet-fed rats.

The results of the study by Reddy *et al.* indicate that feeding a choline-deficient diet impairs the activation of procarcinogens to reactive species which are mutagenic. A similar conclusion was previously reported by Rogers, who studied the effects of feeding a multiple lipotrope-deficient diet on the liver activation of several chemical carcinogens.[100] However, the studies of Reddy *et al.* also indicated that in the case of proximate carcinogens, e.g., HO-*N*-2-AAF, and of direct carcinogens, e.g., MNU and MNNG, the choline-deficient diet possibly had no effect or actually enhanced their carcinogenicity by impairing their conversion to inactive metabolites.

Thiamine

Requirements and Effect of Deficiency. The recommended daily requirement for infants up to 1 year of age is 0.3–0.5 mg; for children aged 1–3, 4–6, and 7–10, 0.7 mg, 0.9 mg, and 1.2 mg, respectively; for males aged 11–51, 1.2–1.5 mg; and for females aged 11–51, 1.0–1.1 mg. Thiamine in the form of pyrophosphate participates as a coenzyme in the oxidative decarboxylation of α-keto acids to aldehydes. The major known deficiency disease of humans is beriberi, which presents clinically as a spectrum of manifestations. One of the early symptoms is a peripheral neuropathy. Initially the deep tendon relfexes are increased, but later they may be absent. The muscles are often tender and may atrophy. Fatigue, decreased attention span, and impaired capacity to work may also occur. This is the clinical picture of so-called dry or atrophic beriberi. If even less thiamine is taken in, cardiovascular sign and symptoms occur. The heart is often enlarged and edema may also be present. Tachycardia occurs with the slightest effort in the so-called subacute or wet beriberi. The most acute type of thiamine deficiency is Wernicke's encephalopathy, which occurs mainly in alcoholics, or vomiting associated with pregnancy, or surgery on the gastrointestinal tract. Wernicke's encephalopathy is often associated with high morbidity and mortality.

Effect on Carcinogenesis in Animals. An early study showed that thiamine deficiency did not suppress growth of AAF-induced liver tumors when the effect of lower food intake was taken into consideration.[101]

Effect on Cancer Patients. Significant numbers of cancer patients with advanced malignant disease may be thiamine deficient, as evidenced by their lower transketolase activities.[102] Thiamine pyrophosphate is a coenzyme required for transketolase activity. About 30% of cancer patients tested have a thiamine pyrophosphate uptake greater than 25%, which is indicative of thiamine deficiency. The urinary thiamine excretory levels of these patients are greater than normal, perhaps reflecting the lower serum levels.

There is a possibility that a thiamine deficiency may be due to a reduced ability of cancer patients to convert thiamine to thiamine pyrophosphate, as there is no evidence that the dietary intakes of thiamine were suboptimal. In three treated patients with a generalized invasion by a tumor of the lymphoid-hematopoietic systems, the neuropathologic findings were consistent with Wernicke's encephalopathy.[103] It is likely that this neurological complication was due to a thiamine deficiency caused by severe malabsorption. In 35 patients receiving 5-FU as a chemotherapeutic agent, thiamine deficiency has been observed.[104]

Vitamin B$_{12}$

Requirements and Effect of Deficiency. The recommended daily intake for vitamin B$_{12}$ is 0.5–1.5 μg for infants up to 1 year of age; for children 1–10 years, 2.0–3.0 μg; and for adult men and women, 3.0 μg. The amount of intake that might have an effect on human cancer is unknown. Both vitamin B$_{12}$ and folic acid are required for thymidylate synthesis, and therefore of DNA. A vitamin B$_{12}$-containing enzymes removes a methyl group from methyl folate and transfers it to homocysteine, thereby converting homocysteine to methionine, and in the process regenerating tetrahydrofolic acid, from which the 5,10-methylene tetrahydrofolic acid is synthesized. In addition to the methyl transfer from methylfolate, vitamin B$_{12}$ deficiency results in neurological damage to the myelin, as well as the neuropathies and cerebral manifestations that arise from myelin disorders. Vitamin B$_{12}$ is also required for the hydrogen transfer and isomerization whereby methylmalonate is converted to succinate. Vitamin B$_{12}$ is involved in carbohydrate, fat, and protein metabolism. Vitamin B$_{12}$ is important in the synthesis of the amino acid methionine and appears important in maintaining sulfhydryl groups in the reduced form necessary for the function of many SH-activated enzyme systems. Deficiency of vitamin B$_{12}$ results in megaloblastic anemia accompanied by leukopenia and thrombopenia.

Effect on Carcinogenesis in Animals. An increase in the activity of four carcinogens has been observed in experimental animals.[105] Vitamin B$_{12}$ supplementation has also significantly enhanced the induction of both hyperplastic nodules and hepatoma by aflatoxin in the groups of rats fed high-protein diets.[105A] In contrast, a lack of vitamin B$_{12}$ may slow the carcinogenic process involving methylation of macromolecules such as that observed with dimethylnitrosamine and dimethylhydrazine.[106] A deficiency of vitamin B$_{12}$ has been shown to be somewhat effective in preventing liver carcinogenesis by dimethylaminoazobenzene.[107] Yamamoto observed that vitamin B$_{12}$ deficiency reduces colon tumor incidence in rats receiving azoxymethane.[108]

Effect on Cancer Patients. Elevation of serum B$_{12}$ has been associated with increased granulocytic proliferation, such as that which occurs in chronic myelogenous leukemia.

Excess mortality from gastric cancer seems to exist among patients with pernicious anemia.[109] Ruddell *et al.* postulated a mechanism to explain the increased incidence of gastric cancer. The nitrite concentration of the gastric juice from 13 fasting pernicious anemia patients was found to be nearly 50-fold greater than that of age-matched controls. If nitrosation does occur *in vivo*, the intragastric production of carcinogenic *N*-nitroso compounds might explain the higher incidence of gastric cancer in patients with pernicious anemia. Arvanitakis *et al.* observed an association between pernicious anemia and several other neoplasma during a period of 3–20 years after the diagnosis of pernicious anemia.[111]

Other investigators have observed a coexistence between pernicious anemia and blood malignancies, such as leukemia, erythremic myelosis, polycythemia vera, and multiple myeloma. Carmel and Eisenberg observed in nonhematologic malignancies that a high serum B_{12} level, with or without an unsaturated transcobalamin 1 elevation, usually implies a poor prognosis in cancer patients.[112]

Folic Acid

Requirements and Effect of Deficiency. The recommended daily intake for folic acid for infants up to the age of one year is 30–45 μg; children 1 to 11 years of age, 100–300 μg; and adults, 400 μg. Folic acid as well as vitamin B_{12} are required for the synthesis of thymidylate and therefore DNA. Lack of adequate DNA synthesis causes many hematopoietic cells to die in the bone marrow. Megaloblastosis (the presence of giant germ cells) is the end product of deranged DNA synthesis. The underlying biochemical defect that translates poor thymidylate synthesis into morphological megaloblastosis may be failure to elongate DNA chains in the presence of a relatively normal capacity to initiate DNA synthesis.

Progressive dietary folic acid deprivation in humans results in a series of biochemical and hematological sequences of cells. Low serum folate will result in hypersegmentation of blood cells in about 6–11 weeks. At about 13 weeks, a high urinary formiminoglutamate is evident; at 17 weeks, low folate is seen in the red blood cells; macroovalocytosis is seen at 18 weeks; and at about 19 weeks, megaloblastic marrow followed by anemia can result from the low serum folate. Folate coenzymes involve transfer of one-carbon unit. These reactions include (1) *de novo* purine synthesis; (2) pyrimidine nucleotide biosynthesis; (3) amino acid conversions, serine to glycine, histidine to glutamic acid, and homocysteine to methionine; (4) generation of formate into the formate pool; and (5) methylation of small amounts of transfer RNA.

Einhorn and Retzenstein have observed an increased requirement for folic acid in cancer patients.[113] This increased need is attributable to the accelerated cell division that occurs in malignant neoplasms and leukemias, and the fact that folate is an important factor in cell division. Patients with malignancies have lower blood folic acid levels than the controls.[114] The decreased blood levels may be related to the increased tumor requirements for folic acid.

Effect of Folic Acid on Tissue Culture and Animal Plasma Levels. The activity of dihydrofolate reductase has been shown to increase following the infection of mouse kidney cell cultures with polyoma virus or monkey kidney cell culture with simian virus 40 (SV40). Lower plasma and liver folate have been observed in mice with Rauscher murine leukemia than in normal mice.[115]

Methotrexate. Methotrexate (MTX) is a potent folic acid antagonist used extensively as an anticancer drug. High-dose MTX followed by citrovorum factor (CVF), or 5-formyltetrahydrofolate, reversal was introduced by Djerassi et al. in children with acute lymphocytic leukemia.[116] These workers subsequently reported its effectiveness in children with lymphomas and in adults with carcinoma of the lung, breast, and pancreas. Jaffe demonstrated the effectiveness of this regimen in metastatic osteosarcoma.[117] High-dose MTX treatment is necessary, as low doses may yield an inadequate intracellular drug concentration. Methotrexate has been shown to enter cells primarily by diffusion, but it is also actively excreted. In mixed cellular populations with overlapping cell-division cycles, prolonged high-dose infusions of drug may be required to ensure high intracellular concentration during susceptible phases of the cell cycle.[116] Methotrexate has generally been considered to act primarily by inhibiting the enzyme dihydrofolate reductase, and thereby biosynthesis of thymidylate.

Other Folate Antagonists

Diaminodichlorophenyl methylpryimidine/Diaminodichlorophenyl methylpyrimidine (DDMP) has been observed to act as a folate antagonist. DDMP is apparently not as toxic as methotrexate and was used by Alberto *et al.* in a clinical trial on 128 patients with partial responses.[118] Supplementary citrovorum factor rescue could also be given in case of toxicity.

10-Deazaaminopterin/The folate analogue, 10-deazaaminopterin was substantially more active than methotrexate, after subcutaneous administration in mice, against three of five ascites tumors and two of three solid tumors.[119] The data indicate that because of a broader spectrum of effective antitumor action in mice than exhibited by methotrexate, this compound may also have greater clinical usefulness than methotrexate.

Pyridoxine (Vitamin B_6)

Requirements and Effect of a Deficiency. The recommended daily intake of pyridoxine in infants up to 1 year of age is 0.3–0.6 mg; for children aged 1–10, 0.9–1.6 mg; for adult men, 1.8–2.2 mg; and for adult women, 1.8–1.0 mg. Patients on pyridoxine-deficient diets have been characterized by weakness, irritability, nervousness, insomnia, and difficulty in walking. Convulsive seizures and nervous irritability have been observed in infants fed a commercial liquid milk formula low in vitamin B_6. Clinical improvement observed on supplementation was confirmed by a return of the abnormal electroencephalographic (EEG) patterns to normal.

Effect on Carcinogenesis in Animals. Pyridoxine deficiency has been reported to produce regression of mouse sarcoma 180 as well as other tumors.[120,121] A deficiency of dietary pyridoxine brings about a reduction in the growth of several Morris hepatomas.[122] Pyridoxine deficiency may be effective against tumor growth by reducing serine dehydratase activy. Tryfiates observed greatly reduced serine dehydratase activity in normal liver and in livers containing hepatomas 5123A, 7316B, and 7800 from rats fed pyridoxine-deficient diets.[123] Tumor growth of transplantable Morris hepatoma 7288 (transplantable cancer was also found to be inhibited by pyridoxine-deficient diets).

Effect on Cultured Cells. Pyridoxine in the millimolar range is toxic to cultured Fu5-5 rat hepatoma cells.[124] Although the mechanism by which vitamin B_6 inhibits cell growth has not been determined, cells cultured 6 hr in vitamin B_6-enriched medium have been shown to take up and incorporate less [^{3}H]thymidine than is observed in control cultures. In addition, elevated levels of ATP have been found in the cultures exposed to the vitamin for short periods of time. A pyridoxine-resistant Fu5-5 rat hepatoma cell line has been established by a stepwise increase in the concentration of pyridoxine in the medium.[125]

Effect on Immunity. Pyridoxine is also an important factor in immune reactions. In impairment of antibody response in human erythrocytes, diptheria toxoid and influenza virus have been observed in albino rats fed pyridoxine-deficient diets.[126,127] Similar observations were made by inducing vitamin B_6 deficiency by the administration of the antagonist deoxypyridoxine. In nutritionally deprived animals inoculated with *Mycobacterium tuberculosis* BCG vaccine, delayed cutaneous hypersensitivity to purified protein derivative was depressed, even though the *in vitro* correlates of sensitization were demonstrable.[128] In addition, rejection of skin homotransplants across the major histocompatibility barrier was delayed in pyridoxine-deficient animals.[129] Morover, specific tolerance to donor antigens and consequent acceptance of skin grafts could be achieved by injection of the donor's spleen cells into vitamin B_6-deficient recipient mice.[130]

Effect on Cancer Patients. Seventeen patients with carcinoma of the breast, larynx, and lung were treated with a pyridoxine-deficient diet for 10–80 days. Nine patients also received 4-deoxypyridoxine, a pyridoxine antagonist, for varying intervals, but no inhibitory effects were observed.[131] Deoxypyridoxine alone or in combination with other agents has significantly affected the growth of lymphosarcoma and acute leukemia both in human subjects and in cultured tumor cells.[132,133]

Potera *et al.* measured the plasma pyridoxal phosphate concentration in 30 cases of early breast cancer, in 21 patients with locally recurrent disease, and in 43 patients with systemic metastases.[134] The two groups of patients with advanced breast cancer had significantly lower plasma pyridoxal phosphate levels than were found in 36 healthy women of similar ages.

Niacin

Requirements and Effect of a Deficiency. The recommended daily intake of pantothenic acid is 6–8 mg for infants up to 1 year of age; for children aged 1–10, 9–16 mg; for adult men, 16–19 mg; and for adult women, 13–15 mg. Although pellagra has been endemic in corn-eating areas of the world for more than 200 years, it was not until 1908 that the diagnostic symptoms were recognized. The early symptoms of pellagra are weakness, lassitude, anorexia, and indigestion. These symptoms are followed by the classical three D's: dermatitis, diarrhea, and dementia. The mental symptoms that often accompany the early stages of pellagra are irritability, headaches, sleeplessness, loss of memory, and emotional instability. Toxic confusional psychosis, acute delirium, and catatonia have also been observed in advanced cases of niacin deficiency. The deficiency of dietary intake of nicotinic acid, or tryptophan-containing proteins, can be obtained by analyzing the urine for its *N*-methylnicotinamide content.

Effect on Animal Carcinogenesis. Rakieten *et al.* reported that the combined administration of streptozotocin and nicotinamide to rats resulted in the induction of pancreatic islet tumors containing high concentrations of immunoreactive insulin.[135] Pretreatment of rats with large doses of nicotinamide appeared to promote the development of kidney neoplasias in rats given several doses of diethylnitrosamine.[136]

Barra *et al.* observed that inhibitors of poly(ADP-ribose)synthetase influence DNA synthesis and examined the possibility that nicotinamide or isonicotinamide might potentiate the effect of bleomycin on DNA replication and repair.[137] Both nicotinamide and isonicotinamide caused an approximately 50% inhibition of total [^{3}H]thymidine incorporation in HTC cells. In addition, significant inhibition by both nicotinamide and isonicotinamide on unscheduled DNA synthesis was observed after preincubation of hepatocytes and HTC cells with bleomycin.

Inhibitors of poly(ADP-ribose)synthetase activity have been reported to enhance the cytotoxicity of alkylating agents.[138] However, there was only a small enhancement of the toxicity to L1210 cells of γ-radiation by inhibitors of poly(ADP-ribose)synthetase. Smulson *et al.* observed that nicotinamide increases the enhancement of survival times of mice bearing L1210 cells treated with *N*-methyl-*N*-nitrosourea.[139]

Effect of 6-Aminonicotinamide. Shapiro *et al.* showed that a potent niacin antagonist, 6-aminonicotinamide (6-AN), has potent antitumor activity against mammary adenocarcinoma in mice.[140]

Administration of nicotinamide can reverse the antitumor activity of 6-AN. Many antitumor agents have been shown to cause a marked decrease in tumor cell nicotinamide adeninedinucleotide (NAD).[141] The decrease of NAD levels may be responsible for the antitumor activity of these compounds. Shimoyama *et al.* demonstrated that the tryptophan-NAD pathway and the activity of nicotinic acid mononucleotide pyrophoshorylase was decreased by the antitumor agent.[142]

Interrelationships with Tryptophan Metabolism. Studies of tryptophan metabolism in cancer patients have also been of considerable interest. The kynurenine pathway in patients with bladder cancer has been found to be altered.[143] Bladder cancer patients, as well as patients with cancer of the larynx and bronchus, showed more 5-hydroxytryptamine and 5-HIAA excretion than did cancer-free patients.[144] Basu *et al.* showed that patients with various malignancies have 5-HIAA levels that were sixfold higher and conversely the N^1-methylnicotinamide levels were about fourfold lower than those of control subjects.[145] The results suggest that the greater proportion of tryptophan is metabolized in the cancer patients via the hydroxyindole pathway.

VITAMIN C

During the mid-eighteenth century, James Lind demonstrated that the juice of fresh citrus fruits cures scurvy. The active agent was the enolic form of 3-keto-L-gulofuranlactone and was named ascorbic acid, or vitamin C, which was later isolated during the late 1920s by Albert Szent-Gyorgyi.[146] Methods had been devised by the mid-1930s to synthesize the compound, and it soon became widely available at low cost. Ascorbic acid is an α-ketolactone, the empirical formula of which is $C_6H_8O_6$ (Fig. 4-2). Ascorbic acid contains a double bond between the α- and β-carbon atoms as well as an acid-ionizing group. The relationship between ascorbic acid and some of its metabolites is summarized in Figure 4-2.

A vitamin C deficiency can cause serious problems, the worst being scurvy. The present recommended dietary allowance of the Food and Nutrition Board of the U.S. National Academy of Sciences–National Research Council is 50–60 mg/day for an adult. This amount is adequate to prevent scurvy in most normal adults. The onset of scurvy can be detected 60–90 days on a diet containing no ascorbic acid. Baker *et al.* reported that scurvy can be prevented with doses of ~ 10 mg/day, which corresponds to a plasma level of 0.7 mg/dl.[147] An intake increased to 50 mg/day of ascorbic acid will maintain a pool size of ~ 1500 mg, which will roughly half-saturate tissues with ascorbic acid, corresponding to a

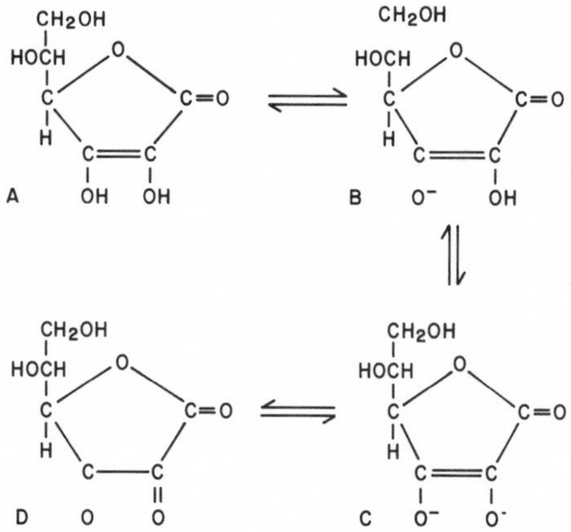

Figure 4-2. Ascorbic acid and some of its metabolites. (A) ascorbic acid; (B) ascorbate anion; (C) ascorbyl radical; (D) dehydroascorbic acid.

plasma level of 0.7 mg/dl. This amount of tissue saturation will protect a healthy person suddenly deprived of ascorbic acid against scurvy for 60 days. Hornig *et al.* believes that full saturation of the body with ascorbic acid will provide a body pool size of 3000 mg.[148] This level of tissue saturation can be accomplished on a daily intake of 200 mg/day. There is no evidence, however, that this intake level, which leads to full saturation of tissues, improves the health of normal persons. There are marked increases in urinary excretion, oxidation, and general catabolism of ascorbic acid as the pool sizes exceed 1500 mg.

Even so, there is a possibility that a larger intake could lead to better health and greater control of disease. This question was raised as soon as the pure compound became freely available. However, administration of larger amounts of vitamin C to biological systems has led to genotoxic effects in several different test systems. This section summarizes the beneficial genetic effects of vitamin C as well as the genotoxic effects.

Anticarcinogenic Effects of Vitamin C

Preventative Effects in Animals

Skin Cancer. Vitamin C prevents carcinogenesis through a variety of mechanisms. Vitamin C may prevent tumorigenesis through its antioxidant action. The antioxidant effect may be through the prevention of peroxidation, which produces free radical damage to various cellular components. When ascorbic acid (0.2%) was applied concomitantly with croton oil to mouse skin previously treated with 7,12-dimethylbenzanthracene (DMBA), the total number of mouse skin papillomas was reduced.[149] However, vitamin C did not seem to be as effective as selenium and vitamin E in the same experiments. Slaga and Bracken observed a decrease in the number of skin tumors induced by DMBA-phorbol carcinogenesis in mice also treated with ascorbic acid.[150] Sadek and Abdelmegid observed skin tumors in most toads they had painted with DMBA.[151] Animals injected with ascorbic acid into the dorsal lymph sac showed tumor inhibition when painted with same level of DMBA. In contrast, high doses of ascorbic acid administered orally in the drinking water had no effect on mammary tumor induction and tumor incidence, nor could ascorbic acid prolong the survival time of rats treated with DMBA.[152] Shoyab studied the effect of vitamin C on the binding of tritiated DMBA to murine epidermal cells DNA in culture. Vitamin C and its salt significantly reduced the binding of DMBA to DNA.[153] The number of squamous cell carcinomas induced by UV light was reduced, and the onset of the malignant tumors was delayed in mice fed standard diets containing vitamin C.[154]

Bladder Cancer. Schlegel *et al.* observed that vitamin C reduces uroepithelial carcinoma in mice and also suggested that a similar mechanism may exist in humans.[155] The tryptophan metabolite 3-hydroxyanthranilic acid (3-HOA) is thought to be stabilized by ascorbic acid, thereby preventing carcinogenicity when 3-HOA is implanted in the bladder. In one study 10 bladder tumor patients were found to excrete urine with a higher concentration of 3-HOA and 3-HOK (3-hydroxykyurenine) than was found in urine excreted by normal subjects.[156] Price *et al.* found elevated levels of various chemiluminescent tryptophane metabolites such as 3-HOA in the urine of patients with bladder cancer.[157] Another study reported that only about 50% of tumor patients excreted urine with high concentrations of 3-HOK.[158] In contrast to these two studies, Benassi *et al.* found lower than normal rather than elevated concentrations of 3-HOA in the urine of bladder tumor patients.[159]

In an attempt to explain the differences in the three experiments, Schlegel investigated the stability of 3-HOA in the urine of normal patients and patients with bladder tumors.[160] About 90% of the 3-HOA was recovered in normal patients after an incubation at 37°C for 6 hr. In patients with bladder tumors, recoveries below 50% occurred.[161] The difference in the recovery level of normals and bladder patients suggests a variability in the redox environment of the urine. However, when ascorbic acid was given orally, urinary 3-HOA was stabilized. In contrast, Soloway *et al.* found ascorbic acid to have no effect on the occurrence of neoplasia in the rat bladder after administration of *N*-[4-(5-nitro2-furyl)-2-thiazoly1]formamide (FANFT).[162]

Effect on Nitrosation. Ascorbic acid has also been found to block the *in vitro* formation of carcinogenic *N*-nitroso compounds by the reaction between nitrous acid and oxytetracycline, morpholine, piperazine, *N*-methylaniline, methylurea, and dimethylamine. The extent of blocking depends on the compounds nitrosated and the experimental conditions.[163]

In subsequent *in vivo* studies, Mirvish *et al.* showed that ascorbic acid inhibits formation of nitroso carcinogens in mice.[164] In their study, Swiss and strain A mice were fed amines or amides in their diet, and nitrite was given in their drinking water. Under these conditions, pulmonary tumors developed, but when ascorbic acid was added to the diet, there was a marked reduction of these tumors. Ascorbic acid also consistently produced an inhibitory effect when nitrite and amino compounds were administered by the same routes.[165,166]

Historically, salt or saltpeter has been used for the preservation of food; the crude salt frequently contains considerable amounts of nitrate. A high nitrate content is also present in fertilizers, and the nitrate is incorporated into foodstuffs, especially into such vegetables as spinach and carrots. In addition, nitrite is frequently added to pork to prevent the oxidation of its high content of unsaturated fat that leads to the formation of rancid products. Nitrite was also extensively added to meat to make it look redder and therefore more desirable for purchase. However, this practice has generally been curtailed. In an experiment with boiled potatoes, the added nitrite levels were blocked by the addition of ascorbate.[167] The species formed from nitrous acid responsible for the oxidation of ascorbic acid is the same species effecting nitrosation of secondary amines.[168] Between pH 1.5 and 5.0, the nitrosation of secondary amines in the absence of oxygen and the presence of ascorbic acid can be summarized by two competitive parallel second-order reactions:

$$\text{Amine} + N_2O_3 \xrightarrow{k_1} \text{nitrosamine} + NO_2^- + H^+ \tag{1}$$

$$\text{Ascorbate} + N_2O_3 \xrightarrow{k_2} \text{dehydroascorbate} + 2NO + 2H_2O \tag{2}$$

If $k_2 > k_1$, then reaction (2) is mostly complete before (1) starts. Large doses of vitamin C have protected rats from liver tumors induced by aminopyrine and sodium nitrite.[169] The mechanism is thought to result, in part, from blockage of *in vivo* nitrosation, which forms dimethylnitrosamine. However, ascorbic acid does not completely protect against lung and kidney tumor production. Perhaps the concentration of ascorbic acid is insufficient in the kidney and the lung to block *in vivo* nitrosation.

Effects in Man

Most patients with malignant disease seem to have minimal tissue stores of vitamin C.[170–172] Ascorbic acid is known to be involved in the hydroxylation of proline to form hydroxyproline, an amino acid necessary for collagen synthesis.[173] In addition, patients with breast tumors or skeletal metastasis have been shown to have low leukocyte vitamin C and elevated urinary hydroxyproline values.[171] In one experiment, the diets of cancer patients were supplemented with vitamins, yet the blood levels of vitamin C remained low. This experiment suggests that perhaps cancer patients have a greater requirement for vitamin C.

The clinical and biochemical observations suggest that megadoses of vitamin C may slow the rate of collagen breakdown. Cameron and Pauling postulated that cells are normally restrained from proliferation by the highly viscous intracellular glycosaminoglycans.[174] To remove this restraint, the glycosaminoglycans must be depolymerized by the cells in their immediate environment. This process can be accomplished by the release of hyaluronidase and kept in check by a physiological hyaluronidase inhibiter. The inhibiter may be oligoglycosaminoglycan, which requires ascorbic acid for its synthesis. However, DeClerck and Jones tested tumor-induced hydrolysis against extracellular matrices both with and without added ascorbic acid.[175] The matrix containing glycoproteins and underhydroxylated elastin was particularly susceptible to hydrolysis by the tumor proteases.

Large doses of ascorbic acid have a palliative effect on terminal cancer patients.[176] Patients treated with ascorbate have been found to have a mean survival time of ~ 300 days longer than that of controls.[177] After 1 year, 22% of the ascorbate-treated patients and 0.4% of controls were alive. This study was conducted in Scotland, where it is rare for patients to undergo extensive chemotherapy and irradiation, which might alter their immune status. The considerable interest and controversy that resulted from this study led Creagen *et al.* to repeat the study at the Mayo Clinic with a 150-patient double-blind study.[178] Seven weeks was the median survival time for all patients, and the survival curves essentially overlapped. No significant differences were observed in symptoms, performance studies, appetite, or weight between the two groups. It is possible that in contrast to the Scottish study, in which patients had not undergone extensive irradiation and chemotherapy, the patients at the Mayo Clinic study had been subjected to such aggressive treatment, which may have altered their immune response to vitamin C.

In several patients with familial polyposis, ascorbic acid reduced rectal polyps.[179] A daily dosage of 3 gm vitamin C reduced the number of rectal polyps in five of eight patients and a major reduction of polyps in three cases. Bussey *et al.* conducted a randomized trial of ascorbic acid in polyposis coli.[180] Over a 2-year period, this hypothesis was tested in a randomized, double-blind study of 49 patients. Of 36 patients who were evaluable at completion, 19 received ascorbic acid 3 gm/day and 17 received a placebo. A significant reduction was found in the polyp area in the ascorbic acid-treated group at 9 months' follow-up as well as trends toward reduction in both number and area of rectal polyps during the middle of the trial. However, by 18 months, the area counts of evaluable patients were about the same in the ascorbic acid-treated and the placebo groups. The results of Bussey *et al.* suggest that ascorbic acid temporarily influences polyp growth or turnover even though the results had no current therapeutic value.[180] A labeling study of rectal epithelium with [³H]thymidine for those patients followed for 18 months or more was significantly lower in the ascorbic acid group. Since the labeling index identifies those cells entering DNA synthesis during the 1 hr exposure to [³H]-TdR, the results are suggestive of a suppression of DNA synthesis by ascorbic acid.

Epidemiological Relationships

Several studies have suggested inverse relationships between vitamin C intake from fresh fruits, vegetables, and salads and several types of cancer. Meinsma noted that the consumption of citrus fruits by patients with gastric cancer was lower than that by controls.[181] Similar inverse associations between fresh fruit consumption or vitamin C intake and gastric cancer have been reported by Higginson,[182] Haenszel and Correa,[183] and Bjelke.[184] Weisburger *et al.*[185] suggested that the prevalence of gastric cancer is greater in the Northern Hemisphere or in mountainous regions providing relatively little everyday access to fresh fruits, vegetables, and salads. Vitamin C was also shown to block experimental nitrosation of the Japanese Sanma fish which is consumed in a Japanese region with high risk of gastric cancer, and to block completely the formation of mutagens in the reaction mixture. Their results suggest that the risk of gastric cancer in humans can be decreased by ensuring the intake of foods containing vitamin C on a year-round basis.

Stomach cancer incidence rates were compared among four groups: Japanese in Japan, Japanese in Hawaii, Caucasians in Hawaii, and all American whites.[186] When the Japanese and Caucasians in Hawaii were divided by place of birth, the Japanese migrants to Hawaii were found to have greater age-adjusted incidence rates than the Japanese born in Hawaii, while the Caucasian migrants to Hawaii from the United States had lower rates than the Caucasians born in Hawaii. Examination of dietary data in relationship to place of birth showed positive associations of stomach cancer with rice consumption, pickled vegetables, and dried/salted fish and a negative association with vitamin C intake. These results are consistent with the theory that stomach cancer is caused by endogenous nitrosamine formation from dietary sources and that vitamin C may protect against the disease. Dungal and Sigurjonsson suggested that the greater incidence of gastric cancer in Iceland may be related to the large intake of smoked food, especially in conjunction with a low intake of vitamin C.[187]

Epidemiological studies by Hirayama,[188] Bjelke,[189] Maclennan *et al.*,[190] Mettlin *et al.*,[191] and Graham *et al.*,[192,193] have shown risk reductions for lung, stomach, colon, rectum, and bladder cancers among persons who more frequently ingested those vegetables that are important sources of β-carotene as well as vitamin C and other nutrients. Mettlin *et al.* found inverse associations of both the indices vitamin A and vitamin C consumption with esophageal cancer, based on the frequency of consumption of selected food items by male cases and controls.[194] This relationship was stronger for vitamin C than for vitamin A, however, and only the association with vitamin C was statistically significant after controlling for smoking and alcohol use. A relatively low intake of leafy green vegetables was observed in the high esophageal cancer rate area of the Caspian littoral of Iran.

Cancer of the larynx has been associated with smoking and alcohol ingestion.[195] The study also found that males ingesting low amounts of vitamin A or vitamin C have about twice the risk of those ingesting large amounts. Graham *et al.* made a similar dietary study in regard to breast cancer. There was no difference in the risk of breast cancer associated with ingesting diets containing various levels of either vitamin C or the cruciferous vegetables.[196] However, risk of breast cancer in women over 55 years of age increased somewhat with decreases in ingestion of foods containing vitamin A.

A case-control study of women with cervical abnormalities identified through Papanicolaou smears was conducted in the Bronx, New York, to explore the relationship between nutritional intake and cervical dysplasia.[197] The computer analysis of 3-day food records showed a mean vitamin C intake per day of 107 mg for the controls, compared with 80 mg for cases. Analysis of matched pairs yielded a 10-fold increase in the risk of cervical dysplasia for those on low vitamin C intakes. If other studies confirm these findings, it may be important to explore a possible protective effect of supplementary vitamin C for women at high risk of cervical cancer.

Ziegler *et al.* also evaluated esophageal cancer mortality in a case-control study conducted among Black male residents of Washington, D.C.[198] Indicators of their general nutritional status were found by interviewing their next of kin. The least-nourished one-third of the study population had nearly twice the mortality risk of esophageal cancer. Estimates of the intake of vitamin A, carotene, vitamin C, thiamine, and riboflavin were inversely associated with relative risk, but each micronutrient index was less strongly associated with risk than were the broad food groups from which the micronutrients were derived.

In contrast, Jain *et al.* found no association between vitamin C consumption and colon cancer in a case-control study based on quantitative data obtained from dietary histories.[199]

Effect on Cell Division and Growth

Ramirez *et al.* studied the direct effects of ascorbic acid and dehydroascorbic acid *in vitro* on human lymphocyte proliferation to phytohemagglutinin

(PHA) and concanavalin A (con A) stimulation.[200] When the cells were exposed to physiological and high concentrations of ascorbic acid and dehydroascorbic acid, the cells showed dose-dependent poorer [3H]thymidine incorporation than did the controls without the vitamin. Even when supraoptimal concentrations were used, there was no return of the mitogen response, indicating that ascorbic acid did not inhibit the response by direct competition. Viability studies of cells in culture showed that concentrations of ascorbic acid and dehydroascorbic acid that inhibited the mitogenic stimulation of lymphocytes were not toxic throughout the culture period. Inhibition of [3H]thymidine incorporation occurred when ascorbic acid was added as late as 96 hr after initiation of the culture. The greatest inhibitory effect, however, was observed when ascorbic acid was added at initiation or early in culture. It is likely that the high physiological and high concentrations of ascorbic and dehydroascorbic acid affect the early metabolic events in the process of mitogen-stimulated lymphocyte activation. When macromolecular synthesis was measured, RNA, protein, and DNA synthesis was significantly inhibited. The early inhibiting effect exerted by ascorbic acid and dehydroascorbic acid may be on early cell membrane associated events (i.e., molecular transport, phospholipid metabolism, sodium and potassium ion exchanges, and calcium influx), which are important factors in mitogenesis. For example, both ascorbic and dehydroascorbic acid may be interfering with glucose transport across the lymphocyte membrane, rendering the cell metabolically inactive after PHA stimulation.

The mitotic activity of the transplantable mouse tumors, sarcoma 37, Krebs-2, and Ehrlich carcinomas, in the ascites form, was inhibited after treatment with a mixture of vitamins C and B_{12}.[201] When the vitamins were administered alone, at the same dosage, however, they did not have any apparent effect on mitosis or cell morphology. Apparently a synergistic action or some type of interaction between the two vitamins may be involved. Microscopic examination of the stained ascites fluid taken from the mice treated with the vitamin mixtures showed few tumor cells in various stages of disintegration. There was also an increase in lymphocytes, monocytes, and neutrophils. However, no tumor cells could be found later in the experiment, and monocytes and macrophages were abundant. It appears that the vitamin mixture ascorbic acid and B_{12} has a specific effect, in that it inhibits the mitotic activity of neoplastic cells while it does not inhibit mitoses of normal cells.

Dixit and Rao studied the influence of a pharmacological dose of ascorbic acid on the action of DMBA on DNA, RNA, and protein levels in young adult (10–12 weeks of age) female mice that had been subjected to partial hepatectomy.[202] Both DMBA and ascorbic acid inhibited the level of DNA in regenerating liver, and their combined action was additive. This action of DMBA could be due to decreased DNA polymerase activity and/or increased DNAase activity. The fallen DNA content in regenerating liver after ascorbic acid treatment might wholly or partly be due to a DNA breaking action of this vitamin. In addition, DMBA treatment of partially hepatectomized mice suppresses the RNA and protein content in liver, but this action of DMBA can be counteracted by ascorbic acid treatment. It is not certain whether ascorbic acid and DMBA act on RNA polymerase activity or act directly on RNA molecules themselves.

Ascorbic acid, at monotoxic concentrations, causes a substantial reduction in the ability of RNA avian tumor viruses to replicate in both avian tendon cells and chicken embryo fibroblasts.[203] Less transformation was observed in the virus-infected cultures in the presence of ascorbic acid as evidenced by morphology, reduced glucose uptake, and decreased collagen synthesis. Ascorbic acid does not appear to act by altering the susceptibility of the cells to initial infection and transformation, but instead appears to interfere with the spread of infection due to a reduction in virus replication and virus infectivity. This observed effect is reversible and requires the continuous presence of vitamin C in the culture medium. It is conceivable that ascorbic acid under these culture conditions could increase interferon production by Rous sarcoma virus-infected cultures and hence retard further virus spread. Ascorbic acid has been shown to increase interferon production in mouse embryo fibroblasts by poly(rI)-poly(rC) and in human embryo lung fibroblasts infected with Newcastle disease virus. There is also a possibility that some of the cells that appear to be normal may be infected. Because ascorbic acid causes the production of some defective units, cells could become infected by the transformation-defective subpopulation, thereby becoming resistant to further infection by the transforming virus. Schwerdt and Schwerdt showed that ascorbic acid reduces rhinovirus replication in cultured human cells after the first cycle of virus replication.[204]

Bullough and Rytomaa showed that certain tissues contain and produce tissue-specific proteins termed chalones, which are able to promote the functional activity of the tissue cells, and that mitotic dormancy is a secondary outcome of chalone action.[205] Edgar suggested that hydrolytic enzymes activated by dehydroascorbic acid release mitotically dormant cells from chalone-like influence and that dehydroascorbic acid then assumes control over cell division.[206] The concentration of dehydroascorbic acid may be increased by the various stimuli that activate mitotically dormant cells, thereby provoking the release and activation of hydrolytic enzymes that may dedifferentiate the affected cells by destroying mitotic repressors (e.g., chalones), which help turn over cellular constituents associated with the tissue function of the cells. Ascorbate has been shown to stimulate RNA synthesis in wheat nuclei by assisting in the removal of histone from inducible chromatin, thus aiding in the dedifferentiation process.[207] If a decrease in the concentration of dehydroascorbic acid were to occur, there would be a burst of mitotic activity, but this would eventually lead to mitotic dormancy as chalones reestablish the tissue function of the cells.

Freidel et al. studied the in vitro effect of D-isoascorbic acid and betaine hydrate, both alone and in combination, on normal and malignant cells.[208] D-isoascrobic acid, an isomer of vitamin C, as well as betaine hydrate (quaternary amine) were found to inhibit mitosis of sarcoma 37, Ehrlich carcinoma, and L-1210 leukemia cells *in vitro*. There was greater inhibitory activity when these compounds were combined than when either was administered individually. When D-isoascorbic acid and betaine hydrate are combined, it is likely they have a blocking action at certain cell membrane receptor sites, possibly preventing the entrance of materials responsible for the increased ability to divide, but having no effect on normal cell division, as evidenced by the failure of normal cell division to be affected.

Preferential Toxicity of Vitamin C on Cancer Cells

Ascorbic acid has been shown to inhibit cells in tissue culture. This inhibition may be due to either a toxic effect or to an anticarcinogenic effect. L-Ascorbic acid has been shown to suppress the growth of bone marrow cells from patients with acute nonlymphocyte leukemia.[209] In simultaneous cultures for leukemic and normal marrow cells, the suppression of the leukemic cell colony was noted with a concentration of L-ascorbic acid as low as 0.1 mM (an achievable concentration *in vivo*), but normal myeloid colonies were not suppressed until the concentration of L-ascorbic acid reached an extremely high level (1 mM).

The effect of vitamin C on cell proliferation and DNA synthesis has been studied using two tumor lines, Hep. and KB.[210] An increase in the ratio of dead to live cells and a decrease in the rate of DNA synthesis was observed.

Ascorbate, when combined with copper, has been demonstrated to reduce the viscosity of DNA solutions rapidly and has also exhibited some carcinostatic effects on transplanted sarcoma-180 tumors in mice.[211] Melanoma cells have been found to incorporate vitamin C preferentially, and *in vitro* studies show that vitamin C is more toxic to melanotic cells. Melanoma cells were inhibited 20–500 times more than any other cell studied. These concentrations of vitamin C were thought to be attainable in humans.

6-Hydroxydopamine (6-OHDA) is a neurotoxin for catecholaminergic neurons and neuroblasts. Reynolds *et al.* studied the cytotoxic effect of 6-OHDA on 12 human neuroblastoma cell lines as compared with the effect on nonneuroblastoma cell lines.[212] Most neuroblastoma cells were found to be very sensitive to 6-OHDA. Tumor cells that produce catecholamines are more sensitive to 6-OHDA than are those from noncatecholamine producers. However, human fibroblasts, lymphoblastoid cell lines, and normal marrow are relatively insensitive to 6-OHDA. Ascorbate and 6-OHDA are synergistic in toxicity for human neuroblastoma cells. The *in vitro* addition of 6-OHDA and ascorbic is rapidly lethal for human neuroblastoma cells at concentrations that are minimally toxic for hematopoietic cells. This observed differential toxicity may provide a means for selective destruction of neuroblastoma cells in bone marrow harvested for autologous transplantation. It is likely that the cytotoxicity of ascorbic acid for the human neuroblastoma cells and the enhancement of the 6-OHDA effect is due to formation of hydrogen peroxide, which in turn increases intracellular levels of free radicals.

Benade *et al.* showed that ascorbate is highly toxic or lethal to Ehrlich ascites carcinoma cells *in vitro*.[213] This toxicity was found to be greatly increased synergistically by concomitant administration of 3-amino-1,2,4,-triazole (ATA). When given alone, ATA is almost completely harmless to cancer cells, except for specifically inhibiting their catalase (H_2O_2-decomposing) activity. These workers concluded that the cytotoxic effect of ascorbate is due to the intracellular production of hydrogen peroxide and that the enhancement of the ascorbate effect by ATA is due to its inhibition of cellular catalase, thereby reducing the ability of the cells to detoxify hydrogen peroxide.

Mouse neuroblastoma (NB) in cells in culture was found to be more sensitive to sodium L-ascorbate than were rat glioma cells by the criterion of growth inhibition (due to cell death and reduction in cell division). At nonlethal concentrations, sodium ascorbate potentiated the effect of 5-FU, x-irradiation, bleomycin, prostaglandin E_1, and sodium butyrate on NB cells, but produced no effect on glioma cells. The D-ascorbate form was equally effective, indicating that the effect by sodium ascorbate was not due to either its vitamin property or its reducing property, because glutathione did not potentiate the effect of 5-FU. The effect could have been due to an intracellular accumulation of H_2O_2 or free redicals, as the addition of catalase to the external culture medium does not provide protection. The potentiating effect of sodium ascorbate may also be mediated by dehydroascorbate. It is likely that ascorbic acid could be used in conjunction with certain chemotherapeutic drugs. However, if sodium ascorbate is used indiscriminantly, the combined treatment may decrease the effectiveness of certain chemotherapeutic agents. For example, sodium ascorbate can decrease the cytotoxic effect of MTX and 5-imidazole-4-carboxamide on NB cells in culture.

Chemotherapeutic Effect in Animals

The subcutaneous injection of 10 mg benzpyrene dissolved in tricaprylin in five Wistar rats induced localized malignant tumors, including fibrosarcoma, rhabdomyosarcoma, and polymorph cell sarcoma.[214] Tumor growth was relatively rapid, reaching weights of 140–155 gm before the rats died 142–168 days after the carcinogen was administered. Under the same experimental conditions, high doses of vitamin C (525 mg/day) administered orally in drinking water to another five rats inhibited to a great extent the benzpyrene carcinogenesis. In the vitamin C-treated group only one slowly growing rhabdomyosarcoma (13 gm weight) developed, showing characteristic damage of malignant cells as well as partial replacement of the neoplastic area with granuloma tissue.

Yamafuji *et al.* studied the antitumor potency of ascorbic, dehydroascorbic, or 2,3-diketogulonic acid and their inhibition of sarcoma-180 growth.[215] The inhibition by the enediols is enhanced by cupric ions, which enhance the depolymerization of native and denatured DNA. The enediols are able to produce a single-strand scission in the double helix. Tumor suppression by ascorbate derivatives may be due to the abnormality of DNA replication or to that of mRNA synthesis.

The growth of tumors in guinea pigs was observed for 20 weeks after they were placed on various doses of vitamin C.[216] In those animals that received 0.3 mg/kg per day ascorbic acid, complete tumor regression occurred in 55% of cases. The animals given 10 mg/kg per day showed tumor inhibition, but no regression. In animals maintained on 1 gm/kg per day ascorbic acid, the tumors grew without any sign of retardation. When increased amounts of ascorbic acid were restored to the diet of scorbutic tumor-bearing guinea pigs, tumors that had not regressed showed enhanced growth. Animals previously maintained on 10 mg/kg per day ascorbic acid responded in turn to the additional vitamins with increased tumor growth. In contrast, when all tumor-bearing animals were maintained on 1 gm/kg per day ascorbic acid, death resulted within 3 weeks when this dose was replaced with 0.3 mg/kg per day.

The stimulation of tumor growth by megadoses of vitamin C agrees with the findings of earlier reports.[217–219]. It is likely that the rapidly growing tumor tissue has a greater requirement than that of most adult tissue for ascorbic acid. Further evidence that the tumor is dependent on vitamin C for growth is shown by the response seen after reversing the diet. It is likely the immune response is involved in tumor enhancement or regression, but the mechanism is poorly understood. Experimental evidence indicates that vitamin C may reduce the immunological response.[220 −222] These experiments are consistent with the experimental observation of Migliozzi.[216]

Waddell and Gerner studied the effect of indomethacin and ascorbic acid on desmoid tumors in a few patients.[223] After a partial response to radiation, administration of indomethacin caused complete resolution of a desmoid tumor. In another patient, indomethacin caused an immediate response and then became ineffective until large doses of ascorbic acid were also administered. Slow resolution of the tumor began and has continued for 14 months. A third case treated with idomethacin and ascorbic acid from the beginning produced shrinkage of the tumor. Although there is no known mode of action that would account for the observed response of desmoid tumors, there is a possibility that cyclic adenosine monophosphate (cAMP) is lowered by indomethacin in conjunction with an inhibition of cell growth by vitamin C. The molecular mechanism by which indomethacin inhibits tumor growth is unknown, but the prominent action of this drug is inhibition of prostaglandin (PG) synthesis, the consequences of which are many and varied. However, it is possible that both drugs lower cAMP, interrupting the cell cycle and restricting growth. High cyclic nucleotide concentrations have been found necessary for initiation of the growth cycle as opposed to steady levels.[224]

The growth of the solid form of Ehrlich ascites tumor has been found to be significantly slower in mice maintained on distilled water supplemented with 0.1% ascorbic acid than in mice maintained on distilled water alone.[225] Gruber *et al.* studied this process histologically and found several morphological alterations in tissue architecture in solid Ehrlich ascites tumors implanted in the hind limbs of mice drinking distilled water supplemented with 0.1% ascorbic acid.[226] Light microscopic observations of nonnecrotic tumor sections showed cluster of cells and occasional regions of denser connective tissue among tumor cells. Examination of tumors from mice maintained on distilled water did not reveal any clustering of tumor cells. Ultrastructural examination showed tumor cell groupings with evidence of peripheral fibroblast deposition of cellular product between cells, close association of tumor cells within clusters, and a basement membrane. Morphological alterations have been reported in irradiated Chinese hamster ovary cells grown in ascorbic acid-supplemented media[227] and in mesenchymal tumors.[216]

Elvin and Slater studied the effect of novel adducts of ascorbic acid and methylglyoxal (MGA) on the growth of Ehrlich ascites carcinoma (EAC) in male CBA/Ca mice.[228] If MGA was injected twice daily, after injection of tumor cells at day 0, tumor growth was inhibited by 93% and 96%, respectively, when given on days 1–5 post-transplantation. Treatment with MGA on days 5–9 after tumor cell injection was ineffective. A single dose given on days, 1, 3, and 5 after transplantation also significantly increased the survival of EAC-bearing mice. In addition, a number of related ascorbate acetals were tested for antitumor activity using an identical protocol. AsA-acetylacrolein (100 and 200 mg/kg^{-1} twice daily, respectively) was as active a growth inhibitor as MGA, inhibiting the growth of EAC by 97% and 98%. AsA-acrolein and AsA-glyoxal also inhibited the growth of EAC. Under identical conditions, ascorbic acid did not inhibit the growth of EAC, while the aldehydes methylglyoxal and acetylacrolein inhibited tumor growth by 98% and 99%, respectively. If the aldehydes were combined with ascorbic acid, there was a considerable reduction in host toxicity, the LD_{50} for MG being 332 mg/kg and that for MGA 959–1462 mg/kg for a single intraperitoneal dose in mice. Ascorbate is a strong inhibitor of glyoxalase I, and potentiation of the growth inhibitory effects of methylglyoxal through its metabolic inhibition by ascorbate may be important in regard to the distribution of the glyoxalase enzymes in tumors.

In order to increase the antitumor activity of ascorbate, Kimoto *et al.* complexed cupric ion with glycylglycylhistidine and injected this complex along with high doses of ascorbic acid into mice inoculated intraperitoneally with Ehrlich tumor cells.[229] The life span of the mice was increased. This effect was attributed to the ability of this complex to increase peptide-cleaving activity.

Yagishita *et al.* synthesized derivatives of ascorbic acid and studied their effects in Ehrlich ascites carcinoma cells, in regard to the inhibition and the lengthening of survival time, as well as on the morphological degeneration in HeLa cells.[230] In the case of tetra-acetyl-bis-dehydroascorbic acid in dd mice infected with Ehrlich cells, prolongation of survival time was almost double that of the control mice. Abdominal dropsy and body weight were also reduced. However, in the case of dehydroascorbic acid and other derivatives, almost no inhibition and prolongation of survival time were observed. Morphological degeneration of HeLa cells was observed using 2.5–5.0 mg/ml of several derivatives of ascorbic acid. The most effective compound was tetraacetyl-bis-DHA which, at 125 µg/ml, brought about morphological degeneration.

Aqueous solutions of molecular oxygen, or molecular oxygen in combination with either pyrogallol or 6-azauracil increased tumorigenesis in *Nicotiana suaveolens* X *Nicotiana* langsdorffii seedlings relative to control seedlings. Substitution of N_2 for O_2 or degassing solutions of these compounds has eliminated or greatly reduced their tumorigenic effects. Rates of tumorigenesis exceeded 95% for either pyrogallol or 6-azauracil solutions in the presence of oxygen. Seedlings treated with O_2 alone had about a 20% tumor rate. Both dinitrophenol and ascorbic acid, compounds that affect cellular respiration or redox systems, have strongly inhibited the chemically mediated tumorigenesis. Dehydroascorbic acid was found to be much less inhibitory than ascorbic acid. The protective action of ascorbic acid may be related to the tendency of this vitamin to act as a reducing agent and free radical scavenger both *in vivo* and *in vitro*.

Werner *et al.* studied the effect of ascorbic acid on small intestine cancer induced by *N*-ethyl-*N*-nitro-*N*-nitrosoguanidine (ENNG) in rats.[231] The induction of tumors could not be suppressed by amounts as large as 2–3% of sodium ascorbate in food, but the depth of tumor infiltration was restricted by sodium ascorbate.

Reddy *et al.* examined the effect of dietary sodium ascorbate on colon carcinogenesis induced by 1,2-dimethylhydrazine (DMH) or *N*-methyl-*N*-nitrosourea (MNU) in female F344 rats.[232] The incidence of colon and kidney tumors was lower in rats fed 0.25% or 1.0% sodium ascorbate and treated with a single dose of DMH than in the animals fed the diet without sodium ascorbate. However, the tumor incidences did not differ between the sodium ascorbate and control diet-fed animals and then treated with multiple doses of DMH or MNU. Supplementation of 1.2% ascorbic acid to the low-fat diet of Sprague-Dawley rats has also been shown to inhibit DMH-induced colon tumor incidence.[233] In contrast, no significant effect of dietary ascorbic acid on the development of DMH-induced colon tumors has been observed in female CF, mice fed a low-fat diet.[234]

Abul-Hajj and Kelliher observed that high doses of ascorbic acid failed to inhibit the growth of R323OAC and MT/W9α-B transplantable rat mammary tumors.[152]

Effect on Cell Transformation

Benedict *et al.* observed that ascorbic acid at the noncytotoxic concentration of 1 μg/ml could completely inhibit the transformation of mouse C3H/10T ½ cells induced by MCA when added daily as late as 3 weeks after a 24-hr exposure to MCA.[235] Gol-Winkler *et al.*[236] and Rosin *et al.*[237] also observed that ascorbic acid added to the culture medium suppresses the MCA transformation of C3H 10T ½ cells. This experiment was the first indication that ascorbate could influence cellular differentiation at a level beyond the initiation step. Transformation was also completely inhibited if ascorbate was added the day after exposure to MCA and continued for only the first 23 days. These results suggest that the inhibition must be quite stable, unlike that of retinoids, phosphodiesterase inhibitors, and protease inhibitors, which are also able to inhibit chemically induced transformation in C3H/10T ½ cells. These latter agents are able to inhibit only in a reversible manner, however, since the transformed cells seem to reappear once these agents are removed. Transformed cells, however, became resistant to the effect of ascorbate acid if they were initially subcultured several times without ascorbate and were then exposed to the vitamin.

The studies also suggest that differential cytotoxicity to newly transformed cell lines produced by ascorbate is not responsible for the variation in the change of the transformed morphology to a normal phenotype, since no cytotoxicity was produced by ascorbic acid at early passages in any of the cell lines examined.

Sivak and Tu modified the BALB/c-3T3 cell neoplastic transformation to examine the tumor-promoting activity of a set of substances. After initiation of the target cells with MCA, the cultures are treated with PMA.[238] During the following 4-week interval, there was a marked increase in both spontaneous and initiated type III-transformed foci. Saccharin did not influence the occurrence of type III-transformed foci. In contrast, sodium ascorbate and L-tryptophan almost completely inhibited both spontaneous and initiated type III-transformed foci.

Tumor-Enhancing Effect of Vitamin C

Large doses (100 mg/kg body weight daily for 4 months) of vitamin C have been found to promote the induction of sarcomas by a single injection of 20 mg

MCA.[239] The tumors appeared earlier in the group of guinea pigs treated with vitamin C after injection of MCA than in the control group, which was only injected with MCA.

Frith et al. studied the effects of ascorbic acid on the induction of urothelial lesions in mice by 2-acetylaminofluorene (2-AAF). Mice receiving 2-AAF exhibited major histopathological changes at the end of 28 days, including both inflammation of the lamina propria and hyperplasia of the transitional epithelium of the urinary bladder.[240] The most severe lesions were seen in the mice that had received both 2-AAF and vitamin C. Nodular hyperplasia usually occurred in conjunction with the simple hyperplasia and consisted of nodular downgrowths of the transitional epithelium into the lamina proprar. The nodular downgrowths were usually restricted to the fundus of the urinary bladder. The incidence was 54.2% in the mice receiving 2-AAF, but 69.8% in the mice receiving both 2-AAF and vitamin C. The nodular hyperplasia is comparable morphologically to VonBrunn's nests or cystitis cystica in humans.

Antimutagenic Effect of Ascorbic Acid

Antimutagenic Effects in Mammalian Cells

Fecal extracts from many normal individuals contain mutagens that can be detected with the Salmonella tester strains.[244] The occurrence of mutagenically active donors is greater in populations on Western diets than it is with those on Black South African, vegetarian, or Japanese diets. The differences between these population groups suggest that mutagen levels could be affected by dietary factors. Bruce et al. also observed that the levels of fecal mutagens are reduced by > 60% in the feces of all donors when their normal diets were supplemented with 4 gm vitamin C per day.[241]

Dion et al. studied the effect of supplemental ascorbic acid and α-tocopherol on fecal mutagenicity in two separate studies involving 20 healthy human donors, aged 22–55 years.[242] The mutagens were extracted from individual frozen feces samples with dichloromethane and assayed with Salmonella typhimurium tester strain TA100 without microsomal activation. In the first study, with only a single donor on a controlled diet, the fecal mutagenicity decreased ($p < 0.001$) on treatment to 21% of the control. In the second study, with 19 donors on free-choice diets, the mutagenicity decreased on treatment ($p < 0.01$) to 26% of control. It is likely that antioxidants in the diet have a role in lowering the body's exposure to endogenously produced mutagens. The mechanism responsible for the effect of ascorbic acid and α-tocopherol is unknown. Substantial variability in the mutagen levels was observed on a day-to-day basis. Most of this variability is a result of daily physiological changes such as might be associated with transit times, as it appears that the mutagen is a product of colonic bacterial metabolism. The concentration of mutagens in the feces is known to increase with the duration of fecal anaerobic incubation at 37°C. However, as yet there is no direct evidence that fecal mutagenicity is related to large bowel cancer or other human disease. Nor is it known whether a deficiency in antioxidants might lead to an increased malignancy risk.

Leuchtenberger and Leuchtenberger assessed both the morphological and cytochemical effects of L-cysteine and vitamin C on hamster lung cultures exposed to smoke from either tobacco or marihuana cigarettes.[243] Hamster lung cultures, when grown in a normal Eagle-Dulbecco media without L-cysteine and exposed to fresh smoke from either tobacco or marihuana cigarettes for 1–8 weeks, had cytotoxic alterations, loss of lysosomes, and significantly fewer abnormalities in cell division and in the DNA content of chromosomes ($p <$ 0.005). More rapid irregular growth of fibroblasts and/or malignant transformation was observed in the cultures grown in media exposed to smoke (whole smoke or gas vapor phase). Cultures grown with L-cysteine and exposed in the same manner to smoke closely resembled those of nonexposed controls.

Addition of vitamin C to cultures had a similar effect on growth of control and smoke exposed cultures as L-cysteine, but the cultures were less regular and grew more rapidly than with L-cysteine. In addition, there was also occurrence of multinucleated giant cells. The mechanism by which vitamin C protects against the effect of smoke is unknown. However, in these experiments vitamin C is known to block NO compounds and thus prevent formation of carcinogenic and nitroso compounds.

Leuchtenberger et al. found differences in response to vitamin C between marihuana- and tobacco smoke-exposed human cell cultures.[244] Marihuana smoke in normal human lung and human breast cancer cultures (SK-Br-3) caused a significantly greater frequency of mitotic abnormalities than did tobacco smoke, regardless of whether the cultures were grown in the absence or presence of vitamin C.

The response to vitamin C of marihuana smoke-exposed breast cancer cultures was completely different from the response to tobacco smoke-exposed cultures. In the tobacco smoke-exposed cultures, vitamin C caused a reduction of mitotic abnormalities and led to more normal growth of the cells. These features were entirely absent in the marihuana smoke-exposed cultures. Vitamin C accelerates not only the abnormal growth in marihuana-exposed cultures, but also promotes the abnormal growth of the breast cancer cells.

Seiler tested ascorbic acid as well as several other compounds by measuring the inhibition of [^{3}H]thymidine into testicular DNA by the test compound in male mice.[245] Ascorbic acid administered orally at a dose of 1000 mg/kg had no mutagenic effects.

Parshad et al. found that 24-hr exposure to fluorescent light produces chromatid breaks in a line of adult mouse lung cells grown in Dulbecco-Vogt medium supplemented with fetal bovine serum. By increasing the concentration of oxygen in the gas phase of the culture, the light-induced damage appears to be enhanced.[246] The effective wavelengths of light are in the visible range between 400 and 450 nm and it is likely that the mercury emission peaks at 405 or and 436 nm. If catalase or glutathione is added with ascorbic acid to the culture medium, the number of chromatid breaks is reduced to a level not significantly different from that in the shielded cultures. It is likely that the production of H_2O_2 in the culture medium or in the cell is responsible for the chromatid breaks. In long-term culture of mouse cells, most of the chromosomal abnormalities result from exposure of cells or medium to fluorescent room lights in the presence of atmospheric oxygen. Minimization of these genetic abnormalities can be obtained by shielding cells and medium from light, lowering the P_{O_2} of the medium, and including in the medium formulation such reducing agents as glutathione and ascorbic acid.

The effect of radiation on the aqueous buffered solutions of salmon sperm DNA has been demonstrated by structural changes in the DNA, as reflected in alterations in solution viscosity.[247] After irradiation, the viscosity is measured at 30°C, where the DNA maintains its double-stranded form, and at 90°C, where DNA is known to exist only in single strands. After radiation exposures as small as 100 R, radiation effects can be demonstrated in single strands. Shapiro and Kollmann studied the potential protective effect of a large number of agents in this system. However, ascorbic acid was found to have no protective effect.[247]

Antimutagenic Effects in Bacteria

The rate of prototroph formation as a result of gene recombination in multiple mutants of *Escherichia coli* strain K-12 was studied by Clark.[248] These mutants were altered by addition of various chemicals to the nutrient substrate in which the recombining strains are grown. Ascorbic acid had no effect, but indole-3-acetic acid lowered the rate of prototroph formation. There is a possibility that a bacteriophage might be involved in the transference of genetic properties in phototroph formation in *E. coli*. It is known that the K-12 strains contain a phage that can be liberated by small doses of UV light. The chemical composition of the substrate may affect the rate of release of the phage from the host cell.

Hexavalent chromium compounds have been found to be mutagenic for his strains of *Salmonella typhimurium* by inducing both frameshifts and base-pair substitutions.[249] Addition of either microsomal fractions from rat liver or of human erythrocyte lysates results in a complete loss of mutagenicity. Reversal of mutagenicity could be ascribed to reduction of the metal to the inactive trivalent form through a simple oxidoreductive reaction. The reducing agents, ascorbic acid and sodium sulfite, and metabolites, GSH, NADH, and NADPH, either directly tested or obtained by mixing glucose 6-phosphate (G6PD) with S-9 mix, have prevented hexavalent chromium mutagenicity.

N-nitrodimethylamine, N-nitrodiethylamine, and N-nitromorpholine and their N-nitroso analogues N-nitrosodimethylamine and N-nitrosomorpholine, were tested in *Salmonella typhimurium* TA100 and TA1530.[250] All the compounds except N-nitrodiethylamine were mutagenic. The assay required the presence of postmitochondrial supernatant from the liver of aroclor-treated rats, oxygen, and reduced NADPH-generating system. Addition of ascorbic acid and disulfiram to the assays efficiently inhibited mutagenesis by all nitro and nitroso compounds.

Wirth *et al.* studied the mutagenicity of phenacetin and acetaminophen and their respective N-hydroxylated metabolites in *Salmonella typhimurium*.[251] Ascorbic acid inhibited the mutation frequency (80–90%) of N-hydroxyphenacetin in both TA100 and TA98 as well as p-nitrosophenetole in TA100 but caused a slight increase in the mutation frequency of N-hydroxy-2-aminofluorene and 2-nitrosofluorene in both TA98 and TA100.

Experiments were conducted to test the radioprotective effects of ascorbic acid, on seeds of barley, *Horedum vulgare*.[252] Seeds were soaked either before or after γ-irradiation or fission neutron irradiation in distilled water or 0.01–1.00 M ascorbic acid solutions. As evidenced by both reduced germination and seedling growth, ascorbic acid was toxic when seeds were soaked for 1 hr at 22°–24°C before irradiation and then planted immediately. When seeds were soaked in ascorbic acid before irradiation and soaked after irradiation in air-bubbled water at 0°C for 18 hr, the toxicity disappeared, and a dose-dependent protective effect with increasing ascorbic acid concentration was observed for γ-irradiation, and to a smaller extent for neutron irradiation. Cells with chromosomal aberrations were also reduced in the seeds when they were soaked in 0.5 or 1.0 M ascorbic acid. Other experiments suggested that the protective effect was related to reduced hydration of the embryos of seeds soaked in ascorbic acid. When the seeds were presoaked for 2 or 16 hr in 0.01 M ascorbic acid solutions at pH 3 or 7, no radioprotective effect was observed. These results are in contrast to those reported by Selimbekova, who observed radioprotective effects in Allium with ascorbic acid concentration as low as 1×10^{-5} μg/ml.[253]

A radioprotective effect was observed for seeds after irradiation in an oxygen-bubbled ascorbic acid solution of 0.5 M, but this effect was not observed for seeds soaked in nitrogen-bubbled ascorbic acid. The radioprotective effect against oxygen-dependent damage may result from an interaction of ascorbic acid with radiation-induced free radicals.

Lin *et al.* tested the mutagenicity of several brands of soy bean sauce *in vitro*.[254] When treated with nitrite at the 2000-ppm level, soy bean sauce produced a mutagenic substance as demonstrated using several strains of *Salmonella typhimurium*/mammalian microsome mutagenicity test. All 21 different brands of soy bean sauce showed similar results. The greatest amount of mutagenic material was formed with a nitrite level of 2000 ppm at pH 3. Ascorbic acid was found to prevent the formation of mutagenic products in nitrite-treated soy bean sauce. Soy sauce is one of the extracts of food materials especially favored by Chinese people in the preparation of food. The mutagenesis observed with soy sauce may be related to the epidemiological observations that carcinomas of the liver and stomach are the most common malignant tumors among Chinese people living in Taiwan.

Munkres found that ferrous ions are both highly lethal and mutagenic to germinated candidia of *Neurospora crassa*.[255] In these experiments, treatment with 0.2 mM ferrous ions was 14- and 50-fold more mutagenic than was UV irradiation or x-rays, respectively, in the reversion of an inositol autotroph. Ascorbic acid at 2 mM was not lethal itself, but inhibited both the lethality and mutagenicity of ferrous ions. The residual lethality of ferrous ions was completely inhibited by bovine superoxide dismutase (SOD). The protection in these experiments by ascorbic acid and SOD indicates that the superoxide radicals generated by the oxidation of Fe^{2+} are directly or indirectly mutagenic and lethal.

Mutations may arise either directly by free radical-mediated oxidative deamidation of DNA bases or indirectly through the reactions of free radicals with DNA polymerases, which may decrease the fidelity of replication or repair. The partial inactivation of the error-prone *E. coli* repair polymerase *in vitro* by superoxide radicals, generated by xanthine oxidase, leads to a marked increase in the incorporation of the wrong nucleotide, dCTP, relative to the correct one, TTP, with synthetic poly(dAT) template. In addition, the inactivation and the alteration of the synthetic fidelity are known to be prevented by bovine SOD.

Shamberger *et al.* observed that ascorbic acid as well as several other antioxidants including butylated hydroxytoluene, vitamin E, and selenium prevents mutagenesis caused by malonaldehyde or β-propiolactone, when several varieties of *Salmonella* strains were tested with the antioxidants.[256] Malonaldehyde seems to affect the strains with a tendency to mutate through frame-shift mutagenesis while β-propiolactone acts on tester strains known to mutate through both frame-shift mutagenesis and base-pair substitution.

The mutagenesis induced by *N*-methyl-*N*-nitrosoguanidine (MNNG) and dimethylnitrosamine (DMN) in *Salmonella* TA 1530 was found to be inhibited by ascorbate.[257] The inhibition of MNNG-induced mutagenesis resulted from a reaction that took place between ascorbic and MNNG that consumed MNNG. This reaction was greatly enhanced by catalytic amounts of Cu^{2+} and Fe^{3+}. No direct reaction was detected between DMN and ascorbate. Mutagenesis by *N*-methyl-*N*-nitrosourea was not inhibited by ascorbate. Using several *Salmonella* tester strains, nitrosated spermidine was found to be mutagenic but the mutagenesis was blocked by ascorbic acid.[258] A mutagenic response was obtained in the *Salmonella* test by preincubating sodium nitrate and cimetidine in human gastric juice from untreated individuals.[259] Ascorbic acid was efficient in preventing the formation of mutagenic nitroso derivatives. Ascorbic acid was found to decrease the aminopyrine/nitrite-induced mutation frequency in *E. coli*.[260] There was no increase or decrease in the dimethylnitrosamine-induced mutation frequency observed in the presence of ascorbic acid.

Lee *et al.* homogenized seven species of raw fish commonly eaten by Koreans and subjected them to *in vitro* nitrosation under simulated gastric conditions both with and without ascorbic acid and then tested them with the *Salmonella* Ames test.[261] Ascorbic acid in an amount three- to fivefold equimolar to the nitrite used almost completely blocked the formation of the mutagenic principle.

Volatile mutagens were produced from normal human and animal feces upon incubation with sodium nitrite in saline at 37°C for 48 hr.[262] The mutagens were detected using the *Salmonella* Ames tester strain TA 1535 without microsomes. Sodium ascorbate and α-tocopherol each reduced the mutagenicity by about 30%.

Mutagenicity of Ascorbic Acid

Effect on Mammalian Cells

When Chinese hamster ovary (CHO) cells were exposed to solutions of ascorbic acid ($2-5 \times 10^{-4}$ M), somatic mutations resulted at the hypoxan thineguanine phosphoribosyl transferase (HGPRT) locus.[263] In the same experiments, mutant cells were resistant to 6-thioguanine (6-TG) and sensitive to a medium containing hypoxanthine, aminopterin, and thymidine. Mutants were identified by their ability to grow in the presence of the toxic purine analogue 6-TG. Doses of ascorbate that were mutagenic were toxic as well. If catalase was added to these high ascorbate concentrations, mutagenesis and toxicity were prevented. These results suggest that mutagenic metabolites of ascorbate probably involve peroxide radicals. Catalase also reduces the chromosome- and DNA-damaging capacity of ascorbate.[264]

In these experiments the concentration range at which ascorbate is active in inducing 6-TG mutants appears to be very narrow. The induction by ascorbate of revertants to histidine prototrophy in *Salmonella typhimurium* strains also occurred over a narrow concentration range of ascorbate.[265] Similarly, induction of chromosomal damage[264] or DNA repair synthesis by ascorbate occurred over a limited concentration range.[266]

There is a possibility that the mutagenic and chromosome-breaking ability of ascorbate in mammalian cells may represent a possible health hazard. The potential hazard of ascorbic acid is increased by the fact that several transition metals [Cu^{2+}, Mn^{2+}, Fe^{2+}, and Fe^{3+}] greatly enhance the mutagenic action of ascorbate.[264,267]

These results were obtained with *in vitro* bioassays, but suggest that ascorbate could well have genotoxic effects *in vivo*. Early results from the same laboratory indicate that the *in vivo* administration of ascorbate to mice does result in fragmentation of stomach mucosal cells. Whether or not this fragmentation would also occur in man is unknown.

Sister-chromatid exchanges (SCE's) are also induced in Chinese hamster cells by a 2–3-hr exposure to ascorbic acid or bisulfite in the concentration range 10^{-4}–10^{-2} M.[268] When cell cultures were exposed to each of two agents for longer time periods, the activity of these two chemicals was intensified. The divalent metal ion of copper was effective in enhancing the ability of ascorbic acid to induce SCE's and toxicity, suggesting that this action involved the autooxidation of ascorbic acid. When the concentration of 5'-bromodeoxyuridine that was used a labeling compound was varied, the ability of sodium bisulfite to induce SCE's was not affected. This supports the possibility that bisulfite, and not a synergistic reaction between bisulfite and 5'-bromodeoxyuridine, was responsible for the elevated SCE levels.

Although the nature of the active species producing SCE is unknown, evidence has been previously presented that indicates that ascorbic acid breaks DNA when hydroxyl radicals are produced in the presence of oxygen, a reaction stimulated by Cu^{2+} ion.[267] In addition, bisulfite has also been shown to break DNA by a free radical mechanism, and it is possible that the hydroxyl radical is also responsible for this activity.[269] The hydroxyl radical may therefore be responsible for the SCE activity of both ascorbic acid and bisulfite. Morgan *et al.*, using an assay that measures the conversion of covalently closed circular DNA to open circular DNA, proposed a mechanism whereby ascorbate reacts with either oxygen or Cu^{2+} ions to generate H_2O_2 and Cu^{2+} ions, which then react to produce hydroxyl radicals.[270] The induction of SCE's by ascorbic acid can occur without added Cu^{2+}. This activity is not reduced when the system is flushed with nitrogen. Since catalase is able to reduce ascorbic acid-induced SCE yields in this system, this suggests that H_2O_2 is produced and participates in the reaction that produces SCE's.[270]

Ascorbate has caused a dose-dependent increase in SCE's in CHO cells and in human lymphocytes.[271] In addition, ascorbate gave results typical of DNA-damaging chemicals, in the DNA synthesis inhibition test with HeLa cells. Catalase reduced SCE induction by ascorbate, prevented cytotoxicity in CHO cells, and prevented its effect in the HeLa synthesis inhibition test. In contrast, ascorbate has reduced the induction of SCE in CHO cells by MNNG through the direct inactivation of MNNG.

In contrast with results *in vitro*, vitamin C did not lead to an induction of

SCE's in the bone marrow of Chinese hamsters in an *in vivo* SCE test.[272] The test dose, which ranged from 200 to 10,000 mg/kg body weight, was administered both orally and by intraperitoneal injection. Sulfhydryl compounds such as cysteine and glutathione inhibited the SCE induction by ascorbic acid *in vitro* due to their reducing ability.

Even extremely high doses of ascorbic acid had no effect on the SCE rate or on cell proliferation in the bone marrow of the Chinese hamster. One likely reason for this observation might be that, in contrast to cell cultures, the mammalian organism seems well protected against damage induced by H_2O_2 and radicals. Intracellular concentrations of glutathione are high, and in the experiments of Speit *et al.* reduced the *in vitro* SCE-inducing effect of ascorbic acid.[272] In addition, glutathione peroxidase catalyzes reactions of glutathione with H_2O_2 and other peroxides. Other enzymes, such as catalase and superoxide dismutase, will also protect the cells by preventing the destructive action of peroxides and free radicals.

Stich *et al.* tested three multiple vitamin tablets with different ascorbic acid contents, three vitamin C pills with a synthetic or natural source of ascorbic acid, seven iron-fortified vitamin tablets, and vitamin C pills plus iron supplement, for their capacity to induce chromosomal aberrations in cultured CHO cells.[273] Chromosomal breaks and exhanges were induced by all these commercially available vitamin pills. The active dilution range as well as the extent of chromosomal damage induced varied among the several pills tested. The observed frequencies of metaphase plates that had chromosomal aberrations ranged up to 42%. The toxic and clastogenic effects of the vitamin preparations were correlated primarily with their contents of ascorbic acid and iron. The maximum frequencies of aberrations produced by the vitamin C pills were high (24–42%) and occurred at concentrations (0.3–1.0 mg/ml) similar to those previously observed with pure ascorbate.[264,267] When the vitamin C pills at comparable concentrations were supplemented with iron (0.3 mg/ml), there was a reduced toxicity and a decreased frequency of chromosomal aberrations. A similar effect was also observed with purified ascorbate and iron.[264] Reduced toxicity was also observed with multiple vitamin tablets fortified with iron. Vitamin C tablets prepared with "natural" ingredients produced both higher and lower responses than did the synthetic ones at similar ascorbate concentrations. These differences are probably due to unspecified components of the natural vitamins.

The effect of freshly prepared ascorbic acid and an ascorbic acid–Cu^{2+} mixture on the genome of cultured human fibroblasts was studied in several different genetic test systems.[267] Cultured human fibroblasts treated with a mixture of ascorbic acid and Cu^{2+} exhibited DNA fragentation, DNA repair synthesis, and chromosomal aberrations, including chromatid breaks and exchanges. When the ascorbic acid solution was flushed with N_2 immediately before addition to cell cultures, both the DNA-damaging and chromosome breaking were virtually eliminated. The active concentrations of ascorbic acid–Cu^{2+} are relatively high when they were compared with the potent mutagen and carcinogen MNNG.[267]

The reducing agents cysteine, glutathione, cysteamine, ascorbic acid, and H_2O_2 with and without the addition of Cu^{2+}, at nontoxic concentrations, triggered a marked DNA repair synthesis and induced a relatively high frequency of chromosome aberrations in cultured human fibroblasts.[266] The latter effects were reduced by the addition of catalase to solutions of the reducing agents plus Cu^{2+}.

In another experiment, several types of cultured fibroblasts, including chick embryo, human, and mouse, were killed by the addition of sodium ascorbate at concentrations of 0.05–0.25 mM to cultures at inoculation time.[274] Glutathione and cysteine were also toxic. The lethal effect of both ascorbate and glutathione was prevented by the addition of calatase to the medium, suggesting that H_2O_2 formed by intracellular reactions and then excreted into the medium was the cytotoxic agent. Their conclusion was supported by the results that showed 0.05 mM H_2O_2 was lethal and that the effect of this compound on cellular morphology was almost identical to that of sodium ascorbate.

Reducing agents such as 2-mercaptoethanol, ascorbic acid, and hydroquinone brought about a decrease in the sedimentation coefficient of DNA of L·P3 cells, which are a substrain of L-929 mouse fibroblasts, as evidenced by sucrose-density gradient centrifugation.[275] Radical scavengers such as cysteamine and ethanol did not alter the effect of the reducing agents. 2-Mercaptoethanol did not induce double-strand scissions in the linear forms of λ DNA, but it introduced slight single-strand scissions in the twisted circular duplex λ DNA under the conditions used. The sedimentation coefficient of the treated DNA was quite similar to that obtained by treatment with proteolytic enzymes. These results suggest that DNA from L·P3 contains some minor proteins with disulfide bridges in them.

Effect on Bacteria

Using the Ames testing system, significant frequency of his$^+$ revertants per surviving bacterial population was induced by a short (15-min) exposure of *Salmonella typhimurium* (TA 100) to the ascorbic acid–Cu^{2+} mixture. At equimolar concentrations, freshly prepared ascorbic acid does not show a detectable mutagenic effect. This result is in contrast to that of Ames *et al.*, who found ascorbic acid to be weakly positive in the Ames test.[276] In other experiments at nontoxic concentrations, the reducing agents cysteine, cysteamine, glutathione, ascorbic acid, and H_2O_2 with and without the addition of Cu^{2+} did not significantly increase the frequency of mutations using *S. typhimurium* histidine-requiring strains TA 98 and TA 100.[266]

Ascorbic acid inhibits the covalent binding of enzymatically generated 2-acetylaminofluorene-N-sulfate to DNA under conditions in which it increases mutagenesis in *Salmonella* TA-1538.[277] [14]C(acetyl)N-hydroxy-2-acetylaminofluorene (NOH-2-AAF) was found to become covalently bound to DNA during the generation of the reactive N-sulfate ester. Two peaks of radioactivity (fractions A and B) were found when DNA digests were eluted from Sephadex W-20 columns. Fraction B appeared to be a NOH-2-AAF-nucleoside adduct, while fraction A seemed to be more clearly related to protein covalent binding. Ascorbic acid decreased NOH-AAF covalent binding to DNA by nearly 80%. Because ascorbic acid addition increased mutagenesis nearly 12-fold under these conditions, binding to DNA may not account for the increased mutagenesis in these experiments. Enhancement of NOH-2-AAF-induced mutagenesis by ascorbic acid has been observed by Sakai *et al.*[278] Schut and Thorgeirsson,[279] and Thorgeirsson *et al.*[280] In these experiments, the NOH-2-AAF was activated by rat and mouse liver nuclei and rat small intestinal cells. It is likely that free radical formation was enhanced by ascorbic acid through reactions that produce hydroxyl ion free radical. (ArN·). A reaction of the general form

$$ArN· + DNA \rightarrow DNA· + ArNH$$

may be postulated, where ArNH is 2-AAF and DNA· is electron-deficient DNA. The aryl nitrenium ion takes an electron from DNA to produce DNA· and generate 2-AAF. DNA· could then undergo any of a series of rearrangements that may result in a base or strand modification expressed as a mutation.

A number of reductones occur during the processing, storage, or cooking of foodstuffs. Reductones play an important role as intermediates in the aminocarbonyl or Strecker's degradation reaction, which can cause variation in color, odor, or nutritive value of foods. They have many reductone structures, such as enediol, enaminol, enediamine, thiol-enol, and enamine-thiol groups. These reductone structures have significant reducing activity. Some reductones possess antitumor activity as well as nucleic acid-breaking activity, which is enhanced by cupric ion.

Omura *et al.* investigated the mutagenic action of reductones both with and without cupric ion using *Salmonella typhimurium* TA100 strain. In these experiments, triose reductone, which has the simplest enediol structure among reductones CHO-C(OH) = C(OH)H, induced a notable frequency of his$^+$ revertants at 2.5 or 5 mM.[281] Cupric ion added to the triose reductone at a molar ratio of 1:1,000 lowered the most active concentration of triose reductone to 1 mM. Another more typical enediol reductone, ascorbic acid, had no detectable mutagenic action by itself. However, in bacteria treated with a freshly mixed solution of 5 mM ascorbic acid and 1 or 5 μM cupric ion, considerable mutagenic action was observed. The mutagenicity of the two reductones occurred at a relatively narrow range of concentrations.

The frequency of mutations was low when compared with that by MNNG or the mixture of ascorbic acid and cupric ion previously used by Stich *et al.*[267] In these experiments, ascorbyl-3-phosphatal, in which 3-OH groups of ascorbic acid were esterified with phosphate, had no effective mutagenic function even in the presence of cupric ion. These results indicate that the enediol structure of reductones plays an important role in mutagenesis. Higher concentrations of reductones or mixtures with cupric ion seemed to cause a lethal effect on the bacteria. Cupric ion addd to controls exerted no mutagenic action.

The mutagenicity of *trans*-4-acetylaminostilbene (AAS) to *Salmonella typhimurium* TA 98 was studied by testing various metabolites as well as related compounds and by comparison of the mutagenicity in the presence of various subcellular fractions, co-factors and enzyme inhibitors.[282] For the activation of AAS, both the microsomal fraction and an NADPH-generating system were necessary. The cytosolic fraction enhanced the mutagenicity. An inhibitor of deacetylases reduced the mutagenicity to almost zero.

Ascorbate increased the mutagenicity of *N*-hydroxy-2-AAF and potentiated the mutagenicity of the 5-AAS compounds. The effect of ascorbate, which produces one-electron oxidation–reduction reactions and stimulates the cytosolic activation of *N*-acetoxy-AAS by both reduced and oxidized NADP(H), suggests that the ultimate mutagen might be formed by either a one-electron oxidation of the aryl hydroxylamine or by a one-electron reduction of the arylnitroso compound.

Effect on Nucleic Acids

Omura *et al.* also compared the effect of ascorbic acid and two types of ascorbate-related reductones on nucleic acids.[281] Both amino reductone and thiol reductone caused strand scissions in nucleic acids. This finding was confirmed by observations that reductones lowered the viscosity of DNA solution and also shifted the peaks of DNA and RNA to the low-molecular side in their centrifugal profile. Cu^{2+} enhanced their action as in the case of enediol reductones. The thiol reductone showed relatively weak breaking activity compared with that of amino and enediol reductones. Apurinic acid was preferentially degraded by both amino and thiol reductones, suggesting that pyrimidine clusters in nucleic acids are susceptible to breakage.

The viscosity of DNA solution was lowered by the action of ascorbic acid or erythorbic acid.[283] The presence of Cu^{2+} enhanced the decrease of viscosity of DNA. Using sucrose-density gradient centrifugation, it was observed that both single- and double-strand scissions of DNA were produced by ascorbic acid or erythorbic acid and enhanced with Cu^{2+}, while only a single-strand scission was caused by ascorbyl-3-phosphate and Cu^{2+}. Similar action of ascorbic acid or ascorbyl-3-phosphate was also observed for RNA. The result seems to indicate that the enediol group of ascorbic acid has an essential role in the breakage of nucleic acids and that Cu^{2+} increases the action.

Apurinic acid was also decomposed by ascorbic acid, whereas apyrimidinic acid was not, indicating that some pyrimidine cluster may be one of the regions attacked by ascorbic acid. The priming activity of DNA for DNA polymerase was altered after treatment with ascorbic acid under the conditions of the experiment. When DNA is altered or cleaved, its priming activity for DNA polymerase should change, leading to a variation of DNA synthesis.

The damages in DNA arising from irradiation have been measured by the change in the intrinsic viscosity of DNA denatured in alkali and the transforming activity (TA) of DNA, where the DNA-recipient culture was *Bacterium subtilis* 168 try-.[284] Either Fe^{2+} or ascorbic acid enhanced the TA caused by radiation. Apparently the added free radicals caused by Fe^{2+} or ascorbic acid can promote an increase in radiation damages in DNA. Part of the breaks induced by ascorbic acid in DNA is repaired by DNA ligase. The restoration of the TA of DNA after treatment with ligase is evidence that part of the breaks in DNA that arise under the action of products of oxidation by ascorbic acid have $5'-PO_4 - 3'-OH$ ends.

Kuhnlein *et al.* described a simple technique for detecting DNA-modifying agents.[285] In this procedure, the double-stranded covalently closed circular DNA of phase PM2 is exposed to the agent to be tested and then analyzed for DNA damages by assays involving only incubation steps and filtration through nitrocellulose. This procedure permits measurement of DNA modifications that lead to local denaturation of the DNA double helix, interstrand crosslinks, and single- and double-strand breaks. These breaks render the phosphodiester bonds of the DNA sensitive to hydrolysis and damage labilizing the glycosylic bond between base and sugar moieties and increasing the depurination or the depyrimidination rate of DNA.

Single- and double-strand breaks (DNA nicking assay) can be measured by exposing DNA to pH 12.4 for 2 min and then neutralized. The treatment denatures nicked DNA circles but will leave covalently closed circles double stranded. The denatured DNA can then be measured by filtration through nitrocellulose filters that will retain the single-stranded DNA. Cysteine and ascorbic acid both increased the nicking reaction with cysteine the most efficient nicking agent. It is likely hydroxyl radicals are generated that are known to cleave phosophodiester bonds efficiently. The autooxidative process and the DNA nicking can be inhibited by EDTA or by catalase.

Effect on Phage Transformation

Smith induced phage lysis in lysogenic cultures of *Salmonella thompson* by means of nitrogen mustard, mustard gas, sulfathiazole, glutathione, and sodium thiol-acetate.[286] The liberation of phage particles by these cultures was inhibited by urethane, much higher concentrations of thiolacetate than necessary to induce lysis, and by incubating either at $41°$–$43.5°$ or at pH 5.5. The optimal temperature was $37°C$, but in some cases incubation at $22°C$ also had a slight inhibitory action. Cultures did not become nonlysogenic as a result of prolonged passage in broth containing either sodium citrate, ascorbic acid, or urethane. Vitamin C also has a virucidal effect on phage J1 of *Lactobacillus casei,* although it does not inhibit the growth of host bacteria.[287] *D*-Isoascorbic acid (erythorbic acid) also shows virucidal activity, indicating that the phage-inhibiting activity is independent of the stereoisomerism.

Murata and Kitagawa investigated the mechanism of inactivation of a double-stranded DNA, phage J1 of *Lactobacillus casei* by ascorbic acid.[288] Bubbling air, oxidizing agents such as H_2O_2 and $KMnO_4$, and transition metal ions such as Cu^{2+}, Fe^{2+}, Cd^{2+}, Mn^{2+}, Ni^{2+}, and Zn^{2+} enhanced the rate of inactivation of the phage by ascorbic acid. Cu^{2+} and Fe^{2+} were the most effective of the transition metals. Citrate and versene enhanced the survival of the phages five to eight times that of the control. In addition, bubbling nitrogen gas, other reducing agents, and radical scavengers such as hydroquinone and amino ethylisothiuronium bromide · hydrobromide prevented the inactivation. These results suggest that the inactivating effect of ascorbic acid was oxygen dependent and caused by free radicals formed during the autooxidation of ascorbic acid.

Dehydroascorbic acid, an oxidized form of ascorbic acid, was much less effective to phage inactivation than was ascorbic acid. The survival percentages of phage by the treatment with dehydroascorbic acid and ascorbic acid at an identical concentration of 1×10^{-4} M was 85% and 10%, respectively, when the incubation time for the phage was 30 min.

The target of ascorbic acid in the phage particle appeared not be the tail protein, but DNA. Single-strand scissions in phage DNA were caused by ascorbic acid, as exhibited by alkaline sucrose-density gradient centrifugation analysis, and caused a slight decrease in the viscosity of DNA.

The breaks in phage DNA are likely responsible for the loss of infectivity in the inactivated phage particle. However, the inactivated phage particle by ascorbic acid is still able to absorb to host bacterial cells and to inject its DNA into the cells. The injected DNA is biologically inactive and does not lead to the formation of mature phage. Murata *et al.* studied the inactivation of both single-stranded DNA and RNA phages by ascorbic acids and thiol-reducing agents such as glutathione and dithiothreitol.[289] The patterns of inactivation of single-stranded DNA and RNA phages by reducing agents are similar to those of inactivation of double-stranded DNA phages.

Murata *et al.* studied the mechanism of inactivation of a single-stranded DNA phage, δ A of *Escherichia coli* by ascorbic acid as a part of another study on the mechanism of inactivation of viruses by ascorbic acid.[290] When oxygen gas was bubbled through the reaction mixture and oxidizing agents or transition metals were added to the reaction mixture, the inactivation of the phage by ascorbic acid was enhanced. On the other hand, nitrogen gas bubbling and the addition of reducing agents, chelating agents, or radical scavengers prevented inactivation. When the ascorbic acid was preincubated for several minutes, the rate of inactivation was faster than when freshly prepared ascorbic acid solution was used. Dehydroascorbic demonstrated little effect on phage activity. However, hydrogen peroxide concentrations theoretically produced by the autoxidation of ascorbic acid had no effect on the phage. Apparently the free radical intermediates produced during the course of the autoxidation of ascorbic acid participated in the inactivation. The radicals that attacked the DNA of the phage introduced strand scissions in the DNA, which might be mainly responsible for the inactivation. The number of strand scissions was proportional to the concentration of ascorbic acid and the length of incubation. When Cu^{2+} and hydrogen peroxide were present, ascorbic acid caused marked strand scissions.

The DNA isolated from the ascorbic acid-inactivated phage was also analyzed by sucrose-density gradient centrifugation and found to be degraded to smaller molecules. The smaller molecules are evidence that the scission of strand can occur within the virion. The target molecule attacked by ascorbic acid may be DNA, and the scission of DNA strands seems to be mainly responsible for the loss of infectivity.

Wong et al. studied the controlled cleavage of phage R17 RNA within the virion by treatment with ascorbate and cupric ion. Their method permits the controlled cleavage of the phage genome without affecting the properties of the phage-structural proteins or of the secondary structure of the RNA.[291] Large losses of infectivity of the order of 6–7 log were readily obtained without any detectable changes in the attachment capacity of phage or the structural integrity of the virion. Studies on the effect of oxygen catalase and of superoxide dismutase on this reaction have suggested that the hydroxyl radicals generated from H_2O_2 may be the reactive agents responsible for the cleavage of phage RNA. Hydrogen peroxide itself has no effect on DNA cleavage but in the presence of Fe^{2+} hydroxy radicals is known to be liberated, and DNA is rapidly fragmented. Cu^+ is also known to generate hydroxyl radicals from H_2O_2. Therefore, ascorbate, probably reduces oxygen to H_2O_2 and Cu^{2+} to Cu^+. Presumably the Cu^+ then reacts with H_2O_2 to produce hydroxyl radicals. Evidence for the involvement of the hydroxyl radical has also been indicated by reactions in which various hydroxyl radical trapping agents such as mannitol, benzoate, and iodide have been added. The sensitivity of DNA to radiation sensitivity has also been attributed largely to the effect of hydroxyl radicals.

Single-strand scissions have been induced in circular and linear > DNA by dithiothreitol (DTT) and ascorbic acid.[292] When DNA was incubated with DTT in a nitrogen atmosphere, significantly fewer chain scissions were found to occur. Although DTT was not as effective as ascorbic acid in its ability to cause single-strand breaks in λ DNA, both effects were indirect, in that they required oxygen.

The inactivation of pneumococcal transforming activity by ascorbate and similar reducing agents was studied by McCarty.[293] In this test system, minute amounts of a desoxyribonucleic acid fraction isolated from type III pneumococci are capable of causing unencapsulated varients of *Pneumococcus* type II to acquire the capsular structure and type specificity of *Pneumococcus* type III. However, treatment of the extracts with small amounts of ascorbic acid resulted in a complete loss of biological activity. This effect required oxygen and was dependent on the production of peroxides during the course of ascorbate autoxidation. In these experiments, glutathione reversed and inhibited the ascorbate inactivation.

Effect on Drosophila

Kenyon and Andress studied the effect of vitamin C on the induction of X-linked recessive lethal mutations in *Drosophila melanogaster*.[294] These workers used the Basc (Muller -5) test to screen X-chromosomes transmitted by wild-type males fed for 8, 13, or 29 days on instant medium either supplemented or not supplemented with a single dose of ascorbic acid. Males reared on medium with no added ascorbate had 116 nonlethal and no lethal X chromosomes. However, males reared on medium with ascorbate had 445 nonlethal and four lethal X chromosomes.

Mechanism of Action

Ascorbic acid exerts both a genotoxic effect in several mutagenic testing systems as well as antimutagenic effects in other test systems. The chemical and biological explanations for these seemingly contradictory observations remain for the most part unclear. In tumorigenesis experiments ascorbate inhibition can be explained by the scavenging of carcinogenic precursors. However, the cause of the mutagenic effects is much more complicated and may originate in the enediol reductone structure or the hydrogen peroxide and free radical formed during autoxidation.

The enhancement of the effect by metals, especially Cu^{2+}, and its inhibition by catalase strongly support the latter possibility. This explanation may be oversimplified because the range of active concentrations is narrow and can easily be missed. The chemistry and mutagenicity of the ascorbic acid–Cu^{2+} system can be summarized by the following three reactions:

$$AH_2 \rightleftharpoons AH^- + H^+ \qquad (3)$$

In reaction (3) the production of the chemically active species is shown. The percentages of the various forms in solution depend on the pH value of the solution, since the pK_1 is 4.14. The hydrogen peroxide-generating system is shown in reaction (4):

$$AH^- + O_2 + (Cu^{2+}) \xrightarrow{H^+} A + H_2O_2 + (Cu^+) \tag{4}$$

The reaction is slow at low pH in the absence of Cu^{2+}. The mild mutagenic effect can be removed by prior catalase addition. Reaction (5) shows the hydrogen peroxide destruction reactions:

$$H_2O_2 + AH_2, AH^-, A, \text{ etc.} \rightarrow \text{Radicals } (AH^-\cdot, HO\cdot_x) \text{ and products}$$
$$\text{(reductones, hydroxy-, and carboxylic acids)} \tag{5}$$

This reaction will be favored by higher initial AH_2 and Cu^{2+} concentrations. The mutagenic effect will not be completely removed by prior addition of catalase.

The autoxidation of AH_2 is complex and leads not only to hydrogen peroxide and dehydroascorbic acid (A), but also, at high turnover, to 2,3-diketogulonic acid, threonic acid, and oxalic acid as the primary reductone-type products. Because both ascorbic and dehydroascorbic acids react with hydrogen peroxide, the chemistry of these systems can be very complex. Kalus *et al.* conducted a chemical and toxicological study of the AH_2 autoxidation system and some of its more accessible products.[295] The mutagenicity of the oxidative decomposition products, dehydroascorbic acid, 2,3-diketogulonic acid, and threonic acid, was tested with *S. typhimurium* TA 100 strain. Neither dehydroascorbic acid nor threonic acid was mutagenic. However, 2,3-diketogulonic acid was found to be mutagenic. Increasing concentrations yielded increasingly greater mutagenicities. Their results indicate that 2,3-diketogulonic acid may be an important factor in the mutagenicity by ascorbic acid. Hydrogen peroxide is probably an important intermediate as well, because catalase will reduce the number of revertants to values equivalent to that obtained with the controls. The lack of a measurable mutagenic effect and its inability to produce H_2O_2 probably exclude any contribution from dehydroascorbic acid, threonic acid, or oxalic acid (without Cu^{2+} stimulation) in the AH_2–Cu^{2+} system. However, oxalic acid in the presence of Cu^{2+} gives rise to peroxide during oxidation. The residual mutagenic effect cannot be inhibited by prior addition of catalase to the reagent solutions and therefore must arise from as yet unidentified minor products and/or free radicals specific to the system.

In intact healthy cells of fruit or vegetables ascorbic acid is relatively stable. However, without the cell's protective environment when the vegetable tissues are peeled, sliced, crushed, or otherwise mechanically damaged, the extent and rate of oxidative processes are affected by time, temperature, pH, oxygen content, and the presence of oxidative enzymes or heavy metal ions that may be present as catalysts.

The rate of decay of ascorbic acid semiquinone radicals in fruit or vegetable juices can be strongly influenced by their solution environment. Once the radical has been formed, there seems to be little that can be done to prevent its decay. One of the best ways to prevent decay in fruit juices is to avoid increases in pH over that of the natural value (i.e., pH 2.8–3.3). The oxidation of ascorbic acid shows a strong pH dependence, reaching a maximum rate at pH 9.6. Maintenance of the natural pH value will ensure that at all time less than 5% of the ascorbic acid is present as a reactive monoanion. Juices should be refrigerated to ensure low reaction rates and should be firmly capped to prevent oxygen access. Diluants with the minimum amount of trace metal catalysts should be used, and diluants using alkaline mineral waters should be avoided. If dilution must be done with mineral water, attention should be paid not only to the trace metal contents, but to their relationship to the common anions as well. For example, sodium chloride accelerates the Cu^{2+}-catalyzed oxidation, but retards the iron-catalyzed oxidation. In contrast, sodium sulfate retards the Fe^{3+} reaction, but has little effect on the copper reaction.

VITAMIN D

Requirements and Effect of a Deficiency

The recommended daily intake of vitamin D from infants to age 19 in males and females is 10 μg cholecalciferol (10 μg + 400 IU vitamin D). Males and females, aged 19 to 22 should take in 7.5 μg/day. Vitamin D brings about normal mineralization of bone and endochondral calcification, thus preventing rickets in the young and osteomalacia in the adult. Vitamin D also prevents hypocalcemic tetany, a function it shares with parathyroid hormone.

In chronic renal disease, $1,25$-$(OH)_2$ D_3 is not made in sufficient amounts; the result is vitamin D-deficient intestine and ultimately bone. Malabsorption and steatorrhea result in a diminished absorption of ingested vitamin D. Chronic pancreatitis, celiac disease, and biliary obstruction were found to malabsorb vitamin D. Absorption of vitamin D occurs in the jejunum and/or ileum. Bile is essential, with most of the vitamin D in the chylomicrons of the lymphatic system. Vitamin D is then concentrated in the liver and transferred to an d_1-globulin with a molecular weight of 52,000 and acts as a carrier for the vitamin and its metabolites. Marginal vitamin D deficiency can be followed by observing the slow calcification of bones, which can be determined as a morphological change on x-ray films of bone. Simple chemical methods to monitor vitamin D in blood are not yet available.

Effect on Cytosol Receptors

Murphy *et al.* measured cytosal receptors for 25-hydroxycholecalciferol (25-OHCC), estradiol, and progesterone in human mammary carcinomas.[296] Significant positive correlations were found between the concentrations of estradiol and 25-OHCC and the concentrations of progesterone and 25-OHCC receptors. Eisman *et al.* demonstrated a specific receptor for 1,25-dihydroxycholecalciferol (1,25-di-OHC) in a cultured human breast cancer cell line.[297] These workers postulate that the high incidence of metastatic bone destruction and hypercalcemia in this common malignancy is due to these receptors. Colston *et al.* demonstrated the presence of a specific, high-affinity receptors for 1,25-(di-OHCC) vitamin D_3 in malignant melanoma.[298] Receptors were present in both the cultured melanoma cells in melanoma tumor tissue produced by inoculation of cells into athymic rats. Human melanoma cells were also responsive to D_3 *in vitro*. Inclusion of D_3 in the culture medium produced a marked increase in cell doubling time. The inhibitory effect of the hormone on melanoma cell proliferation was dose related. Specific high-affinity cytosolic receptors for 1,25-dihydroxy vitamin D_3 have also been demonstrated in five human cancer cell lines.[299]

VITAMIN E

Requirements and Effect of a Deficiency

The recommended daily intake of vitamin E is 10 mg in adult males and 8 mg in adult females. In children aged 1–10, 5–7 mg is recommended, whereas infants up to 1 year of age should take in 3–4 mg. The average intake of α-tocopherols by adults is 15 mg/day, but the variation could be quite large. Individuals fed diets high in protein and low in plant fat would consume less than 10 mg/day, whereas diets high in polyunsaturated oils might be 60 mg/day. A greater requirement for vitamin E is thought to be necessary for individuals on a high polyunsaturated fat diet, especially when the fats are oxidized or contain large amounts of fish oil. Fish oils have a high peroxidative potential and low levels of tocopherol.

Although mammals on vitamin E-deficient diets can show a wide spectrum of pathological conditions, there is no evidence to indicate that humans are susceptible to vitamin E deficiency on an average American diet.

Effect on Animal Carcinogenesis

Vitamin E may prevent mouse skin tumorigenesis through its antioxidant effect.[300] In these experiments the number of mouse skin papillomas induced by

DMBA-croton oil was reduced by α-tocopherol and vitamin C. Vitamin E was more effective than vitamin C in these experiments. Jaffe reported that a diet containing wheat germ oil reduced the number of a mixed group of tumors resulting from the intraperitoneal injection of 3-methylcholanthrene (MCA).[301] On the other hand, adding wheat germ oil to the diet of mice apparently did not influence tumor development resulting from painting the skin with benzpyrene.[302] α-Tocopherol and a number of phenolic antioxidants did not suppress the induction of subcutaneous sarcoma in the mouse by injection of 3,4,10-dibenzpyrene.[303] In the latter two experiments, it is possible that the potential anticarcinogenic effect of vitamin E was overwhelmed by large amounts of carcinogen. Haber and Wissler added vitamin E to the diet of mice and found a decreased incidence of subcutaneous sarcomas induced by MCA.[304] Harman studied the possible role of free radical reactions in aging and in a number of pathological processes including neoplasia.[305] Rats fed a diet containing large amounts of vitamin E had fewer mammary tumors (8 of 20) induced by DMBA than did the controls (14 of 19). Ip, however, found vitamin E to have no effect on DMBA carcinogenesis in rats.[306] Narayan observed that vitamin E deficiency did not accelerate the induction of rat liver tumors induced by N-2-fluorenyl-acetamide in rats.[307] Konings and Trieling observed an enhanced inhibition of [³H]thymidine incorporation into DNA of vitamin E-depleted lymphosarcoma cells.[308]

Shklar observed that Syrian golden hamsters given oral vitamin had had fewer and smaller buccal pouch cancers induced by DMBA.[309] Microscopic examination revealed that there was less invasion of underlying tissues and less surface necrosis. Pauling et al. found that vitamin E intake had no effect on the incidence of squamous cell carcinoma in hairless mice irradiated with ultraviolet lights.[310] Weisburger et al. observed a greater incidence of stomach cancer in populations consuming low levels of vitamin E and other selected micronutrients.[311] They suggested that ingested nitrites or nitrates are metabolized to carcinogenic alkylnitrosourea compounds in the stomach of rats. Vitamin E, as well as vitamin C, can inhibit the nitrosation reactions that result in gastric nitrosourea formation. Because vitamin E is lipid soluble and vitamin C is water soluble, they may complement each other as carcinogenic inhibitors. Weisburger et al. suggest that gastric cancer is a preventable disease and that its incidence may be decreased by serving foods containing vitamin C and perhpas vitamin E with each meal.[311]

Effect on Mutagenesis

Shamberger et al. observed that vitamin E reduces the in vitro DMBA-induced mutagenesis of human lymphocytes.[312] Vitamin E has also reduced the percentage of benzpyrene-induced chromosomal aberrations in both Chinese hamster cells and Chinese hamster ovary cells.[313] The effect of 400 mg supplemental ascorbic acid and of α-tocopherol on fecal mutagenicity examined in two studies involving 20 healthy human donors aged 22–55 years has been studied by Dion et al.[314] In this study the mutagen was extracted from individual frozen feces samples with dichloromethane and assayed with *Salmonella typhimurium* tester strains TA100 without microsomal activation. In two different experiments, fecal mutagenicity decreased on treatment to 2% and 26% of the control. When ascorbic acid and α-tocopherol were added directly to feces, no changes in mutagenicity occurred. Apparently, antioxidants in the diet may have a role in lowering the body's exposure to endogenously produced mutagens.

Effect on Fibrocystic Breast Disease

Noncancerous lumpy breast tissue is present in 20% of American women. This disorder has been termed either fibrocystic breast disease, mammary dysplasia, or fibrous mastopathy. Abrams[315] and London et al.[316] reported that vitamin E achieved moderate to complete relief of premenstrual symptoms in several women with palpable softening of the breasts, with reduction in cyst size.

VITAMIN K

Requirements and Effect of a Deficiency

The recommended daily intake of vitamin K in adults is 70–140 μg/. Other recommended daily intakes are as follows: for infants to 6 months of age, 12 μg; for infants 6 months to 1 year of age, 10–20 μg; for children aged 1–3 years, 15–30 μg; for children aged 4–6 years, 20–40 μg; for adolescents aged 7–10, 30–60 μg; and for adolescents over age 11, 50–100 μg. A normal mixed diet in the United States will contain 300–500 μg of vitamin K per day, an amount more than adequate to supply the dietary requirement. The anticoagulant effect in vitamin K deficiency is caused by a reduction in the content of plasma prothrombin. Three other coagulation proteins—Factor VII, Factor IX, and Factor X—are also regulated by vitamin K.

Primary vitamin K deficiency is uncommon in humans because of the widespread distribution of vitamin K in plant and animal tissues. In addition, the microbiological flora of the normal gut synthesize the menaquinones in amounts that may supply the bulk of the requirement for vitamin K. Healthy adult subjects fed diets low in vitamin K (< 20 μg/day) for several weeks show minimal signs of vitamin K deficiency as evidenced by prothrombin values of 60–90%, unless they are given bowel-sterilizing antibiotics such as neomycin. In one study, neomycin was required to lower the vitamin K-dependent clotting factors to below 20% of normal in 4 weeks. Apparently the microorganisms synthesizing vitamin K must reside in the gut, because up to 500 mg/day instilled into the cecum does not elevate depressed coagulation factors in anticoagulated patients.

Any disorder that hinders the delivery of bile from the small bowel, such as obstructive jaundice in cancer patients or bile fistula, reduces the absorption of vitamin K from the bowel and causes a reduction of plasma concentration of the vitamin K-dependent factors. Malabsorption syndromes associated with sprue, pellagra, bowel shunts, regional ileitis, and ulcerative colitis also cause a secondary vitamin K deficiency. In chronic liver disease, hypoprothrombinemia with bleeding may occur because of a lack of functional hepatic ribosomes to respond to vitamin K.

Effect of Vitamin K Antagonists on Cancer

Vitamin K antagonists (coumarin derivatives) have been reported to be potent antimetastatic drugs.[317] Decreased blood coagulability and direct effects on tumor cells have been considered as the mode of action. Hilgard et al. showed that phenprocoumon, an anticoagulant, slows down the primary growth of Lewis lung carcinoma in C57BL mice.[318] Hilgard et al. studied the effect of phenprocoumon and of vitamin K deficiency on the metastatic potential of the Lewis lung carcinoma in mice.[319] Both phenprocoumon and vitamin K had a marked inhibitory effect on the number of spontaneous lung metastases.

Effect of Vitamin K on Mutagenesis

Vitamins K_3 and K_1 both inhibit the conversion of benzpyrene to its more polar metabolites in an in vitro rat liver microsomal system.[320] In addition, vitamin K_3 inhibits benzpyrene metabolism in rat liver explants and reduces the mutagenicity of both benzpyrene and aflatoxin in the Ames test. High-pressure liquid chromatography analysis of the products of microsomal benzopyrene metabolism shows a uniform reduction of all the metabolic products.

Effect of Vitamin K on Carcinogenesis

Soft tissue sarcomas of the peritoneum, mediastinum, and subcutaneous tissues were induced in ICR/Ha female mice by intraperitoneal injection of benzpyrene.[320] Mice maintained on a vitamin K-deficient diet for 2 weeks pre-

and postbenzpyrene administration had a lower incidence of tumor and tumor death. Mice that received vitamin K_1 before benzpyrene had an accelerated tumor death rate as compared with the benzpyrene controls. The *in vitro* and *in vivo* findings, although seemingly discordant, are consistent with the proposed concept that vitamins K_3 and K_1 are probably acting as electron acceptors in the microsomal NADPH-dependent mixed-function oxidase reactions in which benzpyrene is converted to its multiple metabolites. The reduction or retardation of benzpyrene metabolism by vitamin K may slow the evolution and also reduce the excretion of the water-soluble metabolites, thus producing higher levels and longer exposure to the proximate and ultimate carcinogens.

REFERENCES

1. Lasnitzki, I. 1963. Growth pattern of the mouse prostate gland in organ culture and its response to sex hormones, vitamin A, and 3-methylcholanthrene. *Natl. Cancer Inst. Monogr.* 12:381–403.

3. Lasnitzki, I. 1976. Reversal of methylcholanthrene-induced changes in mouse prostates *in vitro* by retinoic acid and its analogues. *Br. J. Cancer* 34:239–246.

2. Crocker, T., and Sanders, L. 1970. Influence of vitamin A and 3,7-dimethyl-2,6-octadienal (citrol) on the effect of benzopyrene on hamster trachea in organ culture. *Cancer Res.* 30:1312–1318.

4. Davies, R. E. 1967. Effect of vitamin A on 7,12-dimethylbenzanthracene-induced papillomas in rhino mouse skin. *Cancer Res.* 27:237–241.

5. Bollag, W. 1972. Therapeutic effects of an aromatic retinoic acid analog on chemically induced benign and malignant epithelial tumors by vitamin A acid (retinoic acid). *Eur. J. Cancer* 10:731–737.

6. Shamberger, R. J. 1971. Inhibitory effect of vitamin A on carcinogenesis. *J. Natl. Cancer Inst.* 47:667–673.

7. Saffiotti, U., Montesano, R., and Sellakumar, A. R. 1967. Experimental cancer of the lung. Inhibition by vitamin A on the induction of tracheobronchial squamous metaplasia and squamous cell tumors. *Cancer Res.* 20:857–864.

8. Cone, M. V., and Nettesheim, P. 1973. Effects of vitamin A on 3-methylcholanthrene-induced squamous metaplasia and early tumors in the respiratory tract of rats. *J. Natl. Cancer Inst.* 50:1599–1604.

9. Nettesheim, P., and Williams, M. L. 1976. The influence of vitamin A on the susceptibility of the rat lung to 3-methylcholantherene. *Infrect. J. Cancer* 17:351–357.

10. Smith, D. M., Rogers, A. E., Herndon, B. J., and Newberne, P. M. 1975. Vitamin A (retinyl acetate) and benzopyrene-induced respiratory tract carcinogenesis in hamsters fed a commercial diet.*Cancer Res.* 35:11–16.

11. Cohen, S. M., Wittenberg, J. F., and Bryan, G. T. 1976. Effect of avitaminosis A and hypervitaminosis A on urinary bladder carcinogenicity of *N*-{4-(5-nitro-z-furyl)-2-thiazoly1} formamide. *Cancer Res.* 36:2334–2339.

12. Narisawa, T., Reddy, B. S., Wong, C. Q., and Weisburger, J. H. 1976. Effect of vitamin A deficiency on rat colon carcinogenesis by N-methyl-N-nitro-N nitrosoguanidine. *Cancer Res.* 36:1379–1383.

13. Rogers, A. E., Herndon, B. J., and Newberne, F. M. 1973. Induction by dimethylhydrazine of intestinal carcinoma in normal rats and rats fed high or low levels of vitamin A. *Cancer Res.* *33:*1003–1009.

14. Newberne, P. M., and Rogers, A. E. 1973. Rat colon carcinomas associated with aflatoxin and marginal vitamin A. *J. Natl. Cancer Inst.* *50:*439–448.

15. Chu, E. W., and Malmgren, R. A. 1965. An inhibitory effect of vitamin A on the induction of tumors of forestomach and cervix in the Syrian hamster by carcinogenic polycyclic hydrocarbons. *Cancer Res.* *25:*884–895.

16. Levine, N. S., Salisbury, R. E., Seifter, E., Walker, H. L., Mason, A. D., Jr., and Pruitt, B. A., Jr. Effect of vitamin A on tumor development in burned, unburned, and glucocorticoid-treated mice inoculated with an oncogenic virus. *Experientia 15:*1309–1312.

17. Retura, G., Schittek, A., Hardy, M., Levenson, S. M., Demetriou, A., and Seifter, E. 1975. Antitumor action of vitamin A in mice with adenocarcinoma cells. *J. Natl. Cancer Inst.* *54:*1489–1491.

18. McMichael, H. 1975. Inhibition of growth of Shope rabbit papilloma by hypervitaminosis A. *Cancer Res.* *25:*1309–1312.

19. Anton, E., and Brandes, D. 1968. Lysosomes in mouse mammary tumors treated with cyclophosphamide. Distribution related to the course of disease. *Cancer 21:*483–500.

20. Cohen, M. H., and Carbone, P. P. 1972. Enhancement of the antitumor effects of 1,3-bis-(2-chlorethyl)-1-nitrosourea and cyclophosphamide by vitamin A. *J. Natl. Cancer Inst.* *48:*921–926.

21. Tomita, Y., Himeno, K., Nomoto, K., Endo, H., and Hirohata, T. 1982. Combined treatments with vitamin A and 5-fluorouracil and the growth of allotransplantable and syngeneic tumors in mice. *J. Natl. Cancer Inst.* *68:*823–827.

22. Prutkin, L. 1973. Antitimor activity of vitamin A acid and fluorouracil used in combination on the skin tumor, keratoacanthoma. *Cancer Res.* *33:*128–133.

23. Tani, E., Morimura, T., Kaba, K., and Itagaki, T. 1980. Preliminary study of the effects of vitamin A on antineoplastic activities of chemotherapeutic agents in glioma. *Neurol. Med. Chir. (Tokyo) 20:*665–677.

24. Komiyama, S., Hiroto, I., Ryu, S., Nakashima, T., Kuwano, M., and Endo, H. Synergistic combination therapy of 5-fluorouracil, vitamin A and cobalt-60 radiation upon head and neck tumors. *Oncology 35:*253–257.

25. Merriman, R. L., and Bertram, J. S. 1979. Reversible inhibition by retinoids of 3-methylcholanthrene-induced neoplastic transformation in C3H/10T ½ clone 8 cells. *Cancer Res.* *39:*1661–1666.

26. Todaro, G. J., DeLarco, J. E., and Sporn, M. B. 1978. Retinoids block phenotypic cell transformation produced by sarcoma growth factor. *Nature 27:*272–274.

27. Lotan, R., and Nicolson, G. L. 1977. Inhibitory effeects of retinoic acid or retinyl acetate on the growth of untransformed, transformed, and tumor cells *in vitro*. *J. Natl. Cancer Inst.* *59:*1712–1722.

28. Huang, C. C., Hsueh, J. L., Chen, H. H., and Batt, T. R. 1982. Retinol (vitamin A) inhibits sister chromatid exchanges and cell cycle delay induced by cyclophosphamide and aflatoxin B-1 in Chinese hamster V 79 cells. *Carcinogenesis 3:*1–5.

29. Busk, L., and Ahlborg, U. G. 1980. Retinol (vitamin A) as an inhibitor of the mutagenicity of aflatoxin B-1. *Toxicol. Lett.* *6:*243–249.

30. Busk, L., and Ahlborg, U. 1982. Retinol (vitamin A) as a modifier of 2-aminofluorene and 2-acetyl-aminofluorene mutagenesis in the Salmonella/microsome assay. Arch. Toxicol. 49:169–174.

31. Sporn, M. B., Dunlop, N. M., Newton, D. L., and Henderson, W. R. 1976. Relationship between structure and activity of retinoids. *Nature 263:*110–113.

32. Bollag, W. 1975. Therapy of epithelial tumors with an aromatic retinoic acid analog. *Chemotherapy (Basel) 21:*236–247.

33. Port, C. D., Sporn, M. B., and Kaufman, D. G. 1975. Prevention of lung cancer in hamsters by 13-cis-retinoic acid. *Proc. Am. Assoc. Cancer Res. 16:*21.

34. Grubbs, C. J., Moon, R. C., and Sporn, M. B. 1976. Suppression of DMBA-induced mammary tumorigenesis by retinyl methyl ether. *Proc. Am. Assoc. Cancer Res. 17:*68.

35. Todaro, G., DeLarco, J., and Sporn, M. Retinoids block phenotypic cell transformation produced by sarcoma growth factor. *Nature 276:*272–274.

36. Sporn, M. B., Dunlop, N. M., Newton, D. L., and Smith, J. M. 1976. Prevention of chemical carcinogenesis by vitamin A and its synthetic analogs (retinoids). *Fed. Proc. 35:*1332–1338.

37. Peto, R., Doll, R., Buckley, J. D., and Sporn, M. B. 1981. Can dietary beta-carotene materially reduce human cancer rates? *Nature 290:*201–208.

38. Mathews-Roth, M. M., Pathak, M. A., Fitzpatrick, T. B., Harber, L. H., and Kass, E. H. 1977. Beta carotene therapy for erythropoietic protoporphyria and other photosensitivity diseases. *Arch. Dermatol. 113:*1229–1232.

39. Shamberger, R. J. 1971. Inhibitory effect of vitamin A on carcinogenesis. *J. Natl. Cancer Inst. 47:*667–673.

40. Seifter, E., Rettura, G., Podawer, J., and Levenson, S. M. 1982. Moloney murine sarcoma virus tumors in CBA/J mice: Chemopreventative and chemotherapeutic actions of supplemental β-carotene. *J. Natl. Cancer Inst. 68:*835–840.

41. Sporn, M. B., Clamon, G. H., Dunlop, N. M., Newton, D. L., Smith, J. M., and Saffiotti, U. 1975. Activity of vitamin A analogues in cell cultures of mouse epidermis and organ cultures of hamster trachea. *Nature 253:*47–49.

42. Wilkoff, L. J., Peckham, J., Dulmadge, E. A., Mowry, R. W., and Chopra, D. P. 1976. Evaluation of vitamin A analogs in modulating epithelial differentiation of 13-day chick embryo metatarsal skin explants. *Cancer Res. 36:*964–972.

43. Sani, B. P. 1977. Localization of retinoic acid-binding protein in nuclei. *Biochem. Biophys Res. Commun. 75:*7–12.

44. Wiggert, B., Russel, P., Lewis, M., and Chader, G. 1977. Differential binding to soluble nuclear receptors and effects on cell viability of retinol and retinoic acid in cultured retinoblastoma cells. *Biochem. Biophys. Res. Commun. 79:*218–225.

45. Sani, B. P., and Hill, D. L. 1974. Retinoic acid: A binding protein in chick embryo metatarsal skin. *Biochem. Biophys. Res. Commun. 61:*1276–1281.

46. Sani, B. P., and Donovan, M. K. 1979. Localization of retinoic acid-binding protein in nuclei and the nuclear uptake of retinoic acid. *Cancer Res. 39:*2492–2496.

47. Huber, P. R., Geyer, E., Kung, W., Matter, A., Torhorst, J., and Eppenberger, U. 1978. Retinoic-acid binding protein in human breast cancer and dysplasia. *J. Natl. Cancer Inst. 61:*1375–1378.

48. Basu, T. K., Rowland, L., Jones, L,, and Kohn, J. 1982. Vitamin A and retinol-binding protein in patients with myelomatosis and cancer of epithelial organ. *Eur. J. Clin. Oncol. 18:*339–342.

49. Hill, D. L., and Shih, T. W. 1974. Vitamin A compounds and analogues as inhibitors of mixed-function oxidases that metabolize carcinogenic polycyclic hydrocarbons and other compounds. *Cancer Res. 34:*564–570.

50. Carruthers, C. 1942. The effect of carcinogens on the hepatic vitamin A stores of mice and rats. *Cancer Res. 2:*168–174.

51. Genta, V. M., Kaufman, D. G., Harris, C. C., Smith, J. M., Sporn, M. B., and Saffiotti, U. 1974. Vitamin A deficiency enhances the binding of benzopyrene to tracheal epithelial DNA. *Nature 247:*48–49.

52. Verma, A. K., Shapas, B. G., Rice, H. M., and Boutwell, R. K. 1979. Correlation of the

inhibition by retinoids of tumor-promotor-induced mouse ornithine decarboxylase activity of skin tumor promotion. *Cancer Res. 39:*419–425.

53. Lowe, N. J., and Breeding, J. 1982. Retinoic acid modulation of ultraviolet light-induced epidermal ornithine decarboxylase activity. *J. Invest. Dermatol. 78:*121–124.

54. Conner, M. J., Lowe, N. J., Breeding, J. H., and Chalet, M. 1983. Inhibition of ultraviolet-B skin carcinogenesis by all-trans-retinoic acid regimens that inhibit ornithine decarboxylase induction. *Cancer Res. 43:*171–174.

55. O'Brien, T. G. 1976. The induction of ornithine decarboxylase as an early possibly obligatory, event in mouse skin carcinogenesis. *Cancer Res. 36:*2644–2653.

56. Levine, L., and Ohuchi, K. 1978. Retinoids as well as tumour promotors enhance deacylation of cellular lipids and prostaglandin production in MDCK cells. *Nature 276:*274–275.

57. Hill, D. L., and Grubbs, C. J. 1982. Retinoids as chemopreventive and anticancer agents in intact animals. (Review.) *Anticancer Res. 2:*111–124.

58. Bjelke, E. 1975. Dietary vitamin A and human lung cancer. *Int. J. Cancer 15:*561–565.

59. MacLennan, R., DaCosta, J., Day, N. E., Law, C. H., Ng, Y. K., and Shanmugaratnam. 1977. Risk factors for lung cancer in Singapore Chinese, a population with high female incidence rates. *Int. J. Cancer 20:*854–860.

60. Gregor, A., Lee, P. N., Roe, F. J. C., Wilson, M. J., and Melton, A. 1980. Comparison of dietary histories in lung cancer cases and controls with special reference to vitamin A. *Nutr. Cancer 2:*93–97.

61. Smith, P. G., and Jick, H. 1978. Cancers among users of preparations containing vitamin A. *Cancer 42:*808–811.

62. Mettlin, C., Graham, S., and Swanson, M. 1979. Vitamin A and lung cancer. *J. Natl. Cancer Inst. 62:*1435–1438.

63. Basu, T1K., Donaldson, D., Jenner, M., Williams, D. C., and Sakula, A. 1976. Plasma vitamin A in patients with bronchial carcinoma. *Br. J. Cancer 33:*119–121.

64. Shekelle, R. B., Liu, S., Raynor, W. J., Lepper, M., Maliza, C., and Rossof, A. H. 1981. Dietary vitamin A and risk of cancer in the Western Electric study. *Lancet 2:*1185–1189.

65. Graham, S., Mettlin, C., Marshall, J., Priore, R., Rzepka, T., and Shedd, D. 1981. Dietary factors in the epidemiology of cancer of the larynx. *Am. J. Epidemiol. 113:*675–680.

66. Wynder, E. L., and Bross, I. J. 1961. A study of etiological factors in cancer of the esophagus. *Cancer 14:*389–413.

67. Mettlin, C., Graham, S., Priore, R., Marshall, J., and Swanson, M. 1981. Diet and cancer of the esophagus. *Nutr. Cancer 2:*143–147.

68. Hormozdiari, H., Day, N. E., Aramesh, B., and Mahboubi, E. 1975. Dietary factors and esophageal cancer in the Caspian littoral of Iran. *Cancer Res. 35:*3493–3498.

69. Cook-Mazaffari, P. J., Azordegan, F., Day, N. E., Ressicand, A., Sabai, C., and Aramesh, B. 1979. Oesophageal cancer studies in the Caspian litterol of Iran: Results of a case-control study. *Br. J. Cancer 39:*293–309.

70. Hirayama, T. 1967. The epidemiology of cancer of the stomach in Japan with special reference to the role of the diet. in R. J. C. Harris (Ed.) *Proceedings of the 9th international congress. UICC Monograph Series.* Vol. 10. pp. 37–48. New York: Springer-Verlag.

71. Hirayama, T. 1977. Changing patterns of cancer in Japan with special reference to the decrease in stomach cancer mortality. in H. H. Hiatt, J. D. Watson, and J. A. Winsten (Eds.) *Origins of human cancer.* pp. 55–57. Cold Spring Harbor, New York: Cold Spring Harbor Laboratory.

72. Graham, S., Schotz, W., and Martino, P. 1972. Alimentary factors in the epidemiology of gastric cancer. *Cancer 30:*927–938.

73. Haenszel, W., Kurihara, M., Segi, M., and Lee, R. K. C. 1972. Stomach cancer among Japanese in Hawaii. *J. Natl. Cancer Inst. 49:*969–988.

74. Bjelke, E. 1978. Dietary factors and epidemiology of cancer of the stomach and large bowel. Aktuel Ernaehrungsmed. *Klin. Prax. Suppl. 2:*10–17.

75. Schuman, L. M., Mandell, J. S., Redke, A., Seal, U., and Halberg, F. 1982. Some selected features of the epidemiology of prostatic cancer: Minneapolis-St. Paul, Minnesota case-control study, 1976–1979. in K. Magnus (Ed.) *Trends in cancer incidence: Causes and practical implications.* pp. 345–354. New York: Hemisphere.

76. Romney, S. L., Palan, P. R., Duttagupta, C., Wassertheil-Smollery Wylie, J., Miller, G., Slagle, N. S., and Lucido, D. 1981. Retinoids and the prevention of cervical dysplasias. *Am. J. Obstet. Gynecol. 141:*890–894.

77. Cambien, F., Ducimetierre, P., and Richard J. 1980. Total serum cholesterol and cancer mortality in a middle-aged population. *Am. J. Epidemiol. 112:*388–394.

78. Kark, J. D., Smith, A. H., and Hames, C. G. 1980. The relationship of serum cholesterol to the incidence of cancer in Evans County, Georgia. *J. Chronic Dis. 33:*311–322.

79. Wald, N., Idle, M., Boreham, J., and Bailey, A. 1980. Low serum vitamin A and subsequent risk of cancer—Preliminary results of a prospective study. *Lancet 2:*813–815.

80. Kark, J. D., Smith, A. H., and Hames, C. G. 1982. Serum retinol and the inverse relationship between serum cholesterol and cancer. *Br. Med. J. 284:*152–154.

81. Tannenbaum, A., and Silverstone, H. 1952. The genesis and growth of tumors. V. Effects of varying the level of B vitamins in the diet. *Cancer Res. 12:*744–749.

82. Boutwell, R. K., Brush, M. K., and Rusch, H. P. 1949. The influence of vitamins of the B complex on the induction of epithelial tumors in mice. *Cancer Res. 9:*747–752.

83. Kensler, C. J., Sugiura, K., Young, N. F., Halter, C. R., and Rhoads, C. P. 1941. Partial protection of rats by riboflavin with case in against liver cancer caused by dimethylaminoazo-benzene. *Science 93:*308–310.

84. Miller, J. A., and Miller, E. C. 1953. The carcinogenic aminoazo dyes. *Adv. Cancer Res. 1:*339–396.

85. Morris, H. P. 1947. Effects on the genesis and growth of tumors associated with vitamin intake. *Ann. N.Y. Acad. Sci. 49:*119–140.

86. Chan, P. C., Okamoto, T., and Wynder, E. L. 1972. Possible role of riboflavin deficiency in epithelial neoplasia. III. Induction of microsomal aryl hydrocarbon hydroxylase. *J. Natl. Cancer Inst. 48:*1341–1345.

87. Pacernick, L. J., Soltani, K., and Lorincz, A. L. 1975. The inefficacy of riboflavin against ultraviolet-induced carcinogenesis. *J. Invest. Dermatol. 65:*547–548.

88. Lemonnier, F. J., Scott, J. M., and Thuong-Trieu, C. 1975. Influence of riboflavin on disturbances in tryptophan metabolism and hepatoma production after a single dose of aflatoxin B-1. *J. Natl. Cancer Inst. 55:*1085–1087.

89. Stoerk, H. C., and Emerson, G. A. 1949. Complete regression of lymphosarcoma implants following temporary induction of riboflavin deficiency in mice. *Proc. Soc. Exp. Biol. Med. 70:*703–704.

90. Aposhian, H. V., and Lambooy, J. P. 1951. Retardation of growth of Walker rat carcinoma 256 by administration of diethyl riboflavin. *Proc. Soc. Exp. Biol. Med. 78:*197–199.

91. Lane, M. 1971. Induced riboflavin deficiency in treatment of patients with lymphomas and polycythemia vera. *Proc. Am. Assoc. Cancer Res. 12:*85.

92. Morris, H. P., and Lippincott, S. W. 1941. Effect of pantothenic acid and growth of the spontaneous mammary carcinoma in female C_3H mice. *J. Natl. Cancer Inst. 2:*47–54.

93. Petering, L. J., Soltani, K., and Lorincz, A. L. 1975. The inefficacy of riboflavin against ultra-induced carcinogenesis. *J. Invest. Dermatol. 65:*547–548.

94. Newberne, P. M. 1965. Carcinogenicity of aflatoxin-contaminated peanut meals. in G. N. Wogen (Ed.) *Mycotoxins in foodstuffs.* Cambridge, Mass.: MIT Press. pp. 187–208.

95. Lombardi, B., and Shinozuka, H. 1979. Enhancement of 2-acetylaminofluorene liver carcinogenesis in rats fed a choline-devoid diet. *Int. J. Cancer 23:*565–570.

96. Shinozuka, H., Katyal, S. L., and Lombardi, B. 1978. Azaserine carcinogenesis: Organ susceptibility change in rats fed a diet devoid of choline. *Int. J. Cancer 22:*36–39.

97. Takahashi, S., Lombardi, B., and Shinozuka, H. 1982. Progression of carcinogen-induced foci of γ-glutamyltranspeptidase-positive hepatocytes to hepatomas in rats fed a choline-deficient diet. *Int. J. Cancer 29:*445–450.

98. Giambarresi, L. I., Katyal, S. L., and Lombardi, B. 1982. Promotion of liver carcinogenesis in the rat by a choline-devoid diet: Role of liver cell necrosis and regeneration. *Br. J. Cancer. 46:*825–829.

99. Reddy, T. V., Romanathan, R., Shinozuka, H., and Lombardi, B. 1983. Effects of dietary choline deficiency on the mutagenic activation of chemical carcinogens by rat liver fractions. *Cancer Lett. 18:*41–48.

100. Rogers, A. E. 1975. Variable effects of a lipotrope deficient, high fat diet on chemical carcinogenesis in rats. *Cancer Res. 35:*2469–2474.

101. Morris, H. P. 1947. Effects on the genesis and growth of tumors associated with vitamin intake. *Ann. N.Y. Acad. Sci. 49:*119–140.

102. Basu, T. K., Dickerson, J. W. T., Raven, R. W., and Williams, D. C. 1974. The thiamine status of patients with cancer as determined by the red cell transketolase activity. *Int. J. Vit. Nutr. Res. 44:*53–58.

103. De Reuck, J. L., Sieben, G. J., Sieben-Praet, M. R., Ngendahayo, P., Decoster, J. P., and Vancer Eeken, H. M. 190. Wernicke's encephalopathy in patients with tumors of the lymphoid hemapoetic systems. *Arch. Neurol. 37:*338–341.

104. Aksoy, M., Basu, T. K., Brient, J., and Dickerson, J. W. T. 1980. Thiamin status of patients treated with drug combinations containing 5-fluorouracil. *Eur. J. Cancer 16:*1041–1045.

105. Ostryanina, A. D. 1971. Vitamin B_{12} and the neoplastic process. *Vopr. Pitan. 29:*25–31.

105a. Temcharoen, P., Anukarahanonta, T., and Bhamarapratvi, N. 1978. Influence of dietary protein and vitamin B_{12} on the toxicity and carcinogenicity of aflatoxins in rat liver. *Cancer Res. 38:*2185–2190.

106. Pegg, A. E. 1977. Formation and metabolism of alkylated nucleosides: Possible role in carcinogenesis by nitroso compounds and alkylating agents. *Adv. Cancer Res. 25:*195–269.

107. Day, P. L., Payne, L. D., and Dinning, J. S. 1960. Procarcinogenic effect of vitamin B_{12} on p-dimethylaminoazobenzene-fed rats. *Proc. Soc. Exp. Biol. Med. 74:*854–857.

108. Yamamoto, R. S. 1980. Effect on vitamin B_{12} deficiency in colon carcinogenesis. *Proc. Soc. Exp. Biol. Med. 163:*350–353.

109. Elsborg, L., and Masbech, J. 1979. Pernicious anemia as a risk factor in gastric cancer. *Acta Intern. Med. 206:*315–318.

110. Ruddell, W. S., Bone, E. S., Hill, M. J., and Walters, C. L. 1978. Pathogenesis of gastric cancer in pernicious anemia. *Lancet 1:*521–523.

111. Arvanitakis, C., Holmes, F. F., and Hearne, E. A. 1979. Possible associations of pernicious anemia with neoplasia. *Oncology 36:*127–129.

112. Carmel, R., and Eisenberg, L. 1977. Serum B_{12} and transcobalamin abnormalities in patients with cancer. *Cancer 40:*1348–1350.

113. Einhorn, J., and Retzenstein, P. 1966. Metabolic studies of folic acid and malignancy. *Cancer Res. 26:*340–343.

114. Roa, P. B., Lagerlof, B., Einhorn, J., and Retzenstein, P. 1965. Folic acid activity in leukemia and cancer. *Cancer Res. 25:*221–224.

115. Taguchi, H., Sanada, H., Hosei, T., Hara, K., Mizukawa, I., Sezaki, T., Irino, S., Iwasaki, I., and Hiraki, K. 1974. Folic acid metabolism in Rauscher murine leukemia and effect of methotrexate on the blood picture. *Acta Med. Okayama 28:*353–359.

116. Djerassi, I., Farber, S., Abing, E., and Neikerk, W. 1967. Continuous infusion of methotrexate in children with acute leukemia. *Cancer 20:*223–242.

117. Jaffe, N. 1972. Recent advances in the chemotherapy of metastatic osteogenic sarcoma. *Cancer 30:*1627–2631.

118. Alberto, P., Peytremann, R., Medenica, R., and Piccoli, M. B. 1978. Initial clinical experience with a simultaneous combination of 2,4-diamino-5(3,4-dichlorophenyl)-6-methylpyrimidine (DDMP) with folinic acid. *Cancer Chemother. Pharmacol. 1:*101–105.

119. Sirotnak, F. M., DeGraw, J. I., Moccio, D. J., and Dorick, D. M. 1978. Antitumor properties of a new folate analog, 10-deaza-aminopterin in mice. *Cancer Treatm. Rep. 62:*1047–1052.

120. Kline, B. E., Rusch, H. P., Bauman, C. A., and Lavik, P. S. 1943. The effect of pyridoxine on tumor growth. *Cancer Res. 3:*825–829.

121. Mihich, E., and Nichol, C. A. 1959. The effect of pyridoxine deficiency on mouse sarcoma 180. *Cancer Res. 19:*279–284.

122. Tryfiates, G. P., and Morris, H. P. 1974. Effect of pyridoxine deficiency on tyrosine transaminase activity and growth of four mouse hepatomas. *J. Natl. Cancer Inst. 52:*1259–1262.

123. Tryfiates, G. P. 1975. Effect of pyridoxine availability on the activity of serine dehydratase of normal liver, host liver, and three Morris hepatomas. *J. Natl. Cancer Inst. 54:*171–172.

124. DiSarbo, D. M., Paavola, L. G., and Litwack, G. 1982. Pyridoxine resistance in a rat hepatoma cell line. *Cancer Res. 42:*2362–2370.

125. DiDorbo, D. M., and Litwack, G. 1982. B_6 kills hepatoma cells in culture. *Nutr. Cancer 3:*216–222.

126. Pruzansky, J., and Axelrod, A. E. 1955. Antibody production to diphtheria toxoid in vitamin deficiency states. *Proc. Soc. Exp. Biol. Med. 89:*323–325.

127. Axelrod, A. E., and Hopper, S. 1960. Effects of pantothenic acid, pyridoxine and thiamine deficiencies upon antibody formation to influenza virus PR-8 in rats. *J. Nutr. 72:*325–330.

128. Trakatellis, A. C., Stinebring, W. R., and Axelrod, A. E. 1963. Studies on systemic reacitivy to purified protein and derivative (PPD) and endotoxin. 1. Systemic reactivity to PPD in pyridoxine-deficient guinea pigs. *J. Immunol. 91:*39–45.

129. Axelrod, A. E., Fisher, B., Fisher, E., Lee, Y. C. P., and Walsh, P. 1958. Effect of a pyridoxine deficiency on skin grafts in the rat. *Science 127:*1388–1389.

130. Axelrod, E. E., and Trakatellis, A. C. 1964. Induction of tolerance to skin homografts by administering splenic cells by pyridoxine-deficient mice. *Proc. Soc. Exp. Biol. Med. 116:*206–210.

131. Gailani, S. D., Holland, N. F., Nussbaum, A., and Olson, K. B. 1968. Chemical and biochemical studies of pyridoxine deficiency in patients with neoplastic diseases. *Cancer 21:*975–988.

132. Shapiro, D. M., and Gellhorn, A. 1951. Combinations of chemical compounds in experimental therapy. *Cancer Res. 11:*35–41.

133. Korytnyk, W., Hakala, M. T., Potti, P. G. G., Angelino, N., and Chang, S. C. 1976. On the inhibitory activity of 4-vinyl analogs of pyridoxal: Enzyme and cell culture studies. *Biochemistry 15:*5458–5466.

134. Potera, C., Rose, D. P., and Brown, R. R. 1977. Vitamin B_6 deficiency in cancer patients. *Am. J. Clin. Nutr. 30:*1677–1679.

135. Rakieten, N., Gordon, B. S., Beaty, A., Cooney, D. A., Davis, R. D., and Schein, P. S. 1971. Pancreatic islet tumors produced by the combined action of streptozotocin and nicotinamide. *Proc. Soc. Exp. Biol. Med. 137:*280–283.

136. Shoentel, R. 1977. The role of nicotinamide and of other modifying factors in diethylnitrosamine carcinogenesis. *Cancer 40:*1833–1840.

137. Barra, R., Randolph, V., Sumas, M. E., Lanighan, K., and Lea, M. A. 1982. Effects of

nicotinamide, isonicotinamide and bleomycin on DNA synthesis and repair in rat hepatocytes and hepatoma cells. *J. Natl. Cancer Inst. 69*:1353–1357.

138. Nduka, N., Skidmore, C. J., and Shall, S. 1980: The enhancement of cytotoxicity of N-methyl-N-nitrosourea and of γ-radiation by inhibitors of poly (ADP-ribose) polymerase. *Eur. J. Biochem. 105*:525–530.

139. Smulson, M. E., Schein, P., Mullins, D. W., and Sudhakar, S. 1977. A putative role for nicotinamide adenine dinucleotide-promoted nuclear protein modification in the antitumor activity of N-methyl-N-nitrosourea. *Cancer Res. 37*:3006–3012.

140. Shapiro, D. M., Dietrich, L. S., and Shies, M. D. 1957. Quantitative biochemical differences between tumor and host as a basis of cancer chemotherapy. *Cancer Res. 17*:600–604.

141. Barclay, R. K., and Phillips, M. A. 1966. Effects of 6-diazo-5-oxo-L-norleucine and other tumour inhibitors on the biosynthesis of NAD in mice. *Cancer Res. 26*:282–286.

142. Shimoyama, M. S., Yamaguchi, K., and Gholson, R. K. 1967. Enzymic lesions of nicotinamide adenine dinucleotide biosynthesis in hepatomas and in azo dye carcinogenesis. *Cancer Res. 27*:578–583.

143. Brown, R. R., Price, J. M., Freidell, G., and Burney, S. W. 1969. Tryptophan metabolism in patients with bladder cancer. Geographical differences. *J. Natl. Cancer Inst. 43*:295–301.

144. Zeitlin, I., and Smith, A. N. 5-Hydroxyindoles and kinins in the carcinoid and dumping syndromes. *Lancet 2*:986–996.

145. Basu, T. K., Raven, R. W., Bate, C., and Williams, O. C. 1973. Excretion of 5-hydroxyindole acetic acid and N-methylnicotinamide in advanced cancer patients. *Eur. J. Cancer 9*:527–528.

146. Szent-Gyorgyi, A. 1928. Observations of the functions of peroxidase systems and the chemistry of the adrenal cortex. *Biochem. J. 22*:1387–1409.

147. Baker, E. M., Hodges, R. E., Hood, J., Sauberlich, H. E., March, S. C., and Canham, J. E. 1971. Metabolism of ^{14}C and ^{3}H-labeled L-ascorbic acid in human scurvy. *Am. J. Clin. Nutr. 24*:444–454.

148. Hornig, D., Vuilleumier, J. P., and Hartmann, P. 1980. Absorption of large, single, oral intakes of ascorbic acid. *Int. J. Vit. Nutr. Res. 50*:309–314.

149. Shamberger, R. J. 1972. Increase of peroxidation in carcinogenesis. *J. Natl. Cancer Inst. 48*:1491–1497.

150. Slaga, T. J., and Bracken, W. M. 1977. The effects of anti-oxidants on skin tumor initiation and aryl hydrocarbon hydroxylase. *Cancer Res. 37*:1631–1635.

151. Sadek, I. A., and Abdelmegid, N. 1982. Ascorbic acid and its effect on the skin of *Bufo regularis*. *Oncology 39*:399–400.

152. Abul-Hajj, Y. J., and Kelliher, M. 1982. Failure of ascorbic acid to inhibit growth of transplantable and dimethylbenzanthracene induced rat mammary tumors. *Cancer Lett. 17*:67–73.

153. Shoyab, M. 1981. Inhibition of the binding of 7,12-dimethylbenzanthracene to DNA of murine epidermal cells in culture by vitamin A and vitamin C. *Oncology 38*:187–192.

154. Dunham, W. B., Zuckerkandl, E., Reynolds, R., Willoughby, R., Marcuson, R., Barth, R., and Pauling, L. 1982. Effects of intake of L-ascorbic acid on the incidence of dermal neoplasms induced in mice by ultraviolet light. *Proc. Natl. Acad. Sci. (USA) 79*:7532–7536.

155. Schlegel, J. U., Pipkin, G. E., Nishumura, R., and Schultz, G. N. 1969. The role of ascorbic acid in the prevention of bladder tumor formation. *Trans. Am. Assoc. Genitourinary Surg. 61*:85–89.

156. Boyland, E., and Williams, D. C. 1956. Metabolism of tryptophan in patients suffering from cancer of the bladder. *Biochem. J. 64*:578–582.

157. Price, J. M., Wear, J. B., Brown, R. R., Satter, E. J., and Olson, C. 1960. Studies on etiology of bladder carcinoma. *J. Urol. 83*:376–382.

158. Price, J. M., Wear, J. B., Brown, R. R., Satter, E. J., and Olson, C. 1963. Studies on eitology of carcinoma of the urinary bladder. *J. Urol. 83:*376–382.

159. Benassi, C. A., Perissinotto, B., and Allegri, G. 1963. The metabolism of tryptophan in patients with bladder cancer and other urological diseases. *Clin. Chem. Acta 8:*822–831.

160. Schlegel, J. U. 1975. Proposed users of ascorbic acid in the prevention of bladder carcinoma. *Ann. N.Y. Acad. Sci. 258:*432–437.

161. Pipkin, G. E., Nishimura, R., Banowsky, L., and Schlegel, J. U. 1967. Stabilization of urinary 3-hyroxyanthranilic acid by the oral administration of L-ascorbic acid. *Proc. Soc. Exp. Biol. Med. 126:*702–704.

162. Soloway, M. S., Cohen, S. M., Dekernion, J. B., and Persky, L. 1975. Failure of ascorbic acid to inhibit FANFT-induced bladder cancer. *J. Urol. 113:*483–486.

163. Mirvish, S. S., Wallace, L., Eagen, M., and Shubik, P. 1972. Ascorbate–nitrite reaction: Possible means of blocking the formation of carcinogenic compounds. *Science 177:*65–68.

164. Mirvish, S. S., Cardesa, A., Wallcave, L., and Shubik, P. 1975. Induction of mouse lung adenomas by amines or ureas plus nitrite and by N-nitroso compounds: Effect of ascorbate, gallic acid, thiocyanate and caffeine. *J. Natl. Cancer Inst. 55:*633–636.

165. Mirvish, S. S. 1981. Inhibition of the formation of carcinogenic N-nitroso compounds by ascorbic acid and other compounds. in J. H. Burchenal and H. F. Oettgen (Eds.) *Cancer achievements, challenges and prospects for the 1980's.* Vol. 1. pp. 557–587. New York: Grune & Stratton.

166. Ivankovic, S., Preussmann, R., Schmahl, D., and Zeller, J. W. 1975. Prevention by ascorbic acid of *in vivo* formation of N-nitroso compounds. in P. Bogovski and E. A. Walker (Eds.) *N-nitroso compounds in the environment. IARC Scientific Publications #9.* Lyons, France: International Agency for Research on Cancer.

167. Raineri, R., and Weisburger, J. H. 1975. Reductions of gastric carcinogens with ascorbic acid. *Ann. N.Y. Acad. Sci. 258:*181–189.

168. Archer, M. C., Tannenbaum, S. R., Tan, T., and Weisman, M. 1975. Reaction of gastric carcinogens with ascorbic acid and its relaton to nitrosamine formation. *J. Natl. Cancer Inst. 54:*1203–1205.

169. Chan, W. C., and Fong, Y. Y. 1970. Ascorbic acid prevents liver tumor production by aminopyrine and nitrite in the rat. *Int. J. Cancer 20:*268–270.

170. Bodansky, O., Wroblewski, F., and Markardt, B. 1952. Concentrations of ascorbic acid in plasma and white cells of patients with cancer and non-cancerous chronic disease. *Cancer 5:*678–684.

171. Basu, T. K., Raven, R. W., Dickerson, J. W. T., and Williams, D. C. 1974. Leucocyte ascorbic acid and urinary hydroxyproline levels in the patients bearing breast tumor with skeletal metastases. *Eur. J. Cancer 10:*507–511.

172. Krasner, N., and Dymock, I. W. 1974. Ascorbic acid deficiency in malignant diseases: A clinical and biochemical study. *Br. J. Cancer 30:*142–145.

173. Gross, J. 1959. Formatin of collagen: IV. Effect of vitamin C deficiency on the natural salt-extractable collagen of skin. *J. Exp. Med. 109:*557–569.

174. Cameron, E., and Pauling, L. 1973. Ascorbic acid and the glycosaminoglycans: An ortho-molecular approach to cancer and other diseases. *Oncology 27:*181–192.

175. DeClerck, Y. A., and Jones, P. A. 1980. Effect of ascorbic acid on the resistance of the extracellular matrix to hydrolysis by tumor cells. *Cancer Res. 40:*3228–3231.

176. Cameron, E., and Campbell, B. 1974. The orthomolecular treatment of cancer. II. Clinical trial of high-dose ascorbic acid supplements in advanced human cancer. *Chem. Biol. Interact. 9:*285–315.

177. Cameron, E., and Pauling, L. 1978. Supplemental ascorbate in the supportive treatment of

cancer: Re-evaluation of prolongation of survival times in terminal cancer patients. *Proc. Natl. Acad. Sci. (USA) 75:*4538–4542.

178. Creagen, E. T., Moertel, C. G., O'Fallon, J. R., Schutt, A. J., O'Connell, M. J., Rubin, J., and Frytak, S. 1979. Failure of high-dose vitamin C (ascorbic acid) therapy to benefit patients with advanced cancer. *N. Engl. J. Med. 301:*687–690.

179. DeCosse, J. J., Adams, M. B., Kuzma, J. F., LoGerfo, P., and Condon, R. E. 1975. Effect of ascorbic acid on rectal polyps of patients with familial polyposis. *Surgery 78:*608–612.

180. Bussey, H. J. R., DeCasse, J. J., Deschner, E. E., Eyers, A. A., Lesser, M. L., Morson, B. C., Ritchie, S. M., Thomson, J. P. S., and Wadsworth, J. 1982. A randomized trial of ascorbic acid in polyposis coli. *Cancer 50:*1434–1439.

181. Meinsma, L. 1964. Nutrition and cancer. *Voeding 25:*357–365.

182. Higginson, J. 1966. Etiological factors in gastro-intestinal cancer in man. *J. Natl. Cancer Inst. 37:*527–545.

183. Haenszel, W., and Correa, P. 1975. Developments in the epidemiology of stomach cancer over the past decade. *Cancer Res. 35:*3452–3459.

184. Bjelke, E. 1978. Dietary factors and the epidemiology of cancer of the stomach and large bowel. *Akt. Ernaehrungsmed. Klin. Prax. Suppl. 2:*10–17.

185. Weisburger, J. H., Marquardt, H., Mower, H. F., Hirota, N., Mori, H., and Williams, G. 1980. Inhibition of carcinogenesis: Vitamin C and the prevention of gastric cancer. *Prev. Med. 9:*352–361.

186. Kolonel, L. N., Nomura, A. M. Y., Hirohata, T., Hankin, J. H., and Hinds, M. W. 1981. Association of diet and place of birth with stomach cancer incidence in Hawaii, Japanese and Caucasians. *Am. J. Clin. Nutr. 34:*2478–2485.

187. Dungal, N., and Sigurjonsson, J. 1967. A pilot study of dietary habits in two districts differing markedly in respect of mortality from gastric cancer. *Br. J. Cancer 21:*270–276.

188. Hirayama, T. 1979. Diet and cancer. *Nutr. Cancer 1:*67–81.

189. Bjelke, E. 1976. Dietary vitamin A and human lung cancer. *Int. J. Cancer 15:*561–565.

190. MacLennan, R., DaCosta, J., Day, N. E., Law, C. H., Ng, Y. K., and Shanmugaratnam, K. 1977. Risk factors for lung cancer in Singapore Chinese, a population with high female incidence rates. *Int. J. Cancer 20:*854–860.

191. Mettlin, C., Graham, S., and Swanson, M. 1979. Vitamin A and lung cancer. *J. Natl. Cancer Inst. 62:*1435–1438.

192. Graham, S., Dayal, H., Rohrer, T., Swanson, M., Sulty, H., Shedd, D., and Fischman, S. 1977. Dentition, diet, tobacco, and alcohol in the epidemiology of oral cancer. *J. Natl. Cancer Inst. 59:*1611–1618.

193. Graham, S., Schotz, W., and Martino, P. 1972. Alimentary factors in the epidemiology of gastric cancer. *Cancer 4:*927–938.

194. Mettlin, C., Graham, S., Priore, R., Marshall, J., and Swanson. 1981. Diet and cancer of the esophagus. *Nutr. Cancer 2:*143–147.

195. Graham, S., Mettlin, C., Marshall, J., Priore, R., Rzepka, T., and Shedd, D. 1982. Dietary factors in the epidemiology of cancer of the larynx. *Am. J. Epidemiol. 113:*675–680.

196. Graham, S., Marshall, J., Mettlin, C., Rzepka, T., Nemoto, T., and Byers, T. 1982. Diet in the epidemiology of breast cancer. *Am. J. Epidemiol. 116:*68–75.

197. Wassertheil-Smoller, S., Romney, S. L., Wylie-Rosett, J., Slagle, S., Miller, G., Lucido, D., Duttagupta, C., and Palan, P. R. 1981. Dietary vitamin C and uterine cervical dysplasia. *Am. J. Epidemiol. 114:*714–724.

198. Ziegler, R. G., Morris, L. E., Blot, W. J., Pattern, L. M., Hoover, R., and Fraumeni, J. F. 1981. Esophageal cancer among black men in Washington D.C. II. Role of Nutrition. *J. Natl. Cancer Inst. 67:*1199–1206.

199. Jain, M., Cook, G. M., Davis, F. G., Grace, M. G., and Howe, G. R., and Miller, A. B. 1980. A case-control study of diet and colo-rectal cancer. *Int. J. Cancer 26:*757–768.

200. Ramirez, I., Richie, E., Wang, Y., and Van Eys, J. 1980. Effect of ascorbic acid in vitro on lymphocyte reactivity to mitogens. *J. Nutr. 110:*2207–2215.

201. Poydock, M. E., Fardon, J. C., Gallina, D., Ferro, V., and Heher, C. 1979. Inhibiting effect of vitamin C and B_{12} on the mitotic activity of ascites tumors. *Exp. Cell Biol. 47:*210–217.

202. Dixit, A., and Rao, R. 1980. Influence of ascorbic acid on action of DMBA on DNA, RNA and protein levels in mouse liver following partial hepatectomy. *Indian J. Exp. Biol. 18:*1494–1496.

203. Bissell, M. J., Hatie, C., Farson, D. A., Schwarz, R. J., and Soo, W. 1980. Ascorbic acid inhibits replication and infectivity of avian RNA tumor virus. *Proc. Natl. Acad. Sci. (USA) 77:*2711–2715.

204. Schwerdt, P. R., and Sthwerdt, C. E. 1978. Effect of ascorbic acid on rhinovirus replication in W1-38 cells. *Proc. Soc. Exp. Biol. Med. 148:*1237–1243.

205. Bullough, W. S., and Ryotomaa, T. 1965. Mitotic homeostatis. *Nature 205:*573–578.

206. Edgar, J. A. 1970. Dehydroascorbic acid and cell division. *Nature 227:*24–26.

207. Price, C. E. 1966. Ascorbate stimulation of RNA synthesis. *Nature 212:*1481.

208. Freidel, J. F., Fardon, J. C., Tsuchiya, Y., and Nutini, L. G. 1979. In vitro effect of D-isoascorbic acid and betaine hydrate alone and in combination on normal and malignant cells. *Exp. Cell Biol. 47:*463–469.

209. Park, C. H., Amare, M., Savin, M. A., and Hoogstraten, B. 1980. Growth suppression of human leukemic cells in vitro by L-ascorbic acid. *Cancer Res. 40:*1062–1065.

210. Bishun, T. K., Basu, T. K., Metcalfe, S., and Williams, D. C. 1978. The effect of ascorbic acid (vitamin C) on two tumor cell lines in culture. *Oncology 35:*160–162.

211. Bram, S. Froussard, P., Guichard, M., Jasmin, C., Augery, Y., SinoussiBarre, F., and Wray, W. 1980. Vitamin C preferential toxicity for malignant melanoma cells. *Nature 284:*629–631.

212. Reynolds, C. P., Reynolds, D. A., Frenkel, E. P., and Smith, R. G. 1982. Selective toxicity of 6-hydroxydopamine and ascorbate for human neuroblastoma in vitro: A model for clearing marrow prior to autologous transplant. *Cancer Res. 42:*1331–1336.

213. Benade, L., Howard, T., and Burk, D. 1969. Synergistic killing of Ehrlich ascites carcinoma cells by ascorbate and 3-amino-1,2,4-triazole. *Oncology 23:*33–43.

214. Kallistratos, G., and Fasske, E. 1979. Inhibition of benzopyrene carcinogenesis in rats with vitamin C. *Folia Biochem. Biol. Graeca 16:*15–30.

215. Yamafuji, J., Nakamura, Y., Omura, H., Soeda, T., and Gyotoku, K. 1971. Anti-tumor potency of ascorbic, dehydroascorbic, or 2,3-diketogulonic acid and their action on deoxyribonucleic acid. *A. Krebsforsch. Klin. Oncol. 21:*270–276.

216. Migliozzi, J. A. 1977. Effect of ascorbic acid on tumor growth. *Br. J. Cancer 35:*448–453.

217. Brunschwig, A. 1943. Vitamin C and tumor growth. *Cancer Res. 3:*550–553.

218. Fodor, E., and Kunos. S. 1934. Die Wirkung der reinen ascorbinsure auf das Wachstum des experimentellen Mausecarcinomas. *Krebsforsch 40:*567–571.

219. Watson, A. F. 1943. The chemical reducing capacity and vitamin C content of transplantable tumors of the rat and guinea pig. *Br. J. Exp. Pathol. 17:*124–134.

220. Kumar, M., and Axelrod, A. E. 1969. Circulating antibody formation in scorbutic guinea pigs. *J. Nutr. 98:*41–44.

221. Kies, M. W., Mueller, S., and Alvord, E. C. 1964. Influence of ascorbic acid deficiency on immunologic mechanisms. *Z. Immun. Allergie Forsch 126:*228–233.

222. Kalden, J. R., and Guthy, E. A. 1972. Prolonged skin allograft survival in vitamin C-deficient guinea-pigs. *Eur. Surg. Res. 4:*114–119.

223. Waddell, W. R., and Gerner, R. E. 1980. Indomethacin and ascorbate inhibit desmoid tumors. *J. Surg. Oncol. 15:*85–90.

224. Chlapowski, F. J., Kelly, L. A., and Butcher, R. W. 1975. Cyclic nucleotides in cultured cells. *Adv. Cyclic Nucleotide Res. 6:*245–338.

225. Tewfik, F. A., Riley, E. F., and Mital, C. R. 1977. The influence of ascorbic acid on the growth of solid tumors in mice and on tumor control by X-irradiation. *Radiat. Res. 70:*660.

226. Gruber, H. E., Tewfik, H. H., and Tewfik, F. A. 1980. Cytoarchitecture of Ehrlich ascites carcinoma implanted in the hind limb of ascorbic acid-supplemented mice. *Eur. J. Cancer 16:*441–448.

227. O'Conner, M., Malone, J., Moriarty, M., and Mulgrew, S. 1977. A radioprotective effect of vitamin C observed in Chinese hamster ovary cells. *Br. J. Radiol. 50:*587–591.

228. Elvin, P., and Slater, T. F. 1981. Anti-tumor activity of novel adducts of ascorbic acid with aldehydes. *Eur. J. Clin. Oncol. 17:*759–765.

229. Kimoto, E., Tanaka, H., Gyotoku, J., Morishige, F., and Pauling, L. 1983. Enhancement of antitumor activity of ascorbate against Ehrlich ascites tumor cells by the copper–glycyglycyl-histidine complex. *Cancer Res. 43:*824–828.

230. Yagishita, K., Takahashi, N., Yamamoto, H., Jinnouchi, H., Hiyoshi, S., and Miyakawa, T. 1976. Effects of tetraacetyl-bis-dehydroascorbic acid, a derivative of ascorbic acid, on Ehrlich cells and Hela cells (human carcinoma cells). *J. Nutr. Sci. Vitaminol. 22:*419–427.

231. Werner, B., Denzer, U., Mitschke, H., and Brassow, F. 1981. Vitamin C and Dunn-darmkrebs. Eine Experimentelle Studie. *Langenbecks Arch. Chir. 354:*101–109.

232. Reddy, B. S., Hirota, N., and Katayama, S. 1982. Effect of sodium ascorbate on 1,2-dimethylhydrazine-or methylnitrosourea-induced colon carcinogenesis in rats. *Carcinogenesis 3:*1097–1099.

233. Jacobs, M. M., and Griffin, A. C. 1979. Effects of selenium on chemical carcinogenesis: Comparative effects of antioxidants. *Biol. Trace Elem. Res. 1:*1–13.

234. Jones, F. E., Komorowski, R. A., and Condon, R. E. 1981. Chemoprevention of 1,2-dimethylhydrazine-induced large bowel neoplasms. *Surg. Forum 32:*435–437.

235. Benedict, W. F., Wheatley, W. L., and Jones, P. A. 1980. Inhibition of chemically induced morphological transformation and reversion of the transformed phenotype by ascorbic acid in C3H/10T ½ cells. *Cancer Res. 40:*2796–2801.

236. Gol-Winkler, R., DeClerck, Y., and Gielen, J. E. 1980. Ascorbic acid effect on methylcholanthrene-induced transformation in C3H10T ½ clone 8 cells. *Toxicology 17:*237–239.

237. Rosin, M. P., Peterson, A. R., and Stich, H. F. 1980. The effect on ascorbate on 3-methylcholanthrene-induced cell transformation in C3H 10T ½ mouse-embryo fibroblast cell cultures. *Mutat. Res. 72:*533–537.

238. Sivak, A., and Tu, A. S. 1980. Cell culture tumor promotion experiments with saccharin, phorbol, myristate acetate and several common food materials. *Cancer Lett. 10:*27–32

239. Bainc, S. 1981. Vitamin C acts as a cocarcinogen to methylcholanthrene in guinea-pigs. *Cancer Lett. 11:*239–242.

240. Frith, C. H., Rule, J., and Kodell, R. L. 1980. The effects of ascorbic acid on the induction of urothelial lesions in mice by 2-acetylaminofluorene. *Toxicology 6:*309–318.

241. Bruce, W. R., Varghese, A. J., Furrer, R., and Land, P. C. 1977. A mutagen in human feces. in H. H. Hiatt, J. D. Watson, and J. A. Winsten (Ed.) *Origins of human cancer.* pp. 1641–1644. Cold Spring Harbor, New York: Cold Spring Harbor Laboratory.

242. Dion, P. W., Bright-See, E. B., Smith, C. C., and Bruce, W. R. 1982. The effect of dietary ascorbic acid or α-tocopherol on fecal mutagencity. *Mutat. Res. 102:*27–37.

243. Leuchtenberger, C., and Leuchtenberger, R. 1977. Protection of hamster lung cultures by L-cysteine or vitamin C against carcinogenic effects of fresh smoke from tobacco or marijuana cigarettes. *Br. J. Exp. Pathol. 58:*625–633.

244. Leuchtenberger, C., Leuchtenberger, R., and Chapius, L. 1978. Difference in response to

vitamin C between marijuana and tobacco smoke exposed human cell cultures. *Adv. Biosci.* *22/23:*209–218.

245. Seiler, J. P. 1977. Inhibition of testicular DNA synthesis by chemical mutagens and carcinogens. Preliminary results in the validation of a novel short term test. *Mutat. Res. 46:*305–310.

246. Parshad, R., Sanford, K. K., Jones, G. M., and Tarone, R. E. 1978. Fluorescent light-induced chromosome damage and its prevention in mouse cells in culture. *Proc. Natl. Acad. Sci. (USA)* *75:*1830–1833.

247. Shapiro, B., and Kollmann, G. 1969. Mechanism of protection of macromolecules against ionizing radiation by sulfhydryl and other protective agents. *Radiat. Damage Sulphydryl Comp. Proc. Panel* 23–43.

248. Clark, J. B. 1953. The effects of chemicals on the recombination rate in *Bacterium coli. J. Gen. Microbiol. 8:*45–49.

249. Petrilli, F. L., and DeFlora, S. 1978. Metabolic deactivation of hexavalent chromium. *Mutat. Res. 54:*139–147.

250. Khudoley, V., Malaveille, C., and Bartsch, H. 1981. Mutagenicity studies in Salmonella typhimurium on some carcinogenic N-nitramines in vitro and in the host-mediated assay in rats. *Cancer Res. 41:*3205–3210.

251. Wirth, P. J., Dybing, E., vonBahr, C., and Thorgeirsson, S. 1980. Mechanism of N-hydroxyacetylarylamine mutagenicity in the Salmonella test system: Metabolic activation of N-hydroxyphenacetin by liver and kidney fractions from rat, mouse, hamster and man. *Mol. Pharmacol. 18:*117–127.

252. Conger, B. V. 1975. Radioprotective effects of ascorbic acid in barley seeds. *Radiat. Biol. 15:*39–48.

253. Selimbekova, D. D. 1969. Radioprotective properties of ascorbic acid. *Dokl. Akad. Nauk. Azerb. SSR 25:*78–80.

254. Lin, J. Y., Wang, H. I., and Yeh, Y. C. 1979. The mutagenicity of soy bean sauce. *Food Cosmet. Toxicol. 17:*329–332.

255. Munkres, K. D. 1979. Ageing of Neurospora crassa. VIII. Lethality and mutagenicity of ferrous ions, ascorbic acid, and malondialdehyde. *Mech. Ageing Dev. 10:*249–260.

256. Shamberger, R. J., Corlett, C. L., Beaman, K. D., and Kasten, B. L. 1979. Antioxidants reduce the mutagenic effect of malonaldehyde and β-propiolactone. *Mutat. Res. 66:*349–355.

257. Guttenplan, J. B. 1978. Mechanisms of inhibition by ascorbate of microbial mutagenesis induced by N-nitroso compounds. *Cancer Res. 38:*2018–2022.

258. Kokatnur, M. G., Murray, M. L., and Correa, P. 1978. Mutagenic properties of nitrosated spermidine. *Proc. Soc. Exp. Biol. Med. 158:*85–88.

259. DeFlora, S., and Picciott, A. 1980. Mutagenicity of cimetidine in nitrite-enriched human gastric juice. *Carcinogenesis 1:*925–929.

260. Neale, S., and Solt, A. K. 1981. The effect of ascorbic acid on the amine-nitrite and nitrosamine mutagenicity in bacteria injected into mice. *Chem. Biol. Interact. 35:*199–205.

261. Lee, K. Y., Choi, H. W., and Park, S. C. 1979. Bacterial mutation test for the detection of potential carcinogenicity of nitrite-treated Korean raw fishes. *Korean J. Biochem. 11:*31–40.

262. Rao, B. G., MacDonald, I. A., and Hutchison, D. M. 1981. Nitrite-induced volatile mutagens from normal human feces. *Cancer 47:*889–894.

263. Rosin, M. P., San, R. H. C., and Stich, H. F. 1980. Mutagenic activity of ascorbate in mammalian cell cultures. *Cancer Lett. 8:*299–305.

264. Stich, H. F., Wei, L., and Whiting, R. F. 1979. The enhancing effect of transition metals on the chromosome-damaging action of ascorbate. *Cancer Res. 39:*4145–4151.

265. Omura, H., Shinohara, K., Maeda, H., Nonaka, M., and Murakami, H. 1978. Mutagenic

action of triose reductone and ascorbic acid on *Salmonella* typhimurium TA 100 strain. *J. Nutr. Sci. Vitaminol. 24:*185–194.

266. Stich, H. F., Wei, L., and Lam, P. 1978. The need for a mammalian test system for mutagens: Action of some reducing agents. *Cancer Lett. 5:*199–204.

267. Stich, H. F., Karim, J., Koropatnick, J., and Lo, L. 1976. Mutagenic action of ascorbic acid. *Nature 260:*722–724.

268. Macrae, W. D., and Stich, H. F. 1979. Induction of sister chromatid exchanges in Chinese hamster cells by the reducing agents bisulfite and ascorbic acid. *Toxicology 13:*167–174.

269. Hayatsu, H., and Miura, A. 1970. The mutagenic action of sodium bisulfite. *Biochem. Biophys. Res. Commun. 39:*156–160.

270. Morgan, A. R., Cone, R. L., and Elgert, T. M. 1976. The mechanism of DNA strand breakage by vitamin C and superoxide and the protective roles of catalase and superoxide dismutase. *Nucl. Acid Res. 3:*1139–1149.

271. Galloway, S. M., and Painter, R. B. 1979. Vitamin C is positive in the DNA synthesis inhibition and sister-chromatid exchange tests. *Mutat. Res. 60:*321–327.

272. Speit, G., Wolf, M., and Vogel, W. 1980. The SCE-inducing capacity of vitamin C: Investigations in vitro and in vivo. *Mutat. Res. 78:*273–278.

273. Stich, H. F., Wei, L., and Whiting, R. F. 1980. Chromosome aberrations in mammalian cells exposed to vitamin C and multiple vitamin pills. *Food Cosmet. Toxicol. 18:*497–501.

274. Peterkofsky, B., and Prather, W. 1977. Cytotoxicity of ascorbate and other reducing agents toward cultured fibroblasts as a result of hydrogen peroxide formation. *J. Cell Physiol. 90:*61–70.

275. Andoh, T., and Ide, T. 1972. Disulfide bridges in proteins linking DNA in cultured mouse fibroblasts, strain L·93. *Exp. Cell Res. 74:*525–531.

276. Ames, B., Durston, W., Yamaski, E., and Lee, P. 1973. Carcinogens are mutagens: A simple test system combining liver homogenates for activation and bacteria for detection. *Proc. Natl. Acad. Sci. (USA) 70:*2281–2285.

277. Andrews, L. S., Fysh, J. M., Hinson, J. A., and Gillette, J. R. 1979. Ascorbic acid inhibits covalent binding of enzymatically generated 2-acetyl-aminofluororene-N-sulfate to DNA under conditions in which it increases mutagenesis in Salmonella TA-1538. *Life Sci. 24:*59–64.

278. Sakai, S., Reinhold, C. E., Wirth, P. J., Thorgeirsson, P. J., and Snorri, S. 1978. Mechanism of in vitro mutagenic activation and covalent binding of N-hydroxy-2-acetylaminofluorene in isolated liver cell nuclei from rat and mouse. *Cancer Res. 38:*2058–2067.

279. Schut, H. A. J., and Thorgeirsson, S. S. 1979. Mutagenic activation of N-hydroxy-2-acetylaminofluorene by developing epithelial cells of rat small intestine and effects of antioxidants. *J. Natl. Cancer Inst. 63:*1405–1409.

280. Thorgeirsson, S. S., Sakai, S., and Wirth, P. J. 1980. Effect of ascorbic acid on in vitro mutagen covalent binding of N-hydroxyl-2-acetylaminofluorene in the rat. *Mutat. Res. 70:*395–398.

281. Omura, H., Tomita, Y., Fujiki, H., Shinohara, K., and Murakami, H. 1978. Breaking action of reductones related to ascorbic acid on nucleic acids. *J. Nutr. Sci. Vitaminol. 24:*263–270.

282. Glatt, H. R., Oesch, F., and Neumann, H. G. 1980. Factors responsible for the metabolic formation and inactivation of bacterial mutagens from trans-4-acetaminostilbene. *Mutat. Res. 73:*237–250.

283. Omura, H., Iiyama, S., Tomita, Y., Narazaaki, Y., Shinohara, K., and Murakami, H. 1975. Breaking action of ascorbic acid on nucleic acids. *J. Nutr. Sci. Vitaminol. 21:*237–249.

284. Fomenko, L. A., Leonteva, G. A., Gaziev, A. I., and Kuzin, A. M. 1974. Radiosensitization of DNA in the radiosensitization on DNA in the presence of reducing agents and a catalyst of radical reactions. *Radiobiology 14:*137–139.

285. Kuhnlein, U., Tsang, S. S., and Edwards, J. 1979. Characterization of DNA-damages by

filtration through nitrocellulose filters: A simple probe for DNA-modifying agents. *Mutat. Res.* *64:*167–182.

286. Smith, H. W. 1953. The effect of physical and chemical changes on the liberation of phage particles by lysogenic strains of *Salmonella. J. Gen. Microbiol. 8:*116–134.

287. Murata, A., Kitagawa, K., and Saruno, R. 1971. Inactivation of bacteriophages by ascorbic acid. *Agr. Biol. Chem. 35:*294–296.

288. Murata, A., and Kitagawa, K. 1973. Mechanism of inactivation of bacteriophage J1 by ascorbic acid. *Agr. Biol. Chem. 37:*1145–1151.

289. Murata, A., Kitagawa, K., Inmaru, H., and Saruno, R. 1972. Inactivation of single-stranded DNA and RNA phages by ascorbic acids and thiol reducing agents. *Agr. Biol. Chem. 36:*2597–2599.

290. Murata, A., Oyadomari, R., Dhashi, T., and Kitagawa, K. 1975. Mechanism of inactivation of bacteriophage δA containing single-stranded DNA by ascorbic acid. *J. Nutr. Sci. Vitaminol. 21:*261–269.

291. Wong, K., Morgan, A. R., and Paranchych, W. 1974. Controlled cleavage of phage R17 RNA within the virion by treatment with ascorbate and copper (11). *Can. J. Biochem. 52:*950–958.

292. Bode, V. C. 1967. Single-strand scissions in circular and linear γ DNA by the presence of dithiothreitol and other reducing agents. *J. Mol. Biol. 26:*125–129.

293. McCarty, M. 1945. Reversible inactivation of the substance inducing transformation of pneumococcal types. *J. Exp. Med. 81:*507–514.

294. Kenyon, A., and Andress, L. 1980. Does vitamin C induce X-linked recessive lethal mutations in *Drosophilia melanogaster? Genetics 94:*552–553.

295. Kalus, W. H., Filby, W. G., and Munzner, R. 1982. Chemical aspects of the mutagenic activity of the ascorbic acid autoxidation system. *Z. Naturforsch. 37:*40–45.

296. Murphy, L. C., Wild, J., Posen, S., and Stone, G. 1979. 25-Hydroxycholecalciferol receptors in human breast cancer. *Br. J. Cancer 39:*531–535.

297. Eisman, J. A., MacIntyre, I., Martin, T. J., and Moseley, J. M. 1979. 1,25-Dihydroxy vitamin D receptor in breast cancer cells. *Lancet 2:*1335–1336.

298. Colston, K. W., Colston, M. J., and Feldman, D. 1981. 1,25-Dihydroxy vitamin D₃ and malignant melanoma: The presence of receptors and inhibition of cell growth in culture. *Endocrinology 108:*1083–1086.

299. Colston, K., Colston, M. J., Fieldsteel, A. H., and Feldman, D. 1982. 1,25-Dihydroxy vitamin D₃ receptors in human epithelial cancer cell lines. *Cancer Res. 42:*856–859.

300. Shamberger, R. J. 1970. Relationships of selenium to Cancer. I. Inhibitory effect of selenium on carcinogenesis. *J. Natl. Cancer Inst. 44:*931–936.

301. Jaffe, W. 1949. The influence of wheatgerm oil on the production of tumors in rats by methylcholanthrene. *Exp. Med. Surg. 4:*278–282.

302. Haddow, A., and Russell, H. 1937. The influence of wheat germ oil in the diet on the induction of tumors in mice. *Am. J. Cancer 29:*363–366.

303. Epstein, S. S., Joshi, S., Andrea, J., Forsyth, J., and Mantal, N. 1967. The null effect of antioxidants on the carcinogenicity of 3,4,9,10-dibenzpyrene to mice. *Life Sci. 6:*225–233.

304. Haber, S. L., and Wissler, R. W. 1962. Effect of vitamin E on carcinogenicity on methylcholanthrene. *Proc. Soc. Exp. Biol. Med. III:*774–775.

305. Harman, D. 1969. Dibenzanthracene induced cancer. Inhibiting effect of vitamin E. *Clin Res. 17:*125.

306. Ip, C. 1982. Dietary vitamin E intake and mammary carcinogenesis in rats. *Carcinogenesis 3:*1453–1456.

307. Narayan, K. A. 1970. Vitamin E deficiency and chemical carcinogenesis. *Experientia 26:*840–841.

308. Konings, A. W. T., and Trieling, W. B. 1977. The inhibition of DNA synthesis in vitamin E-depleted lymphosarcoma cells by x-rays and cytostatics. *Int. J. Radiat Biol. 31:*397–400.

309. Shklar, G. 1982. Oral mucosal carcinogenesis in hamsters: Inhibition by vitamin E. *J. Natl. Cancer Inst. 68:*791–797.

310. Pauling, L., Willoughby, R., Reymonds, R., Blaisdell, B. E., and Lawson, S. 1982. Incidence of squamous cell carcinoma in hairless mice irradiated with ultraviolet light in relation to intake of ascorbic acid and of D, L. α-tocopheryl acetate. *Int. J. Vitam. Nutr. Res. Suppl. 79:*53–82.

311. Weisburger, J. H., Reddy, D. V. M., Hill, P., Cohen, L. A., Wynder, E. L., and Spingarn, N. E. 1980. Nutrition and cancer-on the mechanisms bearing on causes of cancer of the colon, breast, prostate and stomach. *Bull N.Y. Acad. Med. 56:*673–696.

312. Shamberger, R. J., Baughman, F. F., Kalchert, S. S., and Willis, C. E. 1973. Carcinogen-induced chromosomal breakage decreased by antioxidants. *Proc. Natl. Acad. Sci. (USA) 70:*1461–1467.

313. Smalls, E., and Patterson, R. M. 1982. Reduction of benzopyrene induced chromosomal aberrations by DL-alpha-tocopherol. *Eur. J. Cell Biol. 28:*92–97.

314. Dion, P. W., Bright-See, E. B., Smith, C. C., and Bruce, W. R. 1982. The effect of dietary ascorbic acid and α-tocopherol on fecal mutagenicity. *Mutat. Res. 102:*27–37.

315. Abrams, A. A. 1965. Use of vitamin E. in chronic mastitis. *N. Engl. J. Med. 272:*1081–1082.

316. London, R. S., Solomon, D. M., London, E. D., Strummer, D., Bankowski, J., and Mair, P. P. 1978. Mammary Dysplasia; clinical response and urinary excretion of 11-deoxyketosteroids and pregnanediol following α-tocopherol therapy. *Breast 4:*19–22.

317. Hilgard, P., and Thornes, R. D. 1976. Anticoagulants in the treatment of cancer. *Eur. J. Cancer 12:*755–762.

318. Hilgard, P., Schultz, H., Wetzig, G., Schmitt, and Schmidt, C. G. 1977. Oral anticoagulation in the treatment of a spontaneously metastasizing murine tumor (3LL). *Br. J. Cancer 35:*448–453.

319. Hilgard, P. 1977. Experimental vitamin K deficiency and spontaneous metastases. *Br. J. Cancer 35:*448–453.

320. Israels, L. G., Ollman, D. J., Friesen, E., and Israels, E. D. 1982. Vitamin K as a regulator of benzopyrene metabolism, mutagenesis and carcinogenesis. *Clin. Invest. Med. 5:*46B.

Chapter 5

Minerals and Cancer

Only a few epidemiological studies have been conducted to determine the relationship between minerals and the incidence of cancer in humans. This is mainly due to the difficulty of identifying populations with significantly different intakes of the various minerals. In contrast, there have been numerous studies on the carcinogenic effects of many metals, administered at high doses to the animals parenterally. However, the results of these animal studies have shed little light on the potential carcinogenic risk from these elements in the amounts occurring naturally in the diet of humans.

Very few feeding studies have been conducted to test the carcinogenicity of trace elements in animals. This type of animal test is difficult because some of the levels of these elements are toxic levels that far exceed dietary requirements. In addition, synergistic interactions of the element under investigation with other elements are difficult to control.

Schroeder and associates have investigated the carcinogenicity of several trace elements in a series of large-scale experiments extending over 15 years.[1-4] In their experiments, animals were raised in an environment that permitted maximum control of trace element contamination. One diet of known composition was fed to the animals, which were observed throughout their lifetime. The following elements were studied in at least 50 mice and/or rats per treatment: antimony, arsenic, cadmium, chromium, fluorine, gallium, germanium, indium, lead, nickel, niobium, palladium, rhodium, selenium, tellurium, tin, titanium, vanadium, yttrium, and zirconium. These elements were added to the drinking water at levels of 5 mg/liter, except for selenium (3 mg/liter) and tellurium (2 mg/liter). These levels (about 100 times greater than the amounts present normally in the diet) did not significantly affect either growth or survival of the animals. In general, there were no effects or minimally significant effects, only rhodium and palladium (tested in mice only showed any signs of carcinogenicity).

SELENIUM AND CANCER

Observations of chronic selenium toxicity in animals have been made for almost 700 years, but selenium was not identified as the responsible agent until

the 1930s. However, about two decades later, the economic importance of se-
lenosis and selenium deficiency for animal producers became apparent. These
observations have stimulated the mapping of selenium distribution in the soils,
forages, and tissues of people on several continents. Some situations of extreme
differences of exposures were noted, even within individual countries. This
knowledge enabled investigators to make epidemiological correlations of diseases, including cancer and heart disease in humans and animals, and to conduct
laboratory experiments to test the resulting hypotheses. One of the more exciting
effects of selenium on health is the anticarcinogenic effect of selenium against
experimentally induced cancer in several animal systems.

Skin Cancer

Effect on DMBA-Croton Oil Carcinogenesis

In an effort to modify experimental carcinogenesis during its development
and to determine whether free radical damage due to peroxidation might be
involved during carcinogenesis, sodium selenide as well as other antioxidants
were applied concomitantly along with croton oil to female Swiss albino mice
initiated with 7,12-dimethylbenzanthracene (DMBA). In the initial experiment,
sodium selenide greatly reduced the number of the mice with skin tumors ($p <$
0.05).[5] In addition, the total number of tumors was reduced not only by sodium
selenide, but by vitamin E as well. Riley has also observed a reduction in
DMBA-croton oil carcinogenesis by sodium selenide.[6]

In five of six nondietary tumor-promotion experiments, sodium selenide
significantly reduced the number of mice with tumors. In two of these six
experiments, vitamin E also significantly reduced the number of mice with
tumors.[7] Both sodium selenide and vitamin E significantly reduced the number
of mice with tumors induced by DMBA-phenol. In addition, the total number of
tumors was reduced. In this experiment vitamin E was somewhat more effective
than sodium selenide.

The complete carcinogen 3-methylcholanthrene (MCA) was also applied
concomitantly with sodium selenide. After 19 weeks of daily application of
0.01% MCA in acetone, 87% of the control mice had tumors, but in the sodium
selenide group, 68% of the mice had papillomas ($p < 0.10$). The total numbers
of papillomas and cancers were greatly reduced when compared with those in the
controls.

The effect of selenium-deficient and selenium-adequate diets on DMBA-
croton and benzpyrene carcinogenesis was also studied.[7] Dietary sodium selenite
markedly reduced papillomas induced by the tumor promoter DMBA-croton oil.
In the experiment 14 of 35 mice fed 1.0 parts per millions (ppm) sodium selenite

had papillomas at 20 weeks. Of the mice fed selenium-deficient diets, 26 of 36 had papillomas ($p < 0.01$). At 27 weeks there was also a reduction in the number of animals with cancers in the group supplemented with 1.0 ppm sodium selenite.

Effect of Benzpyrene Carcinogenesis

A similar tumor pattern was observed with benzpyrene. At 22 weeks, 31 of 36 mice fed selenium-deficient diets had papillomas, while 16 of 36 mice fed diets containing 1.0 ppm sodium selenite had papillomas ($p < 0.001$)[7] At 27 weeks the numbers of cancers and the size of the cancers were decreased in the mice fed 1.0 ppm sodium selenite.

Malonaldehyde

There is a possibility that malonaldehyde may be increased through the peroxidation of unsaturated fat when selenium and vitamin E levels are low. Skin treated with DMBA and croton oil (more unsaturated fat) exhibited greater peroxidation (malodinaldehyde increase) and more tumors than did skin treated with DMBA and croton resin. In addition, peroxidation in two experiments increased after DMBA initiation, but returned to normal at about day 45. Antioxidants applied on days 2–21 in another experiment, at the same time as the peroxidation increase, decreased the tumor incidence.[8]

Because of the structural similarity of malonaldehyde to the known carcinogens, β-propiolactone and glycidaldehyde and the increase of malonaldehyde levels or peroxidation, malonaldehyde was tested as an initiator and a tumor promotor.[9] One application of malonaldehyde, β-propiolactone, glycidaldehyde or DMBA (initiation) was given to each group of mice. Each was treated with croton oil for 30 weeks. After this period the groups initiated with malonaldehyde, β-propiolactone, glycidaldehyde, or DMBA had an incidence of 52, 44, 40, and 95% tumors, respectively. Applications of DMBA, benzpyrene, and MCA to mouse skin increased malonaldehyde levels.

Liver Cancer

Effect on Methyl-Dimethylaminoazobenzene

In 1949 Clayton and Baumann reported that the inclusion of 5 ppm selenium in a purified diet reduced the incidence of liver tumors in rats induced by 3-methyl-4-dimethylaminoazobenzene (DAB).[10] Selenium as sodium selenite was fed during a 4-week period of interruption between two 4-week periods during which DAB was fed. Two separate experiments showed a reduction of about 50% in the incidence of liver tumors when selenium was fed during the intermediate period. The animals on the selenium diet gained weight at a slower rate than did control animals. The slower gains were due in part to a decrease in food intake. Five ppm of selenium in the diet is considered by selenium researchers to be toxic, with 3 ppm being borderline toxic. In general, cancer researchers avoid toxic levels of a test substance or a carcinogen, because the effect against carcinogenicity may be due to toxicity.

The effects of selenium on DAB-induced hepatocarcinogenesis was determined.[11] Three groups of male Sprague-Dawley rats were fed DAB: one group served as control, one group received 6 ppm Se (Na_2SeO_3) in the drinking water, and one group received 6 ppm of selenium added to the diet in the form of high-selenium yeast. The azo compound was incorporated into the diet for 8 weeks and then removed, and the two types of selenium supplements were continued for an additional 4 weeks. At this time there was a 92% tumor incidence (11 of 12 animals) in the controls. Selenium in the drinking water reduced the incidence to 47% (7 of 15) and the dietary supplementation reduced tumor incidence to 64% (9 of 14).

In another study seven groups of Sprague-Dawley male rats were fed diets containing selenium for 9 weeks.[12] Group 1 served as control. Group 2 received 4 ppm Se as sodium selenite in the drinking water for 9 weeks. Group 3 had only 4 ppm Se in the drinking water for the initial 3 weeks. Group 4 had only 4 ppm Se in the drinking water for the final 4 weeks. Group 5 had 2 ppm Se in the drinking water for 9 weeks. Group 6 received 1% sorbic acid. Group 7 received 0.5% butylated hydroxytoluene for the entire period. The tumor incidence by group was as follows: group 1, 12 of 15; group 2, 2 of 14; group 3, 7 of 13; group 4, 5 of 13; group 5, 6 of 15; group 6, 15 of 15; and group 7, 0 of 15. The experiment confirmed the findings of the inhibition by selenium of azo dye carcinogenesis.[11] It was also of interest that in group 4 there was a reduction of hepatocarcinogenesis when the selenium was given during the later stages of the study.

Effect on Diethylnitrosamine Carcinogenesis

In 1979 Balanski and Hadsiolov fed diethylnitrosamine (DEN) to rats and in one experimental group also fed 1 ppm sodium selenite.[13] In a second experiment these workers also fed 5 ppm or 10 ppm sodium selenite to rats along with the DEN. In rats fed 1 ppm sodium selenite along with the DEN 15 of 20 rats had liver tumors and 2.26 tumors per tumor-bearing rat. In the control group, 17 of 20 of rats had tumors, with an average of 2.9 tumors per tumor-bearing rat. Even though the number of animals with tumors was not significantly different, there were 50 tumors in the control and only 34 tumors in the group fed 1 ppm sodium selenite. There was also a reduction in the number of tumors per tumor-bearing animal in a second experiment, in which the animals were fed 5 ppm or 10 ppm sodium selenite. The control group had 68 tumors, the group fed 5 ppm had 40 tumors, and the group fed 10 ppm had a total of 15 tumors. The tumor-reducing effect in this second experiment may have been due to toxicity. Dzhioev has also tested selenium on diethylnitrosamine carcinogenesis in rats.[14] Selenium treatment reduced the percentage of rats with tumors from 100% to 27%. In another experiment, selenium reduced the percentage of mice with DEN-induced lung tumors from 76% to 54%.

Effect on Acetylaminofluorene Carcinogenesis

Harr *et al.* divided 80 female OSU rats into four groups, with 20 rats per group.[15] The rats, which were supplemented with vitamin E, were selenium deficient and were fed the carcinogen 2-acetylaminofluorene (AAF) along with varying amounts of selenite. A dramatic decrease was observed in the rates of induced hepatic and mammary cancers after increased additions of selenium. The rats fed 0, 0.1, 0.5, and 2.5 ppm selenium had a combined incidence of 60%, 60%, 10%, and 0% of hepatic or mammary cancer. In a preliminary experiment, Harr *et al.* reported that 4 ppm Se (Na_2SeO_3) in water for 14 weeks reduced the number of tumors in rats given dietary AAF.[15] A final incidence of tumors of 9 of 13 rats was observed in the group given the basal diet alone, while 4 of 14 rats developed hepatomas when given the selenium supplement. No tumor or liver changes were observed in the control animals.

Marshall *et al.* studied the effects of the addition of 4 ppm Se as sodium selenite to the drinking water of male albino rats fed diets containing AAF for 14 weeks.[17] There was about a 50% reduction in tumor incidence, with 9 of 13 occurring in the control rats and 4 of 14 in the selenium-supplemented group. Selenium in the drinking water also provided protection against hepatic damage. Oral selenium administration led to a decrease in N-hydroxylation and an increase in ring hydroxylation. When selenium was added to a microsomal assay system, 3-OH-AAF formation increased and N-OH-AAF formation decreased. These changes shifted the balance of metabolism toward the detoxification pathways and away from the carcinogenic pathways.

In vivo, MC has been demonstrated to reduce the carcinogencity of AFF in rats.[18] In the experiment of Marshall *et al.* MC-induced microsomes were used.[17] The *in vitro* reduction in the formation of N-OH AAF seems to parallel the *in vivo* finding of Lotliker *et al.*[18] By contrast, Lotliker *et al.* have reported that MC pretreatment leads to increases in both ring and N-hydroxylation of AAF.[19] Therefore the mechanism of inhibition of AAF carcinogenesis by MC may be a result of lower liver levels of N-OH AAF due to increased biliary excretion of N-OH AFF rather than of decreased formation of N-OH AFF. Dietary selenium also

had no effect on the MC-induced mixed-function oxidase activity, which metabolizes AAF. This result with rat liver microsomes agrees with the previous observation of Rasco et al. that selenium does not affect the induction of aryl hydrocarbon
hydroxylase activity in cultural human lymphocytes.[20]

Wortzman et al. have fed male weanling Charles River CD rats a Torula
yeast-based selenium-deficient diet or the same diet supplemented with selenium
(0.5 ppm) as sodium selenite.[21] The effect of dietary selenium on the interaction
between AAF and rat liver DNA was studied in vivo. There was no difference
between selenium-deficient and selenium-supplemented rats with respect to the
total amount of AAF covalently bound to liver DNA in vivo at 1, 4, 16, 24, 96,
or 168 hr after a single intraperitoneal injection of labeled AAF. However,
alkaline sucrose gradient analysis revealed the production of DNA single-strand
breaks in the livers of selenium-deficient rats at 4 hr after intraperitoneal injection of AAF (10 mg/kg AAF). These lesions were apparently repaired 24 hr after
injection of the carcinogen. Under the same experimental conditions, AAF failed
to produce evidence of DNA damage in the livers of selenium-supplemented
rats. The dose of 20 mg/kg AAF resulted in extensive degradation of hepatic
DNA, which was repaired at 48 and 72 hr after administration and was not
affected by the selenium status of the animals. Neither the selenium-supplemented nor the selenium-deficient animals exhibited any significant alteration in
lipid peroxidation, which was measured by determining the hepatic malondialdehyde content of rats after AAF injection.

Besbris et al. have studied the metabolism of AAF in vitro, and the urinary
excretion of a single intraperitoneal dose of AAF was studied in weanling rats
maintained on an selenium-deficient diet or the same diet supplemented with 0.5
ppm selenium.[22] Hepatic microsomes isolated from selenium-supplemented rats
generated greater amounts of noncarcinogenic phenolic metabolites of AAF than
did microsomes from selenium-deficient animals. In addition, selenium-supplemented animals excreted significantly less N-hydroxy-AAF. These results suggest that the protective effect of dietary selenium against AAF-induced hepatocarcinogenesis may be due, in part, to its ability to inhibit the production of N-
hydroxy-AAF in vivo.

Effect on Aflatoxin Carcinogenesis

Chen et al. fed a low-selenium and vitamin-free semipurified basal diet or
that diet supplemented with graded levels of selenium or vitamin E or both to
day-old single-comb white Leghorn chicks of both sexes maternally depleted in
selenium and vitamin E.[23] Fourteen-day-old chicks were given 1 mg/kg
[^{3}H]aflatoxin B_1 (AFB$_1$) and killed either 2 or 24 hr later. The covalent binding
of AFB$_1$ to liver DNA and RNA in chicks fed the basal diet was significantly
gerater than in chicks supplemented with selenium or vitamin E. Phenobarbital

treatment before administration of AFB_1 decreased adduct formation in most groups and abolished differences in adduct formation due to diet. These experiments suggest that combined selenium–vitamin E deficiency enhances activation or inhibits detoxification of AFB_1 *in vivo*. In the Mongolian gerbil, hepatic protein analysis demonstrated two protein peaks in the sodium selenite + AFB_1 group that were absent in all other groups.[24] It is likely that these proteins were selenoproteins that were directly or indirectly involved in the lower incidence of histopathological damage in this group.

Colon Cancer

Jacobs *et al.* have studied the effect of 4 ppm sodium selenite in the drinking water on colon carcinogenesis. Sprague-Dawley rats were injected weekly with either 1,2-dimethylhydrazine (DMH) or methylazoxymethanol acetate (MAM).[25] After 17 weeks, the total number of tumors was decreased in the selenium-treated groups. The DMH control group had 39 tumors as compared with only 11 tumors in the selenium-treated rats. The control MAM group had 73 tumors versus only 42 in the selenium-treated animals. The incidence of MAM-induced tumors was 93% (14 of 15) with the selenium additive and 100% (14 of 14) without it. However, selenium reduced the incidence of DMH-induced colon tumors by more than 50%. In the DMH-treated group 13 of 15 had tumors, whereas in the selenium-treated group only 6 of 15 had tumors.

Jacobs *et al.* (1981) have also studied the effect of adding a 4 ppm selenium supplement to the drinking water before, during, and after 20 weekly injections of DMH.[26] The incidence of colon tumors in groups provided selenium before DMH, before and during DMH, and only during DMH treatment was reduced to 39% (11 of 28), 43% (13 of 30), and 36% (10 of 28), respectively. The incidence in the DMH-only control was 63% (19 of 30). At 10-week intervals throughout the study, selected blood and tissue components and hematological changes were correlated with DMH treatment: serum glutamic oxalacetic transaminase (SGOT) increased twofold; serum alkaline phosphatase increased 24%, serum protein content decreased 14%, the white blood count increased two- to threefold, and hemoglobin decreased 67%. The enzyme and blood changes likely reflect host–tumor interaction rather than early carcinogenic reactions. Selenium in the drinking water has also been found to inhibit DMH-induced large bowel carcinogenesis but to facilitate the induction of small bowel cancer by the same carcinogen in the same animals.[27]

Soullier *et al.* have studied the effects of selenium supplementation on azoxymethane-induced intestinal cancer in Sprague-Dawley rats given 8 weekly injections of azoxymethane and fed a 30% beef fat diet.[28] There were two groups: one group served as controls and the other received selenium supplementation of 8 ppm H_2SeO_3 in the drinking water. The average number of intestinal tumors was 6.5 in the control group and 3.1 in the selenium-supplemented group. A significant reduction was observed in tumor incidence in the proximal half of the colon of the selenium-treated rats. Increases in the selenium levels of the intestinal and the proximal part of the colon seem to parallel the anticarcinogenic action of selenium. The lack of a protective effect in the distal part of the colon may reflect a decrease of selenium observed in that part of the colon. This segment-specific reduction in tumors correlates well with the observed preferential uptake of supplemental selenium.

Harbach and Swenberg have studied the effects of selenium on DMH metabolism, DNA alkylation, and the rate of cell turnover of colon tissue. The effects of selenium pretreatment consisting of 4 ppm in the drinking water for 2, 4, or 6 weeks on DMH metabolism[29] were monitored in male Sprague-Dawley rats by measuring expired $^{14}CO_2$ and azo [^{14}C]methane over a 12-hr period after a subcutaneous injection of [^{14}C]DMH. Selenium pretreatment as compared with the controls caused an increase in exhaled azomethane (31–69%) and a corresponding decrease in $^{14}CO_2$ (4–33%) as the duration of the treatment increased from 2 to 6 weeks.

When the extent of DNA alkylation was measured as N^7 and O^6-methylguanine formation after selenium pretreatment, a reduction of 20–27% was observed in the liver and alkylation was increased 40–43% in the colon. In addition, metabolic incorporation of carbon = 14 from [^{14}C]DMH into adenine and guanine (presumably via C pathways) was reduced 69–72% in colon DNA of selenium-treated rats, and [^3H]thymidine incorporation was reduced 61–65%. These decreases may have been due to decreased cell turnover. A similar response in regard to DNA alkylation was not observed in the liver. The observations of Harbach and Swenberg suggest that selenium decreases hepatic DMH metabolism and that this decrease may be compensated by an increase in extrahepatic metabolism and alkylation.[29] Although colon alkylation is increased by selenium pretreatment, fewer tumors result. The decrease in the number of tumors may be due to a decrease in DNA synthesis in the colon. Other as yet undetermined mechanisms may be important as well. Banner et al. have observed that MAM acutely inhibits the synthesis of RNA and DNA.[30] Selenium had no effect on the inhibition of RNA and DNA by MAM both in the liver and in the colon. MAM does not require microsomal activation. Their observations suggested that the tumor-preventative effects of selenium on MAM are probably due to a mechanism other than carcinogen activation and interaction.

Breast Cancer

Effect on Virus-Induced Cancer

Schrauzer and Ishmael have given 2 ppm selenium in the form of SeO_2 in the drinking water for 15 months to 30 virgin C3H strong, female mice, which are especially susceptible to virally induced spontaneous mammary tumors induced by the Bittner milk virus.[31] The exposure of the mice lowered the incidence of spontaneous mammary tumors from 82% in the untreated controls to 10% in the selenium-treated mice. In the same experiment another group of mice was given arsenic in the drinking water at levels of 10 ppm. The tumor incidence in this group was reduced to 27%, but the growth rate of spontaneous or transplanted mammary tumors showed significant enhancement. In contrast, the mammary tumors in the control group grew about twice as fast as those in the selenium group.

Selenium and Other Metal Interactions

In a subsequent study the spontaneous tumor incidence was observed in the C3H St mice that were given 2, 5, and 15 ppm selenium and arsenic at the 10- and 80-ppm level.[32] Another group was given a Se/Zn supplement in a ratio of 5 : 200 ppm. The percentage tumor incidence in the 2-, 5-, and 15-ppm selenium groups was 10%, 36%, and 33%, respectively. The 10- and 80-ppm arsenic-treated groups had a tumor incidence of 27% and 40%, respectively. The Se/Zn group had an incidence of 94% (mammary tumor), close to the 82% observed in the nontreated control group. The result in the Se/Zn group might be predicted because of the known antagonistic interaction between selenium and zinc. Similar known antagonistic reactions are known for arsenic and selenium, but arsenic and selenium were not tested together in this experiment. Using a similar experimental design, Schrauzer et al. jointly administered 2 ppm arsenic as arsenite along with 2 ppm selenium as selenite in the drinking water of inbred female C3H/St mice.[33] Arsenic and selenium were also tested alone. The tumor incidence was 41% in the control group, 36% in the arsenic-treated group, 17% in the selenium-treated group, and 62% in the As/Se-treated group. The increase in carcinogenesis with As/Se treatment seems to be consistent with the known interactions between arsenic and selenium.

Concentrations of arsenic and selenium in lung, liver, and kidney tissue from dead smelter workers and from a control group have been measured with the aid of neutron-activation analysis.[34] A sevenfold increase of arsenic was found in lung tissues from the exposed workers compared with the control group. The median value of arsenic in lung tissue from workers who died from lung cancer was not higher than corresponding amounts from workers dead from other malignancies or from cardiovascular or other diseases. As the time of retirement increased, the arsenic content decreased in the liver, but not in the lung tissue. Workers dead from malignancies had a higher As : Se ratio (0.61 ± 0.42) than did workers from other diseases (0.34 ± 0.26). Controls had a value of 0.06 ± 0.05. This result seems to parallel the report of Schrauzer et al.[33] However, accumulation of antimony, cadmium, lead, and lanthanum was observed in lung tissue from the exposed workers. This finding indicates a possible multifactorial cause behind the excess mortality from lung cancer in smelter workers.

Shamberger and Bratush have measured the cadmium, selenium, and zinc levels of the kidney cortex from 123 patients who died from different diseases.[35] Selenium was significantly lower in patients with cancer metastases. Cancer patients also showed a trend toward a lower selenium level. In contrast, zinc was significantly greater in kidneys from patients with cancer or from those with cancer metastases. The Zn : Se ratio had a greater significant difference from controls than did selenium or zinc alone.

Nonsmokers and cigar smokers had a significant lower kidney cadmium content than was found in cigarette smokers. Nonsmoking cancer patients with metastases had a greater kidney cadmium content than did nonsmokers with other diseases. The Cd : Se ratios were greater in cancer patients and in cancer patients with metastases than in the controls. A positive significant correlation was found between zinc and cadmium in 123 patients.

Schrauzer et al. (1981) have also observed that exposing mice to high lead : selenium ratios leads to a lower tumor incidence.[36] The 19 months' exposure to 25 ppm lead caused little if any toxicity and produced an overall tumor incidence of about 20%. Exposure to only 5 ppm lead under identical condtions markedly shortened the tumor latency period and produced high tumor incidence, a pattern similar to that of arsenic when jointly administered with selenium.

Schrauzer et al. have reported that inbred female C3H/St mice exhibit the normal incidence of spontaneous mammary adenocarcinoma of 80–100%, if they are maintained on a standard commercial laboratory diet containing 0.15 ppm selenium with meat and dried skimmed milk as major protein sources.[33] If animals of the same strain are kept on a diet containing 0.45 ppm selenium with fish meal as the main source of protein, the tumor incidence decreased to 42%. The tumor incidence decreases further to 25%, 19%, and 10% if the animals receive an additional 0.1, 0.5, and 1.0 ppm selenium in the drinking water. Selenium-supplemented groups of animals also remained tumor-free for longer periods than did the unsupplemented controls.

Schrauzer et al. have infected four groups of female inbred C3H/St mice with the Bittner milk virus particle.[37] Since selenium is present in most foods in the organic rather than the inorganic form, and drinking water is not a normal source of the element, these workers decided to investigate its effects when added to the diet in the proper nutritional form. One group was maintained on a Torula yeast diet supplemented with 1 ppm selenium (organically bound in yeast) and had a 27% incidence. The mice, which were switched from the 1-ppm selenium diet to a diet containing only 0.15 ppm selenium after reaching the age of 13.8 months, rapidly develop mammary tumors during their remaining life span with the overall tumor incidence reaching 69%. This is not statistically different from the 77% incidence of tumors observed in animals maintained on the 0.15-ppm selenium diet over their entire postweaning life span. In contrast, animals changed from the 0.15-ppm selenium diet to that containing 1.0 ppm selenium at the age of 13.8 months develop mammary tumors with a total incidence of only 46%, which is significantly lower ($p < 0.05$) than in the 0.15-ppm selenium control group. Schrauzer *et al.* demonstrated that dietary selenium prevents and retards tumor development as long as it is supplied in adequate amounts.

Effect on Methyl-N-Nitrosourea-Induced Cancer

Thompson and Becci have tested the effect of two types of diets with or without selenium supplementation on *N*-methyl-*N*-nitrosourea (MNU)-induced mammary carcinogenesis in noninbred female Sprague-Dawley rats.[38] Mammary cancer was induced by a single intravenous injection of MNU. Twenty-three rats fed Purina rodent chow with 5 ppm sodium selenite had a tumor incidence of 85% and 2.30 cancers per rat, whereas 25 controls fed the same diet but with no added selenium had a tumor incidence of 95% and 3.95 cancers per rat. Twenty-five rats fed a *Torula* yeast diet with 1 ppm added sodium selenite showed an incidence of 68% and 1.49 cancers per rat. The control group with 25 rats was fed 0.01 ppm sodium selenite and had an incidence of 68% and 2.11 cancers per rat. Selenium feeding prolonged the latency of mammary tumor appearance. The results of Thompson and Becci's study suggested that dietary selenium had an effect on the postinitiation stage of mammary carcinogenesis.

Thompson *et al.* have used a similar experimental design with either 4 ppm sodium selenite and 300 ppm retinyl acetate or 4 ppm sodium selenite and 300 ppm retinyl actate added to Purina laboratory chow.[39] The effect on the postinitiation stage of mammary carcinogenesis was a reduction in the number of cancers per rat in all three groups. The number of cancers per rat was 3.68 in the control group, 2.84 in the selenium-treated group, 2.44 in the retinoic acid-treated group, and 1.72 in the combined retinoic acid and selenium-treated group.

Effect on 7,12-Dimethylbenzanthracene-Induced Cancer

Thompson and Tagliaferro have studied the effect of selenium on DMBA-induced mammary tumorigenesis. One group of female Sprague-Dawley rats was fed a diet that was unsupplemented, and another group was fed a diet supplemented with 5 mg/kg selenium as sodium selenite.[40] At 35 days of age, the selenium-supplemented rats were randomized into one of two groups and fed the selenium-supplemented diet from 35 to 63 days of age. On day 64, one selenium-treated group was switched to an unsupplemented diet. Rats were maintained on these diets until the study was terminated. At 59 days of age, all rats were administered 20 mg DMBA dissolved in sesame oil via gastric intubation. Rats were palpated twice each week for the detection of mammary tumors. After 90 days post-DMBA, the rats fed unsupplemented diet (control group) had a 95% tumor incidence with an average of 2.9 tumors per rat and mean time to first tumor appearance (MTA) of 50 days. Feeding the selenium-supplemented diet from either 35 to 63 days of age or throughout the study reduced tumor incidence and the average number of tumors per rat and prolonged the MTA (70% and 45%) at 1.5 and 0.9 tumors per rat, and 61 and 71 days, respectively.

Thompson *et al.* repeated and modified their experiment to test either low (7.5 mg) or high (15.0 mg) DMBA. At 28 days of age, the rats were randomized into four groups of 45 rats each and were fed a diet containing either 0.05, 0.15, 1.05, or 2.06 μg/kg selenium.[41] At 50 days of age, 20 rats in each group were given 15 mg DMBA; the remaining rats were given 7.5 mg DMBA intragastrically. All rats were changed to a diet containing 0.21 μg/kg selenium. Most of the rats got tumors, but the number of tumors per rat was reduced by the selenium-supplemented diets. The average number of tumors per rat across treatments was 9.1, 7.4, 7.1, and 5.0 and 5.8, 6.0, 4.5, and 3.8 at the high and low doses of DMBA, respectively. Antineoplastic activity was dependent on the amount of selenium ingested. The data suggested that selenium inhibits some aspect of the initiation stage of DMBA-induced mammary tumorigenesis, which results in a significant reduction in the number of tumor occurrences.

Ip and Sinha have examined the effect of selenium depletion on mammary tumorigenesis after DMBA administration to female Sprague-Dawley rats fed different levels and types of fats.[42] Four selenium-deficient basal diets were used containing either 1%, 5%, or 25% corn oil or 24% hydrogenated coconut oil. Only 0.1 ppm selenium was considered a selenium-adequate diet. In animals that received an adequate supplement of selenium, an increase in fat intake was accompanied by an increased tumor incidence when corn oil was used in the diets. A high saturated-fat diet was much less effective in this regard.

In a third experiment to test the effect of greater amounts of dietary selenium on DMBA-induced mammary carcinogenesis, Ip[43] fed rats 0.1, 0.5, 1.5, or 2.5 ppm (as sodium selenite) along with either a 5% or 25% corn oil diet and 5 mg DMBA. The total number of tumors was as follows (30 rats per group): 26, 23, 19, and 10 in the 5% corn oil group, and 65, 66, 41, and 21, respectively, in the 25% corn oil group. In a second experiment, rats were given 10 mg DMBA, and selenium was added to the diets at 0.1, 2.5, and 5.0 ppm. Tumor yields were found to be 71, 32, and 15, respectively, in the high fat group. In these experiments there was a longer latency period of tumor appearance with selenium supplementation. High dietary selenium levels were able to protect against mammary carcinogenesis, but the rats on a high corn oil diet still developed more tumors than did those on a low corn oil diet at a comparable selenium supplementation.

Ip[44] has also studied the effect of selenium supplementation in the initiation and promotion phase of DMBA-induced mammary carcinogenesis in rats fed a high-fat diet. In this experiment, control animals were fed 0.1 ppm selenium (as sodium selenite), while the experimental groups were supplemented with 5 ppm selenium for various periods of time: -2 to $+24$ weeks; -2 to $+2$, $+2$ to $+24$, $+2$ to $+12$; $+12$ to $+24$; and -2 to $+12$. The time of DMBA administration was taken as zero. Selenium again retarded tumorigenesis to various degrees. Ip made the following conclusions: (1) selenium can inhibit both the initiation and promotion phases of carcinogenesis, (2) a continuous intake of selenium is necessary to achieve maximal inhibition of tumorigenesis (Schrauzer[37] made the same observation in his experiments), (3) the inhibitory effect of selenium in the early promotion phase is probably reversible, and (4) the efficacy of selenium is attenuated when it is given long after carcinogenic injury. Ip also assessed the effectiveness of selenium in inhibiting the reappearance of mammary tumors that had regressed after ovariectomy. In tumor-bearing animals supplemented with 5 ppm selenium immediately after endocrine ablation, the tumors reappeared at a slower rate as compared with the controls. Ip's results suggest that selenium may not only be effective in chemoprevention, but that selenium can also be used as an adjuvant chemotherapeutic agent.

Although Ip's[44] study shows an association between the susceptibility of the mammary tissue to carcinogenesis and its lability to peroxidation as a result of increased fat intake similar to that observed with croton oil and croton resin on DMBA-initiated mouse skin,[8] this does not necessarily mean that lipid peroxidation is the primary mechanism by which dietary fat promotes cancer development. Other factors that might be involved include elevated circulating prolactin, lymphocyte dysfunction, and the involvement of prostaglandins through the cellular immune system. Pharmacological levels of selenium have been reported to potentiate the immune response of the host.[45] It remains to be seen whether the immune response exerts an influence on the promotion of chemical carcinogenesis.

Some of the factors that might affect tumor growth have been examined. Ip has found that selenium does not affect the levels of circulating prolactin and estrogens,[43] hormones important to the development of the DMBA-induced mammary tumors.[46] Ip and Ip[47] have fed rats diets containing 1%, 5%, and 25% of tocopherol-stripped corn. The rats were fed either 0.1 ppm selenium in the form of sodium selenite added to the basal diet or just the basal diet, which contained less than 0.02 ppm selenium. Mammary tumors were induced by intragastric administration of 5 mg DMBA. There was a marked increase of liver glutathione peroxidase in the groups given the 0.1-ppm selenium supplement. The groups fed the basal diet became rapidly depleted in liver glutathione peroxidase activity. There was a marked increase in the number of tumors per rat in the selenium-depleted animals fed the 25% corn oil diet. There was also a significant increase in the thiobarbituric acid values (malodinaldehyde) in the selenium-depleted animals fed the 25% corn oil diet.

Ip's results suggest that there is an association between the susceptibility of the mammary gland to carcinogenesis and its lability to peroxidation, and that both parameters are regulated by fat intake in conjunction with the selenium status of the animal. Ip and Ip[47] have fed rats both retinyl acetate and selenium and markedly suppressed DMBA-induced mammary cancer formation. The final tumor yield was reduced to 8% of the control as compared with 51% and 36%, respectively, for selenium and retinyl actate. A continuous intake of both agents was necessary to sustain the chemopreventive effect.

Young and Milner have studied the effect of 0.1, 2.5, and 5.0 ppm of selenium in a 30% *Torula* yeast diet on DMBA-induced mammary tumors.[48] Tumor incidence 8 weeks after intubation with DMBA was 53%, 14%, and 27% for the three diets. The total number of tumors at autopsy was significantly decreased from 237 for controls to 92 and 113 for 2.5 and 5.0 ppm selenium, respectively.

Welsch *et al.*[49] divided 147 Sprague-Dawley rats into five groups and treated them at 60 days of age with 5 mg DMBA. Selenium, as selenium dioxide (SeO_2), was administered in the drinking water to four of the five groups (30 rats/group) at two doses (2 and 4 mg/liter) from 30 to 90 days of age (series 1) and from 90 to 150 days of age (series 2) before the onset of palpable mammary tumors. One group of 27 rats served as controls. The total number of carcinomas that developed in each group was as follows: controls, 60 carcinomas; series 1: 2-mg Se dose, 27 carcinomas and 4-mg Se dose, 29 carcinomas; series 2 : 2-mg Se dose, 24 carcinomas and 4-mg Se dose, 32 carcinomas. Each dose level of Se in both series significantly reduced the incidence of mammary carcinomas. In a second experiment, 226 nulliparous and 99 multiparous GR mice were treated daily with estrogen and progesterone for 13–16 weeks. SeO_2 was administered in the drinking water (2 mg/liter) to one-half these mice. The total number of mammary carcinomas in the control nulliparous and multiparous mice were 119 and 90, respectively; in the selenium-treated group the nulliparous and multi-parous mice had 113 and 81 tumors; respectively. The results of this experiment indicated that selenium did not affect mammary carcinoma incidence in hor-mone-treated nulliparous and multiparous GR mice.

Medina and Shepherd[50] studied the effect of SeO_2 on DMBA-induced mammary tumorigenesis in BALB/c, C3H/StWi, and BD2F mice. All mice were fed DMBA once a week for either 2 or 6 weeks (1 mg/week per mouse) when the mice were 8 weeks old. SeO_2 was dissolved in water (SeO_2 = 6 mg/liter) and administered *ad libitum* starting when the mice were 6 weeks old. In one group of BD2F, mice, a pituitary gland was grafted under the kidney capsule in order to stimulate lobuloalveolar differentiation in the mammary glands. The results of this experiment in BD2F mice fed 2 or 6 mg DMBA, in

C3H/StWi mice fed 6 mg DMBA, and in BALB/c mice fed 2 mg DMBA indicated that selenium supplementation markedly inhibited mammary tumor incidence. The percentage inhibition of tumor incidence ranged from 42% to 85%. In the BD2F mice fed 2 mg DMBA and containing a pituitary isograft, the hormonal stimulation exerted by the isograft partially counteracted the inhibition mediated by selenium. In the latter group, the mean latent period of tumor formation was delayed by the presence of selenium even though the tumor incidence was not significantly different between the selenium-treated and - untreated mice.

The effect of selenium on the induction of mammary preneoplastic dysplasias was examined in three groups of mice.[50] The term dysplasia denotes pathological lesions that are not neoplasms. Previous studies have indicated that both alveolar and ductal hyperplasias are precursor states of mammary neoplasms. Selenium supplementation reduced the incidence of mice with ductal hyperplasias from 61% to 15% in 5-month-old BD2F mice and from 75% to 25% in 8-month-old BALB/c mice. In 6-month-old MMTV-positive BALB/c-fC3H mice, selenium supplementation reduced the incidence of hyperplastic alveolar nodules from 45% to 10%.

In a third experiment the effect of selenium on the growth rate of first transplant generation mammary tumors was examined in BALB/c, BD2F, and BALB/c-fC3H mice.[50] Of the 36 mammary tumors examined, selenium supplementation influenced the growth rate of only four tumors. The growth rate of three mammary tumors was inhibited and the growth rate of one tumor was enhanced. The results indicated that selenium did not alter the growth of established mammary tumors.

The results of Medina and Shepherd demonstrate that (1) supplemental selenium inhibits both chemical and virus-induced mouse mammary tumorigenesis, and (2) the development of preneoplastic lesions, an early stage in mammary tumorigenesis, is very sensitive to selenium-mediated inhibition.

Pancreatic Cancer

Wistar-derived MRC rats were fed casein diets supplemented with 0.1 or 2.0 ppm selenium as sodium selenite from 7 weeks of age. At 8 weeks, 50 weekly injections of bis(2-oxopropyl)nitrosamine (BOP) was started.[51] Colon adenocarcinoma yield was reduced in male rats fed the high-selenium level (16 carcinomas in 30 rats) compared with the low-selenium level (28 carcinomas in 29 rats).

Tracheal Cancer

Thompson and Becci[52] studied the effect of graded levels of selenium on tracheal carcinomas induced by 1-methyl-1-nitrosourea (MNU) in male Syrian golden hamsters. No significant differences were observed among the groups in the incidence of either benign lesions or carcinomas.

Effect of Selenium on Preneoplastic Lesions

The effect of dietary selenium on the development of L-azaserine-induced preneoplastic abnormal acinar cell nodules (AACN) has been examined in male Wistar rats. The regression of AACN was inversely related to the level, and the relationship was statistically significant.[53] The effects of dietary fat and selenium have been studied on the formation of aflatoxin B_1 (AFB$_1$) induced γ-glutamyltransferase (GGT) positive foci in rat liver has also been investigated.[54] A low-fat diet produced fewer foci than a high-fat diet, which in turn produced fewer tumors than the high-fat diet minus selenium. Similarly, the effect of dietary selenium (0.1, 3.0, or 6 ppm) on the early postinitiation stages of hepatocarcinogenesis induced by diethylnitrosamine (DEN) has also been studied.[55] Selenium as 3 and 6 ppm in the diet significantly decreased mean GGT foci/cm more than 0.1 ppm Se. When a toxic amount of selenium was fed (6 ppm) before phenobarbital stimulation, enhancement of carcinogenesis was observed.

Effect of Selenium on Transformation of Cells in Organ Culture

The influence of sodium selenite on the transformation of mammary cells induced by 7,12-dimethylbenzanthracene (DMBA) has been studied in organ culture of the whole mammary glands from BALB/c female mice.[56] Transformation was determined by the presence of nodulelike alveolar lesions (NLAL) induced by DMBA in the glands *in vitro*. At selenium concentrations of $10^{-5} M$, a small (18%) inhibition of the frequency of transformed glands was detectable at the initiation stage. However, at the promotional stage, $10^{-6} M$ selenium caused a 37% inhibition of the frequency of transformed glands, and an 84% inhibition was present at $10^{-5} M$ concentration of selenium in the medium. Selenium appears to act by preventing expression of the transformed cells.

Effect of Selenium on Benzpyrene-Induced Sarcoma

Witting *et al.* studied the possibility of a tumor-protective effect of selenium on the growth of benzpyrene-induced sarcoma in BALB/c mice.[57] The mice received 4 ppm selenium in their drinking water for 12 months before subcutaneous injection of benzpyrene to induce sarcomas. Unlike the unpretreated controls, the selenium-exposed animals developed significantly fewer and smaller tumors in a given time.

Chemotherapeutic Effect of Selenium

Effect in Animals

Abdullaev *et al.* observed that sodium selenite even in a single dose (1 mg/kg parenteral) retarded the growth of transplanted Ehrlich ascites, Guérin carcinoma, and sarcoma M-1 neoplasms in rats and mice.[58] The selenium-containing salt was most effective when administered as soon as the tumor was palpable. When the chemotherapeutic effect was combined with x-ray therapy, the growth-retardant effect of Na_2SeO_3 against Ehrlich ascites cells was enhanced. Sarcoma M-1 or Guérin carcinoma suspensions exposed before inoculation to Na_2SeO_3 plus heat (40°C) displayed impaired tumor growth *in vivo*. The immune activity of the blood was increased by Na_2SeO_3 treatment.

Poirier and Milner observed that sodium selenite, selenium dioxide, seleno-DL-cystine, and selno-DL-methionine dramatically decreased the viability of Ehrlich ascites tumor cells (EATC) as measured by dye exclusion.[59] Sodium selenate only marginally decreased EATC viability. Intraperitoneal injections of selenite in mice previously inoculated with EATC significantly inhibited tumor development. When the intraperitoneal injections of selenite were delayed 5–7 days after the mice were inoculated with EATC, the effectiveness of this nutrient on the inhibition of EATC growth was found to be reduced.

Greeder and Milner investigated the effect of selenium dioxide, sodium selenite, sodium selenate, selenomethionine, and selenocystine on groups of 10 mice treated with EATC.[60] All selenium compounds were administered at a dose of 2 μg/gm initial body weight. None of the treated mice had tumors, whereas all control mice developed Ehrlich ascites tumors. In a second experiment, the dosage was lowered to 1.0 or 0.25 μg of the same five selenium compounds per gram of body weight and 5 mice per group were treated with EATC. Selenium dioxide, sodium selenite, sodium selenate, and selenocystine at 1 μg/gm all completely inhibited ascitic and solid tumor incidence. Selenomethionine was ineffective, as all five mice developed ascites tumors. At the 0.25-μg/gm dose, all five of the selenomethionine-treated mice developed ascites tumors, and two of five selenocystine-treated mice had ascites tumors. Some of the mice developed solid tumors.

Selenomethionine may have been ineffective because it is actively transported, whereas selenite and selenocystine are not.[61] Greeder and Milner[60] suggest that permeability may be a factor in the efficacy of the various selenium compounds in reducing tumor growth. Selenium also seemed to alter tumor growth selectively, since it had no significant effect on the growth of the host animals.

Selenopurine has been shown to retard the growth of L1210 leukemic cells.[62] The L1210 cell line is known to be susceptible to antifolics and to purine and pyrimidine analogues. Milner and Hsu[63] studied the effect of other forms of selenium on the L1210 cells both *in vitro* and *in vivo*. Selenium administration as sodium selenite was shown to be more effective in increasing the longevity of L1210-inoculated mice than was treatment with sodium selenate, selenocystine, or selenomethionine. Treatment at levels of 20, 30, or 40 μg/day sodium selenite in mice inoculated with 10^2 cells resulted in 50%, 80%, and 90% cures, respectively. A larger number of cells in the inoculum decreased the cure rate. Longevity of L1210-inoculated mice was increased by about 30% when the drinking water was supplemented 3 ppm selenium as sodium selenite. The death of L1210 cells *in vitro* as indicated by trypan blue exclusion was dependent on the form and concentration of selenium tested. When selenium at 1 μg/ml was incubated with L1210 cells for 1 hr before inoculation into mice, selenium significantly retarded the ability of the cells to propagate *in vivo*. Combined therapy with selenium (30 μg/day) and methotrexate resulted in a significantly longer life span of L1210-treated mice than resulted from either compound administered separately.

Medina and Oborn examined the effect of selenium on the growth potential of normal, preneoplastic, and neoplastic mammary cells grown in primary monolayer cell cultures and on three established mammary cell lines.[64] Selenium, present as Na_2SeO_3 in serum-free Dulbecco's modified Eagle's medium, inhibited all mammary cell cultures at 1×10^{-5} M. The growth of primary cell cultures of normal mammary cells and C4 preneoplastic cells and the established line YN-4 was inhibited by selenium at 5×10^{-8} M. This concentration of selenium did not stimulate the growth of D2 preneoplastic cells and tumors in primary cell cultures and established cell lines CL-S1 and WAZ-2t. The differential responses of cells from preneoplastic outgrowth lines C4 and D_2 as well as D2 primary tumors *in vitro* correlated with the sensitivity when these same cell populations were subjected to selenium-mediated inhibition of growth and tumorigenesis *in vivo*.

Ip[65] studied the effect of dietary selenium deficiency and supplementation on the growth of the transplantable MT-W9B mammary tumor in female Wistar-Furth rats. When the diet was supplemented with 2 ppm selenium, tumor growth was inhibited, and the final tumor weight was reduced by approximately 50% compared with the control rats receiving 0.1 ppm selenium. The inhibitory response was not likely due to toxicity, because no weight loss was induced in the rats. On the other hand, selenium deficiency (< 0.02 ppm) had no influence on the growth of the tumor.

Randleman studied the effect of 1 ppm selenium in the drinking water on the ovarian tumors that develop after normal ovaries are sewn into the spleen of albino laboratory rats (SAF/SD strain).[66] Six of nine rats subjected to the ovary-to-spleen transfer with no selenium supplementation had tumors, a 66.6% incidence. In contrast, 2 of 29 rats, having the same ovary transfer but receiving selenium supplement, had tumors (6.8%). Histological examination showed the tumors to be adenocarcinoma of the ovary. The tumors of both of the selenium fed animals were smaller and less advanced than those of the control rats. The tumors of the control rats were solid masses, averaging 1.5 cm in diameter. The two tumors of the selenium-supplemented rats were less than 0.5 cm in both cases. Sodium selenite has also been observed to inhibit the vascularization induced by amelanotic tumor implants (A-Mel-4B32) in the Syrian hamster cheek pouch membrane.[67]

Exon *et al.* exposed mice to selenium-supplemented or deficient rations and then inoculated them with an oncogenic virus, Rauscher leukemia virus (RLV).[68] Splenic lesions were not altered by dietary selenium supplementation or depletion. Under the experimental conditions, selenium did not affect the neoplasia induced by RLV in mice.

Effect in Humans

Watson-Williams summarized the treatment of inoperable cancer with selenium.[69] She reviewed 90 previous cases treated with colloidal selenium and found considerable or appreciable improvement in 72 cases and no improvement in 18 cases. Eight cases were described as clinical cures. Watson-Williams then described the treatment of 20 additional cases with colloidal selenium-β. Selenium has five allotrophic forms of which two are red and three are black. The brick red selenium-β was first used medicinally for cancer in 1833 and has appeared in various powders and pastes employed by the medical profession for the relief of malignant ulcers. A colloidal suspension of selenium, selenium-β is a coral-red fluid. In the 20 patients that Watson-Williams treated, there was apparent arrest of the malignant process in six cases; five more showed improvement, and the condition of the remaining nine patients was inconclusive. Fourteen patients showed relief of symptoms to varying degrees.

Prowse described two cases of breast carcinoma with widespread metastases.[70] These patients received frequent mild doses of high-voltage x-rays and weekly intravenous injections of a compound colloid of selenium and sulfur. Both patients completely recovered. By contrast, Gillett and Wakeley described 100 cases treated with selenium injections.[71] In general, little or no improvement was observed. Because there was no description of the type of selenium used, and since there are many known forms of selenium, it is possible that Gillett and Wakeley used a different preparation from that employed by either Prowse or Watson-Williams.

Epidemiological Relationship

Two major types of epidemiological relationships have been established in two different populations. Even though both relationships were inverse to selenium bioavailability and paralleled the results from animal studies, this does not necessarily imply a real relationship. A series of epidemiological studies has related selenium bioavailability to the human cancer mortality in American cities and states.[72,73] Statistically significant differences were found in the age-specific cancer death rates among states with high, medium, and low selenium levels. The death rates attributable to several types of cancer showed larger difference in males than in females in the states with high selenium levels. The greater difference between males and females may have been due to sex difference or to the fact that males are heavier smokers and are more likely to be exposed to industrial pollution. In the states with high selenium forage levels, there was significantly lower mortality in both males and females from several types of cancer, particularly the environmental problem indicators, such as the gastrointestinal and urogenital types of cancer. A similar observation was observed in 17 paired large cities and 20 paired small cities.[72] Alberta and Saskatchewan also have a higher selenium bioavailiability and a lower human cancer death rate.

Schrauzer *et al.* correlated the age-corrected mortality from cancer at 17 major body sites with the apparent dietary selenium intakes estimated from food-consumption data in 27 countries.[74] Significant inverse correlations were also observed for cancers of large intestine, rectum, prostate, breast, ovary, lung, and leukemia; weaker inverse associations were found for cancers of the pancreas, skin, and bladder. Another study found similar inverse correlations between cancer mortalities at the above sites and the selenium concentrations in whole blood collected from healthy human donors in the United States and several other countries. Schrauzer *et al.*[74] postulated that the cancer mortalities in the United States as well as other Western industrialized nations would markedly decline if the dietary selenium intakes were increased to about twice the current average amount supplied by the U.S. diet.

The per capita intake of zinc, cadmium, copper, and chromium were also estimated from food consumption data in 28 countries; these intakes were correlated with the age-corrected mortalities from cancers of the intestine, prostate, breast, skin, other organs, and leukemia.[75] These correlations suggest that the anticarcinogenic effect of selenium may be counteracted by other trace elements. Manganese correlated inversely with cancer of the pancreas and arsenic intakes correlated inversely with male lung cancer mortalities. Zinc concentrations in whole blood collected from healthy donors in the United States correlated directly with regional mortalities from cancers of the intestine, breast, and other sites.

Jansson and Jacobs[76] reported that Seneca County in the Finger Lakes region of New York has an incidence of colorectal cancer about 1000 rankings removed from that of the surrounding counties. The mortality rate for white males in Seneca was 125 : 100,000/year, while the other 57 counties in New York state had rates ranging from 145 to 216 : 100,000/year. The mortality rates for white females were 108 : 100,000/year in Seneca County and 118 to 160 : 100,000/year for the other counties.

Selenium might contribute to these low rates, because the selenium level in the community water system in Seneca Falls is about twice the average level in New York. Another more important factor may be the fact that the soil in Seneca is alkaline, while it is acid in most other parts of New York state. In addition, there is a low level of rainfall around Seneca County. These two factors may facilitate the uptake of selenium in plants. Another factor that may be important is the phenomenon that Lake Seneca and Lake Cayuga are both deeper and lower, relative to sea level, than all the other Finger Lakes. Both lakes penetrate the horizontal salt strata underlying the region, resulting in concentrations of Na, K, and Cl ions about 20 times higher in Seneca and Cayuga Lakes than in the other Finger Lakes. With such differences between the levels of the macroelements, it is likely that there are also great differences in the amounts of different trace elements.

Bogden et al. measured selenium, polonium-210, Alternaria spore counts, as well as the tar and nicotine contents of tobaccos from countries with high and low incidences of lung cancer.[77] The tobacco concentrations of polonium-210 were similar in cigarettes from high- and low-incidence countries, as were levels of cigarette smoke tar and nicotine. However, tobaccos from low-incidence countries had significantly lower Alternaria spore counts. In addition, the mean selenium concentrations of tobaccos from the high-incidence countries (0.16 ± 0.05 μg/gm) were significantly lower than those of tobaccos from the low incidence countries (0.49 ± 0.22 μg/gm). The differences in the selenium content of tobacco probably reflect soil levels of selenium. The major tobacco-growing regions in the Southeast United States have relatively low selenium concentrations in the soil. In contrast, Columbia and Mexico have been noted for high selenium levels in soil for several decades.

Selenium Blood Levels in Cancer Patients

Shamberger et al. compared selenium levels in the blood of 48 healthy individuals (27 men and 21 women) with selenium levels in the blood of 87 patients with gastrointestinal cancer, 9 patients with hematologic cancers, and 39 patients with other types of cancers.[78] No significant differences were observed in selenium levels between men and women or between persons below 50 years of age and those above 50 years of age. These results were in contrast to other findings that the selenium level in the blood begins to decrease at about 40–50 years of age.[79]

Measured in micrograms per deciliter (μg/dl), the selenium levels were found to be 22.3 ± 0.6 for normal men and 23.6 ± 0.8 for normal women, compared with 15.8 ± 0.4 for colon cancer patients, 15.3 ± 0.6 for stomach cancer patients, 13.2 ± 1.5 for patients with pancreatic cancer, 15.0 ± 0.7 for patients with liver cancer, and 20.7 ± 1.1 for patients with rectal cancer. However, three rectal cancer patients with liver metastases had very low selenium levels, 13.0 ± 1.1 μg/dl. With the exception of rectal cancer, Shamberger *et al.*[78] found that patients with gastrointestinal cancer had the lowest blood selenium levels.

McConnell *et al.* determined the levels of serum selenium in 110 patients with carcinoma.[80] Thirty-six patients had primary neoplasms of the reticuloendothelial system, 28 patients had medical and surgical nonmalignant disorders, and 18 were healthy nonhospitalized persons. McConnell *et al.* found that the carcinoma patients had significantly lower selenium levels and that patients with gastrointestinal cancer had lower levels than those with primary lesions. They also noted, in agreement with Broghamer *et al.*[81], that the lower the level of selenium among carcinoma patients, the greater the risk of metastases, multiple primaries, recurrence, and early death.

McConnell *et al.* also compared 30 women with breast cancer and 18 controls and found significantly lower serum selenium levels among the breast cancer patients ($p < 0.001$).[82] In another study, McConnell *et al.* compared the serum from 35 women with breast cancer with the serum samples from 27 women to be free of breast cancer.[83] Again, serum selenium was lower in the patients with breast cancer (X, 1.25; SEM, 0.04) and than the control group (χ, 1.57; SEM, 0.08). Capel and Williams measured the plasma selenium and the erythrocyte selenium and glutathione peroxidase in 15 women with breast cancer and compared these values with similar assays done on 14 postmenopausal controls and 11 premenopausal controls.[84] In agreement with the studies of McConnell *et al.*,[82,83] the plasma selenium level of the breast cancer patients was significantly lower than that of the controls ($p < 0.001$). Erythrocyte selenium and gluthathione peroxidase levels were significantly higher than in the controls. In addition, the levels of erythrocyte glutathione peroxidase was significantly higher ($p < 0.05$) in premenopausal women who were using steroidal-oral contraceptives and were more similar to postmenopausal control levels.

Broghamer *et al.* determined serum selenium levels by neutron activation analysis of 59 patients with a variety of reticuloendothelial tumors.[85] The mean serum concentration for the control group of nonhospitalized healthy individuals was 1.48 ± 0.07 mg/gm dry serum, whereas the mean serum level of selenium for the 59 primary reticuloendothelial malignancies was 1.61 ± 0.16 mg/gm dry serum. Chemotherapy, particularly for less than 6 weeks' initiation, produced elevations in serum selenium levels. In contrast, Calautti *et al.* also studied serum levels in malignant lymphoproliferative diseases.[86] Selenium was determined by proton-induced x-ray emission in 34 nonhospitalized healthy individuals and in 38 patients with malignant lymphoproliferative diseases (MLD). The mean serum levels of selenium in Hodgkin's disease and non-Hodgkin's malignant lymphoma were not different from those of the control group. Lowered mean serum concentrations were observed in the group with chronic lymphocytic leukemia (5.2 ± 0.7 mg/dl) as compared with normal individuals (7.9 ± 0.3 mg/dl). The difference was significant ($p < 0.005$). Goodwin *et al.* studied blood selenium levels and blood tissue GSH-Px activities in 50 patients with untreated cancer of the oral cavity and oropharynx.[87] Mean erythrocyte selenium and glutathione peroxidase were significantly depressed as compared with age-matched controls.

Schrauzer *et al.* observed that the methylene blue reduction time (MBRT) of human plasma samples was inversely related to the total plasma selenium content.[88,89] The MBRT of human plasma was introduced in 1947 as a chemical test for malignancy, but was later found to be insufficiently specific or accurate for routine cancer diagnosis. From several of the previously mentioned blood selenium studies in cancer patients, it is apparent that selenium is lowered in many of the patients, but many others have normal levels. Therefore, the MBRT, which relies on selenium levels, would not be a useful cancer marker.

Robinson *et al.* measured the selenium and the glutathione peroxidase activity in whole blood, erythrocytes, and plasma in 66 noncancer surgical patients, 80 patients with cancer, and 104 healthy Otago residents from the South Island of New Zealand.[90] Older residents over 60 years of age had lower blood selenium levels than did the young and middle-aged. Blood selenium levels were lower than comparable United States values and were no lower than those of elderly subjects and patients without cancer. In two cancer patients blood selenium levels were decreasing, and the lower values were obtained for five cancer patients and two noncancer patients after a long period of initiation. These low values were similar to values for patients on parenteral nutrition with negligible intakes. Robinson *et al.* suggested that the low selenium status of cancer patients was more likely a consequence of their illness than the cause of cancer. The lower blood selenium levels were associated with lower serum albumin and glutathione peroxidase activities. Because of the low blood levels expected in New Zealand and the expected variation of selenium analysis, it would be difficult to observe lower values in cancer patients.

Selenium as a Carcinogen

The carcinogenic potential has been claimed by a few researchers, but challenged by others. In general, flaws in the experimental design or the nonphysiological nature of feeding markedly toxic amounts for a long period of time have clouded the results. In an experiment designed to determine the lowest level of selenium to cause chronic toxic effects Nelson *et al.* fed rats 5–10 ppm selenium as seleniferous wheat or corn or 10 ppm ammonium potassium selenide.[91] Seventy-five percent of the animals that survived the first 3 months on a seleniferous diet developed liver cirrhosis. In addition, 15 of 53 rats that survived 18–24 months on the diet developed adenomas or adenomatoid hyperplasia. In control rats, the incidence of spontaneous hepatic tumors was less than 1%. Nelson *et al.* experienced difficulty in distinguishing between hyperplasia and true carcinomas, because it was difficult to distinguish just when the borderline between nonmalignant and malignant tumor has been passed and just when hyperplasia has passed into tumor. Shapiro postulated that these changes may have represented one phase of hepatic regeneration rather than neoplasia.[92] The inability of these "tumors" to metastasize, impling a lack of malignancy, was also noted.

A group of Russian researchers also claimed that selenium induced hepatic tumors.[93] In their first experiment, these workers noted that 10 of 23 male rats fed 4.3 ppm selenium developed tumors, while 5 out of 19 rats fed 8.6 ppm showed cancerous growths. Because these investigators did not mention any controls, no reliable conclusions can be made. In a second experiment, they were unable to support their prior claim. In one group 5 of 60 rats given selenium as selenate developed tumors and none of 100 rats on the same selenium treatment developed tumors in the second group. Volgarev and Tscherkes noted that the normal spontaneous cancer rate for the strain of rats used was 0.5%, and this rate was used as a basis for comparison with the selenate-treated rats.[93] Because of the lack of proper controls, no conclusions can be drawn from this report.

Schroeder and Mitchener also reported on an experiment designed to show the carcinogenicity of selenium.[94] In this experiment, 418 Long-Evans rats were divided into four groups and then further subdivided by sex. The groups received 2 ppm selenite, selenate, or tellurite. Two problems developed. An initial high mortality rate among the selenite-treated males (50% mortality at 58 days) led the investigators to substitute selenate for selenite. In addition, after 12 months, the investigators raised the selenate (males and females) and selenite (females) treatments from 2 to 3 ppm for the experiment. A second experimental difficulty was a virulent pneumonia that struck the colony of rats when they were 21 months old. Penicillin brought it under control after 3 weeks, but losses were immense: 36% male controls, 49% selenate males, 37% female controls, and 15% selenate females. The investigators used the surviving group in spite of possibly creating statistical bias in their experiment. The following incidence of tumors was reported: 31% controls, 62% selenate, 12% selenite (females), and 36% tellurite. From these results, Schroeder and Mitchener concluded that selenium was carcinogenic and that selenium predominantly induced mammary and subcutaneous fibrous cancers and not hepatic carcinomas.

In addition to the two experimental problems the investigators could have come to a different conclusion about the carcinogenicity of selenium. First, the 31% incidence in the controls and 12% in the selenite is statistically significant, indicating that selenite significantly reduced cancer incidence in the rats. The 62% incidence and the 31% incidence are not statistically significant. Second, Schroeder and Mitchener failed to take into account the importance of age as a contributing factor in the development of cancer. In the selenate-fed male rats, 50% mortality was observed at 962 days and at 1014 days in the selenate-fed female rats. However, 50% mortality in the controls occurred much earlier at only 853 days in males and at 872 days in females. Older rats have a greater cancer incidence, which may have been a factor in their experiment. No attempt for age adjustment was made.

Schroeder and Mitchener also evaluated the effects of 3 ppm selenate and selenite in the drinking water of 427 Swiss mice.[95] They reported that both selenate and selenite were ineffective tumor-inducing agents.

Harr et al. studied extensively the effect of chronic toxicity in rats. They reported no excess of neoplasms in rats fed selenite and selenate at levels up to 16 ppm, even though hepatic toxicity was observed.[96]

Seifter et al. observed multiple thyroid adenomas and "adenomatous hyperplasia of liver" in rats fed bis-4-acetoaminophenyl selenium dihydroxide for 105 days.[97] This compound also has inherent goitrogenic activity. Its sulfur-containing counterpart is also carcinogenic.

The National Cancer Institute Carcinogenesis Test Program has bioassayed SeS for possible carcinogenicity.[98] SeS was administered by gavage to rats and mice of each sex for 105 weeks. The animals were administered SeS suspended in 0.5% aqueous carboxmethylcellulose 7 days/week. The same vehicle without SeS was administered to the control animals. The animals that were administered SeS had decreased body weight; increased tumor formation was observed in female mice and in rats of either sex. Dosed rats and female mice had an increased incidence of hepatocellular carcinomas and adenomas. Female mice dosed with SeS also had an increased incidence of alveolar/bronchiolar carcinomas and adenomas. Because large toxic amounts were administered by gavage, it is unlikely that this experiment is of physiological value.

SELENIUM AND MUTAGENESIS

Selenium appears to have both antimutagenic and mutagenic activities. Ordinarily selenium is present in blood at about $1.25–2.50 \times 10^{-6}$ M. It is hoped that experiments will be designed using this physiological concentration as a starting point. Otherwise toxic or nonphysiological levels might confound the interpretation of the results.

Antimutagenicity

Barley

Sodium selenite and selenoamino acids interfere with crossing-over in barley.[99] Walker and Ting provide cytological evidence for the deformation of the chromatin content of the meiocyte as a result of selenium treatment. This observation suggests that selenium may reduce crossing-over by a relaxation of the chromosomal protein which may lead to a relaxation stress in the chromosomal fibril. The selenohydryl group is less reactive than the sulfhydryl *group*.[100] Consequently this and associated differences in bond strength and distance might introduce alterations in the physicochemical properties of seleno-substituted proteins.

Drosophila melanogaster

Similarly, selenocystine and selenomethionine interfere with the crossover distribution along the X chromosome of *Drosophila melanogaster*.[101] These results were attributed in proteins by the error incorporation of selenocystine residues, supporting a mechanism of pre-exchange DNA breakage induced by stress in an associated protein.

Bacteria

Sodium selenite also acts as an antimutagen if applied together with some known mutagens in *Salmonella*.[102–105] Using the *Salmonella typhimurium* TA1538 bacterial tester, system-graded decreases in mutagenicity with increasing selenium concentrations were observed for each of the three mutagens, i.e., AAF, N-OH-AAF, (N-OH-AF), and DMBA. Selenium decreased the mutagenicity of AAF, N-OH-AAF, and N-OH-AF to 65%, 68%, and 61% of their respective controls with mutagen alone. Shamberger et al.[103] tested the direct alkylating agents, malonaldehyde and β-propiolactone, and the antioxidants vitamin C, vitamin E, selenium, and butylated hydroxytoluene (BHT) on seven mutants of *Salmonella typhimurium*, five of which mutated by a frameshift mechanism and two of which mutated through base-pair substitution. The antioxidants vitamin C, vitamin E, selenium, and BHT at three logarithmic concentrations markedly reduced mutagenesis in those strains that mutated by a frameshift mechanism. Using tester strain TA 100, Adams et al.[104] tested the mutagenicity of DMBA and sodium nitrite alone and with selenium. Selenium addition significantly reduced the mutagencity of both the DMBA and the sodium nitrite. Martin et al.[105] tested the antimutagenic effects of selenium as sodium selenite on the mutagenicity of acridine orange and DMBA. Eight ppm selenium reduced the number of histidine revertants caused by acridine orange and DMBA by 52% and 74%, respectively. When the amounts of selenium added to the plates were increased, the mutagenicity of the test compounds was further suppressed.

Arciszewska et al.[106] tested the antimutagenic effect of selenium as sodium selenite, sodium selenate, selenium dioxide, and selenomethionine using the Ames Salmonella/microsome mutagenicity test with DMBA and some of its metabolites. Selenium progressively decreased the number of revertants caused by DMBA as well as its metabolites, which included 7-hydroxymethyl-12-methylbenzanthracene, 12-hydroxymethyl-7-methylbenzanthracene, and 3-hydroxy-7,12-dimethylbenzanthracene, which were mutagenic for Salmonella typhimurium TA100 in the presence of an S-9 mixture. Selenium supplementation as sodium selenite reduced the number of revertants induced by these metabolites to background levels. Schillaci et al.[107] studied the effects of dietary selenium on the mutagenic activation of DMBA by rat liver 59 using the Ames test. Preparations of S-9 from rats receiving 2.5 ppm Se in their diet produced 46%, 84%, and 70% less revertants than the controls of the 20-, 50-, and 100-mg/kg Aroclor induction levels.

Human Lymphocyte Cultures

Selenium has also been shown to reduce the mutagenicity of known mutagens in human lymphocyte cultures,[108–109] Shamberger et al.[108] incubated blood leukocyte cultures along with DMBA and the antioxidants, ascorbic acid, BHT, sodium selenite, and dl-tocopherol. The reduction of human chromosomal breaks was as follows: ascorbic acid, 31.7%; BHT, 63.8%; sodium selenite, 42%, and dl-tocopherol, 63.2%. More acrocentric-type chromosomal breaks (21.7%) were seen in the untreated controls than in the DMBA-treated group (4.8%). In contrast, the DMBA-treated groups had a higher percentage of meta breaks than did the untreated controls. Ray et al.[109] reported that selenium as sodium selenite, when tested with methylmethanesulfonate (MMS) or N-hydroxy-2-acetylaminofluorene (N-OH-AAF), reduced the sister–chromatid exchange (SCE) by 25–30% and 11–17%, respectively, below the SCE frequencies produced by the individual compounds.[109] However, high sodium selenite concentrations (7.90×10^{-5} M) resulted in a threefold increase in the SCE frequency above the background level of 6–7 SCEs/cell.

Morimoto et al.[110] studied the protective effect of sodium selenite against the cytogenetic toxicity of methylmercury (CH_3HgCl) and mercuric chloride

($HgCl_2$) on human whole-blood cultures in relation to the induction of SCE. The simultaneous addition of selenite (1×10^{-7} to 3×10^{-5} M) to cell cultures containing either methylmercury or mercuric chloride prevented the induction of SCEs by the mercurial in a clear dose-related manner. The formation of bis(methylmercuric)selenide, $(CH_3Hg)_2Se$ from Na_2SeO_3 and Ch_3HgCl, or a high molecular complex consisting of glutathione-Se-Hg from Na_2SeO_3 and Hg Cl_2 involving the participation of glutathione in red blood cells (RBCs) might play an important role in the antagonism between mercury and selenium.

DNA Repair Systems

Russell *et al.* found that selenium compounds are able to induce DNA repair synthesis as a measure of DNA damage in both the isolated rat liver cell system and the Ames *Salmonella* assay.[111] In the liver cells, DNA repair measured by uptake of [^{3}H]thymidine was found to be greater with sodium selenite and selenate than with selenomethionine. Williams[111] previously reported that [^{3}H]thymidine uptake by whole cells may be indicative of DNA repair synthesis. In the bacterial culture system, the repair-deficient variant was inhibited more by selenomethionine than by selenite and selenate.

Lawson and Birt studied that the repair of N-nitrosobis(2-oxopropyl)amine (BOP) induced damage to pancreas DNA in hamsters pretreated with selenium.[112] BOP is a potent carcinogen, preferentially producing pancreatic ductular adenocarcinoma in Syrian golden hamsters. Lawson and Birt examined the initiating phase of BOP carcinogenesis by measuring the production and repair of DNA damage in target (pancreas) and nontarget (liver and salivary gland) tissues of Syrian golden hamsters given a single subcutaneous dose of BOP (20 mg/kg). DNA damage was measured by the alkaline sucrose gradient/fluorometric method. DNA damage repair was slower in the pancreas than in the liver and the salivary gland. Six weeks after dosing, DNA still remained in the pancreas that sedimented at a lower density than pancreas DNA. Selenium was fed at a basal level and added to the diet at levels of 0.1 and 5.0 ppm. DNA damage was measured in the hamsters pretreated for 4 weeks before BOP administration with selenium. There was no apparent difference in the amounts of the DNA damage with any of the different treatments. However, in the hamsters fed 5.0 ppm selenium, DNA damage was repaired faster, so that by 24 hr all the DNA sedimented at the same density as pancreas DNA from control hamsters. The enhancement of repair observed by Lawson and Birt[112] seemed to be similar to that seen by Russell and Nader.[111] Even though the hamsters were fed a toxic 5-ppm level of selenium, they exhibited no overt toxic reactions and maintained a growth rate comparable to that of the control hamsters.

Norppa *et al.* examined the potential mutagenic effect of sodium selenite *in vivo*.[113,114] These workers grew lymphocyte cultures from nine neuronal ceroid lipofuscinosis (NCL) patients who received sodium selenite injections or tablets (0.004–0.05 mg Se/kg body weight daily) for 1–13.5 months and from five healthy persons given sodium selenite tablets (O.025 mg Se/kg body weight daily) for 2 weeks.[113] Whole blood lymphocytes grown in a 72-hr culture from the nine NCL-patients and five healthy persons showed no more cells with chromosomal aberrations than those from five other patients and two normal individuals.

Bone Marrow

Norppa et al. also studied aberrations in mouse bone marrow and primary spermatocytes.[114] Sodium selenite was injected intraperitoneally (0.8 mg Se/kg body weight) into 12 male NMR1 mice. After 24 hr, cytogenetic preparations of bone marrow and testis were made. The bone marrow of the sodium selenite-treated mice contained no more cells with structural chromosomal aberrations than that of the controls. There were no differences between the two groups in the numbers of metaphase–diakinesis stages of primary spermatocytes.

Fecal Mutagenicity

Kuhnlein et al. measured fecal mutagenicity from six healthy male volunteers (24–33 years) who consumed low- and then high-selenium diets. A formula diet containing 19–24 mg Se/day was fed for 45 days, followed by a similar diet containing 203–224 mg Se/day for 24 days.[115] Aqueous extracts of feces from days 1–3, 43–45, and 67–69 were assayed for mutagenicity using S. typhimurium TA100 and TA98. The reduction in fecal mutagenicity for the three periods with TA98 was significant with 20.5, 3.1, and 4.7 revertants. The mean number of revertants corrected for the blank with TA100 was 9.4, 7.8, and 8.8. TA98 is mainly affected by frame-shift mutations. This observation is consistent with those previously made by Shamberger et al., who observed that selenium and other antioxidants mainly affected frame-shift mutagenesis.[103]

Yeast

Rosin found that sodium selenite (1–15 mmol/plate) completely suppressed spontaneous mutagenesis at two independent loci both in wild (YO-300-IC) and in nine mutator isogenic strains of Saccharomyces cerevisiae. The two loci that were studied were the his 1–7, a missence mutation, and lys 1–1, a supersuppressible mutant of the amber variety.[116] The amount of suppression of prototrophic spontaneous reversion at these two loci depended on the concentration of sodium selenite, the yeast strain being studied, and the loci being evaluated. Almost 30-fold greater amounts of sodium selenite were required to suppress the frequency of spontaneous reversion at the histidine locus compared with quantities necessary to show a similar inhibition of lysine spontaneous reversion rates. The histidine and the lysine locus also responded differently to the presence of sodium selenide or sodium selenate. Sodium selenide at 3 μmol/plate completely inhibited spontaneous mutagenesis at the lysine locus for strain YO-800-IC (MUT 1-1). Complete suppression of histidine reversion occurred at 30 μmol/ plate. Sodium selenate suppressed the spontaneous mutagenesis at the lysine, but not the histidine locus. Rosin's results demonstrate the complexity of the effects that environmentally added components can have on mutagenesis.[116]

Mutagenicity

Human Leukocyte Cultures

Nakamuro et al. tested five selenium compounds, Na_2SeO_4, H_2SeO_4, Na_2SeO_3, H_2SeO_3, and SeO_2, for their capacity to induce chromosome aberrations in cultured human leukocytes and for their reactivity with DNA by a rec-assay system and inactivation of transforming activity in Bacillus subtilis.[117] In general, the concentration of the five were at toxic levels and ranged from 1.3 to $5.3 \times 10^{-4} M$. The chromosome-breaking activity was significantly higher for four-valent rather than with six-valent selenium. H_2O_2, H_2SeO_4, and Na_2SeO_4. The rec assay of Kada, which uses B. subtilis with different DNA recombination capacities, suggested that damage to DNA was produced by selenites but not by selenates.[118] In addition, the reactivity of selenites with DNA was also indicated by a significant loss of transformation of the tryptophan marker of B. subtilis DNA treated with H_2SeO_3 and SeO_2. Noda et al. have demonstrated weak base-pair substitution mutagenic activity for both selenate and selenite against S. typhimurium TA100, as well as a slight modifying effect when using recombination repair positive and negative strains of Bacillus subtilus.[119] SeO_2 at 0.01 M was more inhibitory in the recombination-repair-deficient (rec^-) than with wild bacteria (rec^+), indicating that this chemical is damaging cellular DNA.[120]

Ray and Altenburg observed that exposure of whole blood cultures to high sodium selenite concentrations (7.90×10^{-6} to $1.58 \times 10^{-5} M$) resulted in a three- to fourfold increase in the observed average number of SCEs.[121] Analysis of different whole blood components showed that the presence of red blood cells, and specifically red blood cell lysate, was a necessary component for sodium selenite SCE induction in purified lymphocyte cultures. The SCE frequencies of xeroderma pigmentosum as well as those of normal human lymphoblastoid cell lines were found to be unaffected by sodium selenite concentration that produced elevated SCE frequencies in whole blood cultures. If the latter two cell types were incubated with sodium selenite and RBC lysate, increases in the SCE frequencies were comparable to those increases observed in sodium selenite-exposed whole blood cultures.

At higher concentrations of selenium, especially the sodium selenide and sodium selenite form, more SCE's were observed in the presence and absence of S9 mixture.[122] However, selenate at similar concentration did not increase SCE. Because the selenate ion is considerably less toxic than either the selenide or the selenite form, it is likely that the results observed in this experiment are due to toxic effects.

Norppa et al. studied the effect of sodium selenite on the aberrations and SCE's in Chinese hamster bone marrow chromosomes.[123] A clear rise in the number of cells with aberrations (13.0–30.5%) or in the mean number of SCE's/cell (6.7–11.4) was observed when compared with the two control groups (0.9% and 1.0% of cells with aberrations and 3.4–4.4 SCE's/cell. The increase was only seen in the hamsters treated with 3, 4, or 6 mg Se/kg of body weight. The general toxicity of selenium at these high doses, which are near the LD_{50} of selenium, may contribute to the manifestation of observed chromosomal damage. Schwarz observed that the LD_{50} of selenium for mice was about 4.1 mg/kg body weight. The lack of chromosomal changes at selenium doses below 3 mg/kg body weight suggested that a mechanism may exist in vivo that prevents the harmful effects of selenium at low concentration.[124]

Lo et al. added sodium selenite at doses varying 8×10^{-5} to $3 \times 10^{-3} M$ to cultured human fibroblasts and have induced DNA fragmentation, DNA-repair synthesis, chromosome aberrations, and inhibition of mitosis.[125] The response of DNA repair-deficient xeroderma pigmentosum (XP) fibroblasts was similar to that of control cells. The capacity of selenite to induce chromosome aberrations, DNA repair and a lethal effect was enhanced when a mouse liver 5-9 microsomal fraction was incubated with the fibroblasts. XP cells behaved as control cells when they were treated with activated selenite. If sodium selenate at doses ranging from 8×10^{-5} to $3 \times 10^{-3} M$ were incubated with a S-9 preparation, no activation was observed as evidenced by no significant increase in the frequency of chromosome aberrations. One difficulty in uncovering the mutagenic action of selenium compounds is their high toxicity and the relatively narrow range of concentrations that lead to a mutagenic effect, rather than a lethal one. The use of different end points may lead to different results and interpretations. For example, sodium selenite but not sodium selenate gave a positive result when recombination-deficient B. subtilis was used as a test organism in mutagenesis studies,[117] whereas selenate but not selenite gives positive results in the Ames test that used an indicator strain for base-pair substitition.[126] The results presented by Lo et al. for fibroblasts of normal individuals and DNA repair-deficient XP patients were similar to those reported by Nakamuro et al.[117]

Whiting et al. observed that glutathione strongly enhanced the induction of unscheduled DNA synthesis (UDS) in cultured human cells by inorganic selenium compounds. In the presence 10^{-3} M glutathione, high levels of UDS (74–114 grains per nucleus) were observed in cells treated with selenate at 10^{-5}–10^{-3} M, selenite at 10^{-5}–3×10^{-4} M and selenide at 10^{-5}–10^{-3} M.[127] Glutathione also enhanced the clastogenic and cytotoxic effects of selenite and selenate in Chinese hamster ovary cells. Glutathione alone decreased DNA damage and toxicity in both the UDS and the chromosomal aberration assays. In the absence of glutathione, the three inorganic selenium compounds induced low levels of UDS and moderate frequencies of chromosomal aberrations. Whiting *et al.* also examined the effect of three organic selenium compounds on the induction of UDS. No UDS was detected in cells treated with selenocystamine or selenomethionine, with or without added glutathione.[127] However, seleno-cystine at 10^{-4}–10^{-3} M induced a low level of UDS that was enhanced by glutathione.

Whiting *et al.* demonstrated that reduction is involved in the conversion of selenium compounds to mutagenic forms. The active mutagens may be selenols GS-Se$^-$ from inorganic selenium and R-Se$^-$ from organic selenium compounds.[127] The metabolism of inorganic selenium compounds in mammalian tissues has been shown to proceed primarily by interaction with glutathione and glutathione reductase.[128] Selenate, selenite, and selenide might be interrelated by the reactions in Table 5-1. Selenate is slowly reduced to selenite by glutathione and other sulfhydryl compounds [eq. A. (1)], while reduction of selenite [Eq. (2)] and then further reactions occur in seconds. Selenite reduction proceeds via the selenotrisulfide (GS–Se–SG), which is stable and can be isolated (Ganther, 1974), and the selenopersulfide (GSSe$^-$ at neutral pH) which is highly reactive. If excess sulfhydryl is present [Eq. (9)] selenide is protected against oxidation [Eq. (8)].

Whiting *et al.*[127] explained the DNA damage induced by the inorganic selenium compounds on the basis of the above equations. Selenide cannot be oxidized *in vivo* beyond selenotrisulfide (GS–Se–SG), while selenate and selenite can be reduced as far as selenide. In addition, the reactive compounds selenide

Table 5-1. The Metabolism of Inorganic Selenium Compounds in Mammalian Tissues

$HSeO_4^- + 2GSH \xrightarrow{\text{slow}}$	$HSeO_3^- + GSSG + H_2O$	(1)
$HSeO_3^- + 4GSH \longrightarrow$	$GSSeSG + GSSG + OH^- + 2H_2O$	(2)
$GSSeSG + GSH \rightleftharpoons$	$GSSe^- + GSSG + H^-$	(3)
$GS-Se-SG + NADPH \xrightarrow{\text{glutathione reductase}}$	$GSSe^- + GSH + NADP^+$	(4)
$GS-Se^- + H_2O \rightleftharpoons$	$Se^0 + GSH + OH^-$	(5)
$GS-Se^- + NADPH + H_2O \xrightarrow{\text{glutathione reductase}}$	$HSe^- + GSH + NADP^+ + OH^-$	(6)
$GS-Se^- + GSH \rightleftharpoons HSe^- + GSSG$		(7)
$HSe^- + (0) \longrightarrow Se^0 + OH^-$		(8)
$HSe^- + (O) + 2GSH \longrightarrow HSe^- + GSSG + H_2O$		(9)

(HSe⁻) and the selenopersulfide (GS-Se-) are common products of metabolism of the inorganic selenium compounds and may be the ultimate mutagens. These compounds can be easily oxidized and may produce reactive free radicals that could damage DNA. The organic selenium compound selenocystine is reduced to selenocystine by glutathione, and this selenol may also be mutagenic.

Schut and Thorgeirsson tested the effect of selenite on the mutagenicity of N-OH-AAF on the *Salmonella* tester strain TA 1538.[129] Sodium selenite at concentrations up to 0.6×10^{-3} did not affect the N-OH-AFF mutation frequency but was highly toxic to the bacteria. Concentrations of 0.8×10^{-3} to $2 \times 10^{-3} M$ sodium selenite, which killed 67–94% of the bacteria, increased N-OH-AAF mutation frequency up to fivefold.

Tkeshelashvili *et al.* studied the effect of three metals, arsenic, selenium and chromium on the accuracy of DNA synthesis *in vitro*. Neither arsenic nor selenium altered the accuracy of the fidelity assays under the normal conditions of magnesium activation, nor did they affect the mutagenicity of manganese.[130] Chromium in the form of Cr (III) as well as Cr (VI) diminished the fidelity by which *Escherichia coli* DNA polymerase 1 copies polynucleotide templates.

SELENIUM AND IMMUNITY

Many nutritional factors may increase or decrease immunocompetence in experimental animals. Among the nutritional factors affecting immunity are intakes of calories, proteins, vitamins, and minerals. The essential amino acids, the essential fatty acids, minerals, and the vitamins are all required for proper humoral immunity.

Effect of Selenium on Humoral Immunity

The first report of an enhancement of humoral immunity by selenium was made by Berenshtein.[131] In this experiment Berenshtein administered thyroid vaccine to 56 rabbits together with sodium selenite (0.05 mg/kg sc) and vitamin E (0.03 mg/kg) before or during immunization with the thyroid vaccine. Rabbits given the selenium and vitamin E and the vaccine had higher antibody (Ab) titers than in control rabbits given vaccine alone. Vitamin E alone had no effect on antibody titers.

Spallholz *et al.* investigated the effects of dietary selenium on the formation of antibody titers in mice sensitized to sheep red blood cells (SRBC) and on the number of spleen plaque-forming B cells, 4 and 7 days postsensitization.[132] Selenium as sodium selenite added to commercial diets of mice increased titers of circulating antibodies to the SRBC antigens. Especially high anti-SRBC antibody titers (IgM) were observed from a group of mice receiving 2.8 ppm Se in their commercial diets. In addition, higher numbers of plaque forming cells (B cells) were observed, especially from mice receiving about 1–3 ppm dietary selenium.

In another experiment fed mice Purina chow diets with supplemental graded levels of selenite (0–8.5 ppm Se).[133] Anti-SRBC immunoglobulins IgM and IgG were titered 4, 7, and 14 days postimmunization. The higher IgM titers which had been observed on days 4 and 7 postsensitization had fallen by day 14 and were replaced by higher IgG titers. The antibody titers obtained after sensitization with SRBC antigens or tetanous toxoid were dependent on the amount of Se administered by injection or supplemented to diets.

In another study, Spallholz et al. used more than 4000 mice. They studied the effect of the route of administration (intraperitoneal, subcutaneous, or intradermal) as well as the usage of Se and vitamin E (0–100 mg Se and/or 0–5 mg vitamin E) on the primary and secondary immune responses to SRBC antigens or tetanus toxoid (TT).[134] Synergism between Se and vitamin E in increasing antibody titers was observed. Anti-TT titers were not increased in the primary immune response, but were enhanced in both the primary and secondary immune responses. The primary immune response to both antigens was measured over a 21-day period, while following the second immunization–sensitization the secondary response was measured over a 21-day period.

Norman and Johnson have reported on field experiments where MuSe[R] (Burns-Biotec Pharmacutical Company, Omaha, Nebr.) was twice administered to calves (25 cc).[135] Vaccination followed with a commercial L. pomona vaccine for protection against leptospirosis. After 6 weeks, the calved were bled and titered for anti- L. pomona antibodies. The data indicated more than a doubling of the average leptospirosis titers in calves given MuSe.

Aleksondrowicz has studied the stimulation of antibody production in mice and rabbits in response to bacterial and mycotic antigens in mice fed 50 mg selenite/kg body weight/day in a standard ration.[136] If the selenite was increased up to 2 mg/kg body weight per day, no stimulation of antibody synthesis was observed.

Shakelford and Martin, using retired male breeder mice (247 days old) given 1, 2, or 3 ppm Se or sodium selenite in their drinking water, found that there was a statistically significant increase of the anti-SRBC Ab titers of mice receiving 1 ppm Se in the drinking water over the control mice.[137] Mice receiving 3 ppm Se in their drinking water had titers that were significantly decreased from the control mice.

Koller et al. observed that selenium counteracts the immunosuppression that is produced by methylmercury. Mice fed, 1, 5, and 10 ppm methylmercury plus 6 ppm selenium significantly increased antibody synthesis.[138] Because methylmercury singly depresses antibody synthesis and the enhancement was greater than the increase by selenium alone, synergism between methylmercury and selenium occurred. These results indicate that environmental contaminants may not act in combination as anticipated.

Nutritional deficiencies in vitamin E and/or selenium caused impaired immune function, as measured by the humoral response to ovine erythrocytes (SRBC) by young chicks, but only at low antigen doses.[139] In the 2-week-old chick, optimum immune function required both vitamin E and selenium; however, at 3 weeks of age, either vitamin E or selenium was sufficient for optimum immune function. At this stage of development, selenium appeared capable of replacing vitamin E with regard to the immune system. Synergism of vitamin E in the presence of adequate selenium was not observed. The amounts of vitamin E and selenium were within nutritional and nonpharmacological levels. In contrast, high dietary selenium produced significant immune suppression in male but not female chicks.

Sheffy and Schultz have used dogs as their experimental animals and found that the humoral response could be influenced by selenium and vitamin E.[140] In addition, vaccination with a canine distemper infectious hepatitis virus vaccine resulted in lower antibody titers in animals deficient in selenium and vitamin E than in control animals. In the vitamin E and selenium-deficient animals there was a delayed appearance of measurable antibody titers following immunization. In these dogs the primary immune response to SRBC was unaffected, whereas it was the secondary response—the IgG anti-SRBC antibody levels—that were reduced in the deficient animals.

Cell-Mediated Immunity

Measurements of cell-mediated immunity are generally made by delayed hypersensitivity and graft-versus-host reactions *in vivo* as well as by mixed lymphocyte culture, mitogen stimulation, and assessment of helper, suppressor, and cytotoxic activity of T-cell *in vitro*. Sometimes antibody-dependent cell-mediated cytotoxicity, which requires K cells (surface Fe receptors) for cytotoxic expression, is used. Cell-mediated activity is also conveyed by soluble products of T-lymphocytes (lymphokines) of which there are many.

Martin and Spallholz fed female Hartley guinea pigs a commercial diet supplemented with 0, 1, 3, 5, or 7 ppm selenium of 4 weeks.[141] At that time each animal was sensitized intradermally with a 0.1% solution of DNCB in propylene glycol. After 10 days each animal was challenged by a serial dilution of DNCB (0.1–0.003%) in ethanol. Erythema and induration of the second challange was semiquantitatively assessed 24 and 48 hr later. The guinea pigs fed diets with 1–3 ppm selenium were more sensitive than the controls to the DNCB. The group of guinea pigs receiving 7 ppm selenium showed some increase of increased hypersensitivity, but this level of selenium was toxic with two of four guinea pigs dying and the remaining two showed much retarded growth.

High levels of glutathione peroxidase have been demonstrated in peritoneal exudate cells.[142] Phagocytic cells of selenium-deficient rats were capable of ingestion of yeast cells *in vitro*, but were unable to kill them. Boyne and Arthur have confirmed the observations obtained from selenium-deficient rats in selenium-deficient cattle. When the neutrophils were isolated from selenium-deficient rats, they were able to phagocytize *C. albicans*, but were less able to kill the ingested cells.[143] In the neutrophils of the selenium-deficient animals glutathione peroxidase activity was not dectable. In addition, reduced numbers of peritoneal macrophages were also noted in the exudates of rats.

The lymphocytes of vitamin E- and selenium-deficient dogs were found by Sheffy and Schultz to be completely suppressed and unresponsive to stimulation with the mitogens, concanavalin a, phytohemagglutinin, pokeweed mitogen, or streptolysin O.[140]

The addition of 50% mg Na_2SeO_4/kg body weight per day to the diets of mice and rabbits has been reported by Aleksondrovicz *et al.* to not only enhance antibody formation, but the selenium also shortened skin allograft rejection times.[136]

Nonspecific Immune Effects of Selenium

There have been several reports of nonspecific immune effects of selenium. Properdin, complement, and lysozyme, which are indexes of natural immunity, have been reported to be increased in the serum of rabbits administered 0.05 mg/kg selenium per day over a period of 92 days.[144] Leukocytes, phagocytic activity, and the bactericidal indexes were also increased in rabbits receiving subcutaneous selenite.[145] Berenshtein and Zdravoukhi reported increased serum levels of properdin, lysozyme and phagocytic activity of leukocytes after 14 daily subcutaneous injections of sodium selenite or sodium molybate, (0.05 mg/kg) to mice.[146]

Desowitz and Barnwell have demonstrated that selenium, administered in drinking water potentiates to protective effect of a killed *Plasmodium berghei* vaccine for Swiss-Webster mice.[147] In addition, they found that the P. berghei antigen combined with the adjuvant dimethyldioctadecyl ammonium bromide (DDAB) conferred a significantly high level of protective immunity. An additive effect was observed in that the greatest degree of protection was found in the group of mice maintained on selenium and vaccinated with antigen-DDAB. The challenging infection was survived by almost all of the animals treated in this manner.

Mulhern *et al.* (1981) divided C57BL/6J mice into four groups of six mice and fed them graded levels of selenium.[148] *In vitro* spleen lymphocyte stimulation was performed on all the groups with mitogens that selectively activate B cells and specific T-cell subpopulations. In addition, mixed lymphocyte reactions, cell-mediated lympholysis reactions, and direct plaque-forming cell response to sheep erythrocytes were determined on the spleen cells from all groups of mice. Significant differences were not observed in assays among any of the first generation animals. Offspring of the mice on the 0.0 ppm selenium diet had a reduced direct plaque-forming cell response to sheep erythrocytes when this group was compared to either the age-matched chow-fed animals and the first generation 0.0 ppm selenium-*Torula*-reared animals. The results of Mulhern *et al.* indicated that even though the different selenium diets do not affect the immune response of the first generation animals, they do affect their offspring.[148]

ZINC

Zinc is known to be an essential constituent of more than 100 enzymes and is essential for life. Because of its important function in nucleic acid polymerases, zinc plays a predominant role in nucleic acid metabolism, cell replication, tissue repair and growth. Marginal zinc deficiency is suspected to occur in a substantial number of infants and older children in the United States. In some areas of the world severe zinc deficiency can occur.

A pronounced zinc deficiency in both animals and humans results in depressed immune functions. Both tissue-mediated as well as humoral responses are affected. Impairment of delayed hypersensitivity reactions to *Candida albicans* in malnourished children can be made normal by topically applied zinc preparations, but it cannot be determined whether or to what degree immunocompetence is impaired by marginal zinc deficiency.[149]

Epidemiological Evidence

Soil Zinc Levels

Stocks and Davies have correlated cancer mortality with the zinc and copper content of soil in 12 districts of England and Wales.[150] Higher zinc levels as well as higher ratios of zinc to copper were found in the soil of vegetable gardens near houses in which a death from gastric cancer had occurred. Lower zinc levels were found in the soil of gardens near houses in which there was a death attributed to another cause. In addition, zinc levels near houses with deaths from other cancers did not differ from those of the noncancer households. These comparisons of soil zinc were made only when the deceased had resided in the same house for 10 or more years. Because the copper soil levels in the soil varied little, the difference may be attributed to zinc.

Per-Capita Zinc Intake

The per-capita food intake data were studied in 27 countries by Schrauzer *et al.*[151] They observed a direct correlation between the estimated zinc intake and age-adjusted mortality from leukemia and cancers of the intestine, breast, prostate, and skin. Because of these results and the inverse correlation between zinc and selenium concentrations in blood, Schrauzer *et al.* suggested that zinc may be increasing cancer risk by its antagonism of selenium.

Wheat and corn have been observed to be the primary dietary staples in many populations around the world which are at high risk for esophageal cancer.[152] Wheat and corn diets generally contain low concentrations of zinc, magnesium, nicotinic acid, and possibly riboflavin. A deficiency in one or more of these micronutrients may be related to esophageal cancer. In contrast, staples which have adequate levels of zinc are consumed in low-risk populations.

Blood and Other Body Tissue Zinc and Cancer

Blood Levels of Zinc. The mean zinc concentrations in pooled blood from healthy donors in 19 U.S. collection sites correlated directly with the corresponding mortality rates from cancers of the large bowel, breast, ovary, lung, bladder, and oral cavity.[151] Levels of zinc and selenium were correlated inversely with each other.

Marked changes also occur in the zinc content of leukocytes in patients with chronic leukemia. In these patients the zinc concentration of the peripheral leukocytes is greatly reduced and cannot be increased by zinc injection. However, in clinical remission, the zinc levels rise to normal levels. The zinc leukocyte content also decreases in patients with other neoplastic disease. Low serum, red blood cell and granulocyte and leukocyte zinc levels have also been observed in the blood of patients with cancer of the lung, and colon, but not in several other types of cancer.[153,154] Some investigators have even suggested this decrease might be used as a diagnostic test for cancer. However, hypozincemia is a nonspecific observation because decreased serum zinc levels have also been found in cirrhosis, hepatitis, lung infections including tuberculosis, myocardial infarction, renal insufficiency, diseases producing increased muscle metabolism, acute tissue injury, and in pregnant women. Steroid therapy, including administration of certain types of contraceptives, also are able to produce a hypozincemia.

Strain *et al.* compared zinc and copper levels in the serum of patients with bronchogenic cancer and the levels in the serum of controls.[155] Even though zinc levels did not differ between the two groups, the copper levels were lower in the controls, resulting in higher ratios of zinc to copper in the cancer patients.[156] Both serum copper and serum zinc levels were elevated in 19 patients with sarcomas. Patients with primary osteosarcomas had elevated serum zinc, those with metastases had depressed zinc levels, and amputees who were clinically tumor free had nearly normal serum zinc levels.

Lin *et al.* examined serum, hair, and tissues from Chinese men in Hong Kong for levels of zinc and other minerals.[157] The zinc levels in serum and diseased esophageal tissue from esophageal cancer patients were much lower than those in other cancer patients and in normal subjects. In addition, the serum of esophageal cancer patients also contained slightly elevated copper levels as well as much lower iron levels than the serum of normal subjects. The zinc levels of hair were also lower in the cancer patients than in normal patients.

Tissue Zinc Levels. Zinc levels are lower in certain types of human cancer tissue. Zinc levels are lower in malignant prostatic cancer than in normal prostate tissue, but zinc is increased in benign hypertrophied prostatic tissue.[158] The zinc concentration in normal liver in one study found to be about 78 μg/gm net weight, but the zinc content of the primary liver cancer itself was about 18 μg/gm.[159] Low zinc levels have also been reported in hepatic metastases from a variety of sources with greater than normal values in the liver with the cancer. Perhaps the lower amount of zinc may be due to the fact that patients with cancer excrete as much as three times more zinc in their urine than do normal persons.

Zinc levels have been reported to be higher in cancerous lung and breast tissue than normal tissue.[160] In one study the mean zinc concentration of breast cancer tissue was 5.7 times that of normal tissue the values in various patients were extremely variable. Low zinc levels have also been reported in hepatic metastases from a variety of sources with greater than normal values in the liver harboring the cancer.[161] Liver, kidney, and lung harboring metastases have a higher zinc content than does the corresponding normal tissue or the tumor itself. When tibias from normal individuals were compared with those with osteogenic sarcoma tissue significant differences in zinc concentrations were observed.[162] Forty control specimens had a mean value of 147.1 μg/gm dry weight, compared to 465.8 μg/gm in eight osteogenic specimens.

For some unknown reason, cancer in one organ may increase the zinc levels in another organ. Increased liver zinc concentrations have been found in patients with cancer.[163] In another study increased liver and kidney zinc have been found in patients with lung, gastric, and nasopharyngeal cancer.[164] Concentrations of liver zinc from patients dying from noncancerous disease have been reported to be similar to that of individuals dying in accidents. Zinc levels were also found to be greater in the kidney tissue of patients who died of cancer that affected other organs.[165] It is likely that the zinc concentrations in the organs not directly involved by the cancer rises as part of the normal tissues biochemical defense reaction to invasion by malignant cells. During the course of a fatal malignant disease, such an invasion is probably inevitable. Because zinc is necessary for the growth of normal tissue, it is likely a critical factor for tumor growth. Zinc has been demonstrated to be an important factor for the activities of reverse transcriptions as well as DNA-dependent RNA polymerase.

Experimental Evidence

Experiments in animals have demonstrated both enhancing and retarding effects of zinc on tumor growth.

Effect of Zinc Deficiency

Inhibition of Carcinogenesis. Several reports have suggested that a zinc deficiency strongly inhibits the growth of transplanted tumors in animals and also prolongs survival time. The initial studies by Petering et al. with transplanted Walker 256 carcinoma in rats were later confirmed by DeWys et al.[166,167] Zinc deficiency has also depressed the growth of P388 leukemia in weanling mice after the third post-transplantation day.[168] Growth of a transplantable hepatoma induced in rats by 3-methyl-4-dimethylaminoazobenzeme was significantly reduced in rats maintained on a low-zinc diet.[169] Ehrlich ascites tumors and plasmacytoma TEPC-183 have also been inhibited by a zinc deficiency. Beach et al. studied the effect of various dietary levels of zinc on Moloney sarcoma virus (MSV) oncogenesis.[170] Mice fed 2.5 ppm zinc demonstrated a decreased incidence of sarcomas and a reduction of tumor size. Feeding low-zinc diets for 6 weeks resulted in a marked reduction in sarcoma initiation and progression. However, mice fed 9 and 5 ppm zinc showed an increase in sarcoma growth. The results of these studies are consistent with the observation that rapidly growing tumor cells require zinc for growth.[171,172] These results do not suggest zinc deficiency as a therapeutic modality because zinc deficiency by itself, with or without concomitant malignancies, results in death of the animals.

Enhancement of Carcinogenesis. In contrast, there is one experiment showing that zinc deficiency enhances chemically induced carcinogenesis. Fong et al. observed that the incidence of esophageal tumors induced by nitrosomethylbenzylamine (NMBA) was significantly greater in zinc-deficient rats than in control rats. When the NMBA was intubated there was a 43% incidence in rats maintained on a zinc-deficient diet and a 15% incidence of carcinoma in control rats.[173] In two additional experiments the dose of NMBA was lowered. No cancer was produced in the control rats, but 83% and 33% were observed in the zinc-deficient animals in the two experiments.

Effect of Zinc Excess

On the other hand, aqueous zinc acetate injected intraperitoneally prevented tumor growth in 59–70% of BDF male mice previously inoculated intra-peritoneally with L1210 leukemia cells.[174] In a similar way, the subcutaneous injection of zinc has markedly suppressed the initiation of sarcoma 180 in mice.[175] However, aqueous zinc acetate injected subcutaneously did not prevent tumor growth in AKR/J mice inoculated intramuscularly with BW 5147 lymphatic leukemia cells.[176] Only a small but statistically significant increase in survival was noted in the latter mice. Zinc intake greatly exceeding nutritional requirements have inhibited Syrian hamster cheek pouch carcinogenesis induced by DMBA[177] and elevated zinc intake have inhibited the growth of a transplantable hepatoma induced by rats by 3-methyl-4-dimethylaminoazobenzene.[169] In contrast, Schrauzer has demonstrated that high concentrations of zinc (200 mg/liter) in the drinking water of C3H mice countered the protective effect against spontaneous mammary carcinoma and resulted in a significant increase in tumor growth.[178] Large amounts of zinc (10 mg/kg body weight) were added to the diet of mice and were found to protect against the induction of 20-methylcholanthrene (MCA)-induced sarcomas in mice.[179] Tumor incidence was found to be 45% in the MCA group with no supplementation and 15% in the MCA group with high supplementation.

Effect on the Immune Response

Zinc deficiency causes atrophy of the thymus as well as other lymphoid tissue and produces abnormalities in both cellular and humoral immunity.[180] Rats fed a zinc-deficient diet have a reduced antibody forming cell response.

Effect on T-cell Immunity. Zinc deficiency produces progressive thymic involution and progress loss of T-cell immunity in mice and rats.[21] The thymus glands of rats fed with zinc deficient diets weigh less than the controls. This reduction of thymic weight may be related to a reduced level of thymic hormone factor thymique system (FTS) whose levels drop progressively after the second week of zinc restriction. Zinc repletion restores normal FTS and thymphocyte function. In mice and humans, levels of FTS usually decline rapidly after onset of sexual maturation as the thymus involutes. When animals and patients are severely zinc deficient, FTS is suppressed, and delayed cutaneous hypersensitivity and skin graft rejections do not occur. If zinc sulfate is applied locally to the skin, responsiveness is apparently restored by direct absorption.[181]

Effect on Antibody Synthesis. Reduced antibody synthesis relating in part to interference with T-lymphocyte helper function may also occur in zinc deficiency.[182] If there is a nutritional repletion of zinc in zinc-restricted animals, thymus and T-cell-dependent antibody-mediated responses are restored. The thymus also has important regulatory roles in antibody synthesis, especially IgG. Zinc deficiency has been shown to result in the inhibition of the IgG response of A/J mice.[183] Mice that were zinc deficient had significant reductions in IgG and IgM production. However, after 4 days on the zinc adequate diet, mice were able to completely repair both the IgM and IgG responses.

Effect on B-cell Function. Zinc is able to promote B cell function by acting as a mitogen for animal and human lymphocytes.[184] The lymphocyte response to phytohemaglutinin, lipopolysaccharide, and concanavalin A is significantly increased by zinc treatment.[185] The beneficial effect of zinc supplementation on the lymphocytes may relate to DNA synthesis necessary for the production of B cell clones.

In addition, there are a number of patients with combined immunodeficiency related to zinc deprivation.[186] These patients have a combined deficiency in thymus cell immunity as well as antibody production. In some cases zinc supplements will correct the assorted gastrointestinal malfunctions, skin rashes, B- and T-cell abnormalities provided of course they were caused by a zinc deficiency. Zinc is also essential to the immune defense against bacterial infection probably due to its B-cell, T-cell macrophages and granulocytic function.

Effect of Excess Zinc on Immune Function. Excess zinc (and probably low zinc)when tested in in vitro inhibits the bactericidal and phagocytic function of macrophages and neutrophils.[180] Both low and high dosages of zinc inhibit the phagocytic capacity of mouse peritoneal macrophages. A parabolic correlation between leukocyte zinc content and neutrophil phagocytic capacity has been observed. Zinc-deficient animals also have impaired neutrophil phagocytic activity. In addition, some functions of granulocytes in prostatic fluid and prostate tissue are regulated by zinc.

Zinc also has a synergistic effect with the bactericidal action of streptonigrin, an antibiotic.[187] The bactericidal actions of zinc itself have been documented by several investigators. Human amniotic fluid that is rich in zinc is useful as an adjunct in wound healing and zinc is also essential for the activity of bacitracin.

Diminished levels of corticosterone may be responsible for the loss of immune responsiveness in zinc-deficient animals.[183] Whatever the precise mechanism it is clear that zinc is necessary for most functions of the immune system. Acrodermatitis enteropathica, which is an inborn error of zinc metabolism, is characterized by marked depressed T-cell activity, thymic hypoplasia and severe combined immunodeficiency. Serum levels of zinc are quite low but three to four times the normal zinc requirement by mouth corrects the condition.

The contradictory reports of the bimodal effect of zinc are not easily reconciled. There could be two different mechanisms of action by which zinc influences two different phases of carcinogenesis. Zinc, perhaps through its effect on the immune system, may be protective during the early phases of transformation, whereas the demonstrated role of zinc in cell proliferation may explain the protective effect of zinc deficiency against the growth of established tumors.

Few people have adequate zinc nutrition. The average American appears to ingest only 8.5 mg of the needed 15 mg RDA. Does marginal zinc deficiency, which appears to be widespread, especially among children, present a risk or provide protection against carcinogenesis.

COPPER

Copper is an essential nutrient that is widely distributed in foods. Public water supplies may be an additional source of copper. The average copper intake for U.S. adults is about 1 mg/day. About 95% of the copper is found in serum as part of the oxidative enzyme ceruloplasmin, which is an α_2-glycoprotein with a molecular weight of about 150,000. The remaining copper is present in an ionic form loosely bound to albumin.

Epidemiological Studies

Blood Correlations

Schrauzer *et al.* used pooled blood samples from healthy donors in 19 American states to correlate blood levels of copper with corresponding cancer mortality rates.[188] Weak direct associations were found for cancers of the intestine, breast, lung, and thyroid.

Per-Capita Intake Correlations

Schrauzer *et al.* also calculated the average concentrations of copper in major food items and international food consumption data, and correlated the per-capita intake of copper with cancer mortality in 27 countries.[188] Direct associations were found for leukemia and cancers of the intestine, breast, and skin. The apparent carcinogenicity might involve selenium antagonism, since large doses of copper produce symptoms of selenium deficiency in animals.

Serum Levels in Cancer Patients

In a study of 236 patients with a variety of malignant lymphomas (excluding Hodgkin's disease), significant increases in serum copper levels were related to disease activity.[189] The extent of the elevation appeared to be much greater in patients with generalized disease compared to those with localized disease. Higher levels were observed before therapy and if the therapy was successful, levels of copper were reduced to within normal levels during the remission. The elevated serum copper patterns were similar to the serum copper levels reported in 191 adult patients with Hodgkin's disease.[190] Patients whose Hodgkin's disease was in remission also had normal values. Elevations may occur 1–6 months before clinical evidence of relapse had occurred. Wilimas has found that monitoring serum copper levels in children was not that useful due to false elevations from other nonmalignant conditions, which included infection, thyrotoxicosis, congestive heart failure, rheumatic heart disease, and anemia.[191] Because of the increased frequencies of nonspecific infections in children, the measurement of serum copper levels may not be as reliable for children and adolescents as for adults.

Serum copper has also been found to be elevated in other forms of cancer including lung cancer (43 of 71 patients), squamous cell carcinoma of the larynx (10 of 67 patients), cervical and gynecological cancer, gastric, osteosarcoma, bladder, breast cancer (23 of 23 patients), melanoma, and non-Hodgkin's lymphoma, but not in prostate cancer.[192] Ceruloplasmin was also found to be increased in primary lung cancer.

Delves et al. have reported elevated serum copper in acute leukemia and a decline in serum copper associated with a therapeutic response.[193]

Tissue Levels in Cancer Patients

Zinc: copper ratios are decreased in all neoplastic kidney tissues.[194] Copper levels also significantly elevated in malignant cervical and endometrial tumors and in malignant melanomas.[195] Malignant tumors of the cervix and corpus uteri had a significant increase of copper, zinc, and magnesium when compared with normal tissues.[196]

Lefkowitch et al. analyzed tissue from a fibrolamellar liver cell carcinoma by several staining and spectrophotometric methods have demonstrated elevated copper and copper-binding protein (CBP) in malignant hepatocytes. Identification of CBP in liver cell carcinoma indicates that it may be a synthetic product of malignant cells, however, mild CBP elevation may also be observed in various chronic liver diseases.[197]

Effect on the Immune Response of Mice

An impaired humoral-mediated immune response (decreased numbers of antibody producing cells) is observed in mice with severe as well as marginal copper deficiency.[198] The magnitude of this impairment can be correlated with the degree of functional copper deficiency (hypoceruloplasminemia).

Effect on Chemically Induced Liver Tumors

Several studies have demonstrated that high levels of copper salts added to the diets of animals provided various degree of protection against chemically induced liver tumors. By adding 9.25% cupric acetate to the diet, DL-ethionine-induced liver carcinogenesis was inhibited in rats.[199] Copper also protects rat liver from damage resulting from treatment with p-dimethylaminoazobenzene, thioacetamide, 3-methoxy-4-aminoazobenzene or its N-methyl derivatives, 2-acetamidofluorene, α-naphthylisothiocyanate, or dimethylnitrosoamine. Since these effects were obtained with extremely high concentrations of copper (0.3–0.6% copper acetate in the diet) and since similar results were found when manganese or nickel were substituted for copper,[200] the action of copper may be pharmacologic, perhaps toxic in nature and nonspecific.

IRON

There are a large number and diversity of enzymes that contain iron or that depend on the presence of this metal for activity. Some of the better-known groups of enzymes include electron transport proteins, iron flavoproteins, hydroperoxidases, and oxygenases. In addition, iron catalyzes a variety of miscellaneous enzymes such as aconitase and tryptophane pyrrolase. Iron also plays a crucial role in initiation and maintenance of DNA synthesis; for example, iron is a cofactor of ribonucleotide diphosphate reductase. Iron is also necessary in animal systems for erythropoiesis, granulopoiesis, collagen synthesis, corticosteroids and prostaglandins.

Epidemiological Evidence

Iron Deficiency

Cancers of the upper alimentary tract including the esophagus and stomach have been associated with iron deficiency. Iron deficiency in Sweden was associated with Plummer-Vinson (Paterson-Kelly) syndrome, which in turn was associated with an increased risk for cancer of the upper alimentary tract.[201] Improvements in nutrition, especially with regard to iron and vitamins in the diet, has been associated with the almost complete elimination of new cases of Plummer-Vinson disease in areas of Sweden where it had formerly been highly endemic.

Iron-deficient patients with antecedent lesions of gastric carcinoma in an area of Columbia with high risk for gastric cancer have been studied by Broitman *et al.*[202] They associated the chronic atrophic gastritis resulting from iron deficiency with hypochlorhydria and achlorhydria, which permitted bacterial colonization of the stomach and also postulated that these bacteria could reduce ingested nitrate to nitrite, thus leading to the formation of nitrosamines that are known to be carcinogenic in the stomach of laboratory animals and are suspected of being carcinogenic in humans. Ruddell *et al.* suggested a similar mechanism to explain the increased risk of gastric cancer in patients with pernicious anemia.[203]

Iron Excess

Even though there have been no epidemiological reports of cancer associated with increased dietary intake of iron, heavy inhalation exposure to high levels of iron oxide has been related to increased risk for lung and laryngeal cancers in iron ore miners, metal workers, and workers in iron foundries.[204] In addition, sarcomata have developed in patients at sites of injection of iron–dextran solutions.[205] There also have been many clinical reports which have associated hemochromatosis with an increased risk for hepatomas and possibly other hepatic and extrahepatic cancers.[206]

Experimental Evidence

Effect on Carcinogenesis

Mice have been protected from the hepatocellular and porphyric toxicity due to 2,3,7,8-tetrachlorodibenzo-p-dioxin (TCDD).[207] It was not determined whether such protection might extend to the teratogenic or possibly carcinogenic action of TCDD. In another study rats were made severely deficient in iron through manipulation of their diet. These iron deficient rats became anemic and developed fatty livers, but were devoid of any neoplastic lesions.[208] In the same study, iron-deficient rats were given 1,2-dimethylhydrazine. Neoplastic lesions developed in their livers within 4 months, as opposed to 6 months in the iron-sufficient group. The authors suggested that severe lack of iron may possibly function as a cocarcinogen.

Effect on Mutagenesis

Fe(II) as iron sulfate has induced reverse mutations in *Salmonella typhimurium* strains TA1537 and TA1538 with the S9 fraction of various species.[209] In nonactivated suspensions, weak mutagenic activity has also been observed.

Effect on Immunity

Joynson *et al.* tested the peripheral lymphocytes from twelve subjects with iron-deficient anemia.[210] These tests revealed an impairment of lymphocyte transformation and migration inhibition factor production on stimulation with *Candida* antigen and purified protein derivative. The intradermal injection of these antigens produced a delayed hypersensitivity skin reaction in only a small number of iron-deficient subjects. The data of Joynson *et al.* suggest that iron deficiency may be a factor in the production or potentiation of immunodeficient states. On the surface these results seem to justify iron supplementation; however, iron in excessive amounts actually increases infectiousness of pathogens.

MOLYBDENUM

Epidemiological Evidence

A few reports have indirectly implicated molybdenum deficiency in the etiology of cancer, especially cancer of the esophagus. In China, Yang has reported that correlation analyses by county have shown an inverse association of esophageal cancer with the levels of molybdenum and a variety of other metals in the soil.[211] Molybdenum levels in the serum, hair, and urine were low in areas at high risk for this cancer. The molybdenum content in surgically removed esophageal cancer specimens was significantly lower than those in normal esophageal tissues. In addition, low levels of molybdenum in the soil have been observed in a region of Africa with high mortality rates from esophageal cancer.[212] Furthermore, low molybdenum levels in water supplies have been correlated with excess esophageal cancer mortality in the United States.[213]

Supplementation of the soil with ammonium molybdate has been found to increase the molybdenum and ascorbic acid content of locally produced grains and vegetables and to decrease their nitrate and nitrite concentration.[214] Luo *et al.* have proposed that high ascorbic acid and decreased nitrate and nitrite content of vegetables could decrease the high incidence of esophogeal cancer in these areas.

Experimental Evidence

Effect on Carcinogenesis Animals

The effect of molybdenum supplementation on the induction of tumors by *N*-nitrososarcosine in the esophagus and forestomach of Sprague-Dawley rats was studied by Luo *et al.*[214] They observed that tumor incidence in the group supplemented with molybdenum (2 mg/liter drinking water) was lower than that of the control group, whose diet contained a molybdenum concentration of 26-μg/kg diet. Molybdenum added to the drinking water (10 ppm) has significantly inhibited *N*-methyl-*N*-nitrosourea-induced mammary carcinogenesis in female rats.[215] A significant increase in the number of lung adenomas in strain A mice were observed when they were given molybdenum in the form of molybdenum oxide.[216] Molybdenum dichloride has antineoplastic properties that inhibit the growth of Ehrlich ascites tumors in mice.[217] Molybdenum is also a biological antagonist of copper which seems to be increased in many types of cancers.

Effect on Mutagenesis

Molybdenum as potassium molybdate and ammonium molybdate was positive in *Bacillus subtilis rec* assay.[218] In addition, Nishioka has also observed that ammonium molybdate was mutagenic in *Escherichia coli*.[218]

IODINE

Iodine is an essential micronutrient in the diet and is an integral component of thyroid hormones. Dietary deficiency of iodine is associated with enlargement of the thyroid gland and endemic goiter, but this deficiency disease does not occur commonly in the United States.

The average daily intake of iodine in the United States is estimated to range from about 60–680 μg/day. The lower level is adequate to meet the minimum daily requirements of 50 μg, and many diets furnish iodine in excess of the recommended daily allowance of 150 μg. The iodinization of table salt, the use of iodine in disinfectants, and the addition of iodate to dough conditioners have contributed to the marked reduction in iodine deficiency in the United States.

Epidemiological Evidence

Thyroid Cancer

Wahner *et al.* concluded that thyroid cancer occurred more frequently in Cali, Columbia (an area of endemic goiter) than in New York state or Puerto

Rico.[219] Williams *et al.* compared the incidence and histological types of thyroid cancer in two contrasting populations: Icelanders with high-iodine diets and Scots from northeast Scotland with normal levels of dietary iodine.[220] On the basis of a pathological review of all surgical thyroid specimens in both studies, the incidence of papillary carcinoma and the ratio of papillary to follicular carcinomas was higher in the high-dietary iodine areas than in the low-dietary iodine areas.

Two studies have found no associations with exposure to iodine. In Australia there was no difference between the observed and expected deaths from thyroid cancer by state, despite the fact that iodine intakes varied and endemic goiter was particularly prevalent in Tasmania.[221] Thyroid cancer mortality rates by state in the United States have been compared with the corresponding prevalence rates of endemic goiter and no association was found between the two diseases.[222] In this study secular trends in mortality from these two diseases were also examined and a decline was found in the endemic goiter rates but not in thyroid cancer rates in the United States during the previous 30-year period. However, the mortality data used in both studies can be misleading for thyroid cancer and other cancers that have high survival rates.

Breast Cancer

Breast cancer in females is a second type of cancer associated with iodine deficiency. Cancer mortality by state in the United States have also been compared with the prevalence of endemic goiter.[223] A direct association was found between the two diseases. On investigator has noted that breast cancer in females is highly correlated with endometrial and ovarian cancer and postulated that low iodine intake may be etiologically related to all three cancers.[224] However, the results of many other studies did not support this hypothesis. Conflicting data have been reported from sub-Saharan Africa, where these three cancers are rare despite very low levels of dietary iodine.[225] In addition, in Hawaii and Iceland where iodine intake is high, there are also high incidence rates for breast cancer.[226]

Experimental Evidence

Iodine deficiency has been reported to produce hyperplastic changes in the breast tissue of female rats during puberty.[227] Because of the epidemiological associations indicating a higher incidence of mammary carcinoma in areas of endemic goiter, the influence of iodine deficiency, on mammary tissue when the thyroid was maintained in a normal state was studied by Eskin.[228] Displastic changes of the epithelium occurred during deficiency. These changes were aggravated by estrogen treatment and advanced to preneoplastic and neoplastic conditions. Supplementation with inorganic iodine reversed these changes, but high doses of thyroxine increased the dysplastic changes. Eskin concluded that iodine deficiency itself rather than the hypothyroidism was responsible for these effects and also demonstrated similar changes by blocking iodine uptake with perchlorate. When the blockade was terminated or when iodine was supplemented, most but not all the hyperplastic tissue changes returned to normal. When the prepubescent rats were made iodine deficient, they were more susceptible to earlier appearance of DMBA-induced mammary tumors, suggesting a cocarcinogenic effect of iodine deficiency.

The ratios of DNA to RNA have been demonstrated to be much higher in the breast of iodine-deficient rats than those for control rats.[229] In iodine-deficiency alterations have been observed in the estrogen receptor protein which suggests that mammary tumorigenesis may be stimulated in the presence of estrogen and higher physiological levels of its receptor. When iodine-deficient animals have been exposed to a carcinogen such as 2-AAF or to thyroid irradiation increased yields of malignant thyroid tumors have been reported.[230]

MANGANESE

Manganese is involved with glycosyltransferase as well as other enzymes, including those needed for chondroitin sulfate synthesis and connective tissue metabolism.[231] Manganese may also be important in gluconeogenesis through its presence in the metalloenzyme pyruvate decarboxylase.

Levels in Malignant Tissue

Malignant breast tissue has been shown to have much greater manganese concentrations than is found in the corresponding normal tissue.[160] In nine patients, normal tissue ranged from 7.2 to 24 μg/gm, whereas the malignant tissue ranged from 10 to 55 μg/gm. In all cases, the concentration of the malignant tissue was greater than in normal controls. In osteogenic sarcoma manganese was also significantly higher than in normal tibia.

Effect on Carcinogenesis

The effects of Mn dusts on carcinogenesis induced by the polycyclic aromatic hydrocarbons benzpyrene and DMBA have been tested in male Fischer 344 rats.[232] At 100 weeks, sarcomas occurred at the injection site in 17 of 20 rats that received benzpyrene alone, whereas 10 of 19 rats receiving benzpyrene plus manganese dust had tumors ($p < 0.05$). Under identical conditions, however, Mn dust did not affect the carcinogenicity of DMBA. In another study, Mn dust inhibited the carcinogenesis of nickel subsulfide, Ni_3S_2, which was administered intramuscularly to Fischer rats. The incidence of carcinomas within 2 years after injection of Ni_3S_2 plus manganese was 7% compared with 77% in rats that received only Ni_3S_2.[233]

There was significantly less sarcoma incidence in rats receiving intramuscular injections of benzpyrene and manganese dust than in rats receiving benzpyrene alone.[234]

After feeding manganeous acetate to rats, there was an inhibition of the hepatocarcinogenesis induced by 3-methyl-4-dimethylaminoazobenzene (MeDAB).[235] At the end of 5 months the hepatoma incidence was 40% (7 of 18) in rats fed MeDAB alone, versus 0% (0 of 21) in rats fed MeDAB plus manganous acetate. The manganese inhibition of MeDAB carcinogenesis may be mediated through enhanced enzymatic reduction of MeDAB to noncarcinogenic metabolites. Manganese ion may divert MeDAB from its usual metabolic conversion to more electrophilic compounds that bind to macromolecules. Manganese may also have an antitumor effect through an enhancement of aryl hydrocarbon hydroxylase activity which is an enzyme responsible for the conversion of aryl hydrocarbons to less carcinogenic forms.

Mechanism of Action

Manganese may exert its anticarcinogenic effect by activating superoxide dismutase. Without manganese the mitochondrial dismutase would be inactive and would accumulate superoxide anion, which may be mutagenic or carcinogenic.

Manganous ion has also been found to inhibit the *in vitro* binding to macromolecules in microsomal suspensions containing added DNA. Manganous ion also seems to have an apparently specific differential inhibitory effect on lymphocyte activation.

FLUORIDE

There has been a great deal of interest in a possible relationship between community water fluoridation and cancer mortality. Some of the early studies reported on cancer mortality in 20 United States cities, one-half of which fluoridated their water supplies during 1952–1956.[236] In 1950 the crude mortality rates for cities with fluoridated water supplies was almost equal to the rates in the cities with nonfluoridated supplies. By 1970 there was a differential of some 20 deaths per 100,000 with higher rates being in the cities with fluoridated water. Reanalysis of these data pertaining to these cities[237] and a similar study of cancer mortality in selected countries in the United States with fluoridated and non-fluoridated water systems did not support these early data.[238] When age, sex, and ethnic status were considered, the ratio between the observed and expected cancer mortality declined in the fluoridated cities and did not change in the nonfluoridated cities. In addition, the proportion of the non-White population and the proportion of the White population age 65 years and over increased more rapidly in the fluoridated than the nonfluoridated cities.

In another study, mortality trends from all causes in 473 United States cities were studied for the period 1950–1970.[239] Heart, kidney and cancer mortality were specifically evaluated with respect to fluoridation status. The fluoridated cities showed an 8% increase in cancer mortality ratio, while the nonfluoridated cities have a 7% increase. There were no consistent or significant relationships between fluoridation and changes in either cancer, heart, or general mortality during the 20-year period.

Erickson has evaluated 24 fluoridated and 22 nonfluoridated cities from 1969 to 1971 and analyzed the data for all causes of cancer in Blacks and Whites. When data were adjusted for age, sex, race, population density, and medium education, there was no evidence of an association that could be attributed to fluoridation.[240]

Oldham and Newell reported that the two groups of cities in the original study differed in their age–sex–race structure in 1950. In addition, fluoridated cities had an excess of cancer deaths of 10.3 : 100,000 population in 1950. However, in 1970, the demographic structure differ much more than it had in 1950. More non-Whites lived in the fluoridated cities. In addition, when demographic changes were considered, the excess cancer rate increased by 1% during 20 years in the fluoridated cities, but increased by 4% during 20 years in the unfluoridated control cities. They conclude that there is no evidence relating fluoridation of U.S. water supplies with cancer.

Taves has evaluated cancer mortality from ten sites and calculated standardized mortality ratios for the periods 1949–1951, 1959–1961, and 1969–1971 in 10 of the largest fluoridated cities left out of the original study and five nonfluoridated cities omitted from the original 15 largest nonfluroidated cities.[241] There was no difference in the standardized mortality rates between the fluoridated and nonfluroidated cities.

MAGNESIUM

A study of the incidence and fine structure of thymic tumors developing in magnesium-deficient rats showed 19 tumors among 92 rats after an average of 65 days of deficiency.[242] All the tumors were classified as malignant lymphoma or lymphosarcoma and developed initially in the thymus.[243] No tumors developed in any control animal receiving the same diet with added magnesium. The thymus glands from female Wistar rats fed magnesium-deficient diets, were strongly degenerated and the number of lymphocytes was reduced especially in the cortex. Thymus degeneration was associated with a decreased rate of DNA, RNA, and protein biosynthesis and necrosis and phagocytosis of lymphocytes. The degeneration was reversed after feeding a magnesium-rich diet. After 10 or 11 weeks of magnesium deficiency, local cell proliferations of immature lymphocytes with a great number of free ribosomes were found in some thymus glands. The local cell proliferations developed into infiltrating tumors without metastases.

In another study, weanling rats on control diets or a diet deficient in magnesium and/or potassium for 1–3 weeks were transplanted with Yoshida or Walker tumors.[244] Up to 40% reduction in tumor size occurred in magnesium deficiency, potassium deficiency (30–60%), and combined deficiency (45–85%). Tumor size showed the best correlation with the combined concentration of plasma Mg and K or muscle K. Organ weights and tissue biochemistry showed that metabolic differences between control and cation deficient rats were due mainly to cation deficiency and the growth of the tumor rather than other nutritional deficiencies.

Mills *et al.* observed that a preconditioned magnesium deficiency will retard the growth of tumors implanted into rats and also tested whether magnesium depletion initiated after tumors were well established would also effectively inhibit their growth.[245] They implanted mammary adenocarcinoma into Fischer 344 rats divided into two groups, and one group was placed on a magnesium-deficient diet. The magnesium-deficient rats were compared with the magnesium-sufficient rats and had the following: 46% lower tumor weight ($p < 0.05$) and 50% greater tumor necrosis ($p < 0.05$). Concentrations of magnesium in the tumor were 39% lower ($p < 0.0005$) and in the plasma 83% lower ($p < 0.0005$).

POTASSIUM

Potassium-deficient rats transplanted with Yoshida or Walker tumors exhibited a 30–60% reduction in tumor size. In a combined deficiency of magnesium and potassium, a 45–85% reduction in tumor size was observed.

ARSENIC, CADMIUM, AND LEAD

It is unlikely that these metals are carcinogenic at the levels ordinarily found in the diet. However, these metals are carcinogenic if large amounts are administered through other routes. However, both lead and arsenic have been observed to counteract the beneficial effect to selenium against spontaneously induced breast cancer.

MIXTURES OF METALS

Two of the combinations of metals that may be taken in the diet and that are carcinogenic are asbestos and talc.

Asbestos

Nickel, lead, and chromium are all found in high concentration in asbestos and many of their compounds are carcinogenic.[246] The asbestos and meso-thelioma relationship is well defined. Apparently the fibrous silicates of asbestos are the main vehicle carrying the potentially carcinogenic metals into the lungs. However, some asbestos could be taken in the food and the water.

Some of the water-soluble nickel salts have been shown to be carcinogenic. A direct relationship seems to exist between the degree of carcinogenicity and its water solubility. These water-soluble nickel salts inhibit benzpyrene hydroxylase in lungs which may allow accumulation of benzpyrene in these tissues thereby enhancing tumor development. The carcinogenicity of chromium seems to depend on the valence state. Trivalent chromium has not been shown to be carcinogenic and its relatively nontoxic, while the hexavalent chromium has been shown to be carcinogenic in lung tissue. Even though lead is present in large amounts in asbestos, its role in the development of lung cancer has not been established. Dietary lead acetate at relatively high levels has been shown to cause tumors in rats. Due to the heavy environmental pollution with lead, further experimentation with different concentrations of lead should be taking place.

Talc

Chemistry

Talc is a pure chemical compound consisting of hydrous magnesium silicate, $Mg_3Si_4O_{10}(OH)_2$, made up of a brucite sheet containing magnesium ions sandwiched between two silica sheets held together by relatively weak forces. Other elements such as nickel and iron may be included in the talc particle lattice, but are so bound within the particle that they are not free to exert any biological action.

Gastric Cancer

The high gastric cancer rate in Japan may be related to talc-dusted rice.[247] Talc frequently contains asbestos and workmen exposed to asbestos show a marked increase in gastrointestinal cancer. Rice grown in California and meant for the American consumer is milled mechanically. Rice is prepared differently for the Japanese consumer. The rice is milled and treated with glucose, and then talc is added. The talc particle is held to the surface of the grain and is believed to better preserve the flavor and prolong shelf life. Japanese consider rice prepared in this way more tasty, both in the United States and in Japan.

Two percent of all talc produced in California from 1959 to 1963 was used as a rice additive, primarily for export to Japan. Optical microscopy of the ash of such store-bought rice showed about 3.7×10^6 asbestos form fibers per gram.

The incidence of gastric cancer in Japanese males in Japan was 77.9 per 100,000. Japanese men in Hawaii had an incidence of only 45 per 100,000. Dietetic studies on immigrant Japanese show that 50–70% of their diet is Japanese-type food. The longer the immigrant has lived in the West the more western his diet becomes; this increase in Western food in the diet parallels a decrease in the incidence of stomach cancer.

Stemmermann et al. have reputed the earlier study.[248] They found that Hawaiian Japanese do consume coated rice almost exclusively, but indigenous Japanese do not. The authors point out that the sale of talc-coated rice has been prohibited in Japan since enactment of a Food Sanitation law in 1947. In addition, Filipinos consumed the greatest amount of talc-coated rice, but had the lowest gastric cancer rates.

Esophageal Cancer

Millet bran is a component of the diet in the area of highest esophageal cancer incidence in northern China.[249] Millet bran was found to contain as much as 20% by weight of silica; some of this silica occurs as friable sheets or sharply-pointed fibers. These types of silica in millet-bran are the likely source of the silica fragments found in the esophageal mucosa surrounding tumors in patients in northern China. Silica fragments and fibers of similar size originating from other plant species also occur in the diet in the two other regions of greatest incidence of esophageal cancer, the Transkei in Africa, and Iran.

O'Neill et al. have examined the seeds of more than sixty different species of weed known to contaminate the wheat in Northeastern Iran.[250] The fiber was found to originate from the seeds of the common Mediterranean grass Phalaris minor. The fibers are broken off from the seed when the wheat is milled but persist in the flour where up to 3000 are found in each gram.

Ovarian Cancer

The effect of genital exposure to talc has been assessed in 215 White females with epithelial ovarian cancers and in 215 control women from the general population matched by age, race and residence.[251] Ninety-two (42.8%) cases regularly used talc either as a dusting powder on the perinuum or on sanitary napkins compared with 61 (28.4%) controls. When parity and menopausal status was considered, this difference yielded a relative risk of 1.02 ($p <$ 0.003) for ovarian cancer associated with these practices. Women who had regularly engaged in both practices had an adjusted risk of 3.28 ($p < 0.001$) compared with women with neither exposure.

REFERENCES

1. Schroeder, H. A., Balassa, J. J., and Vinton, W. H. 1964. Chromium, lead, cadmium, nickel and titanium in mice: Effect on mortality, tumors and tissue levels. *J. Nutr. 83:*239–250.
2. Schroeder, H. A., Mitchener, M., Balassa, J. J., Kanisawa, M., and Nason, A. P. 1968. Zirconium, niobium, antimony and fluorine in mice: Effect on growth, survival and tissue levels. *J. Nutr. 95:*95–101.
3. Schroeder, H. A., and Mitchener, M. 1971. Scandium, chromium (VI), gallium, yttrium, rhodium, palladium and indium in mice: Effects on growth and life span. *J. Nutr. 101:*1431–1438.
4. Schroeder, H. A., and Mitchener, M. 1972. Selenium and tellurium in mice: Effects on growth, survival and tumors. *Arch. Environ. Health 24:*66–71.
5. Shamberger, R. J., and Rudolph, G. 1966. Protection against cocarcinogenesis by antioxidants. *Experientia 22:*116.
6. Riley, J. F. 1968. Mast cells, cocarcinogenesis and anti-carcinognesis in the skin of mice. *Experientia 15:*1237–1238.
7. Shamberger, R. J. 1970. Relationship of selenium to cancer. I. Inhibitory effect of selenium on carcinogenesis. *J. Natl. Cancer Inst. 44:*931–936.
8. Shamberger, R. J. 1972. Increase of peroxidation in carcinogenesis, *J. Nat. Cancer Inst. 48:*1491–1497.
9. Shamberger, R. J., Andreone, T. L., and Willis, C. E. 1974. Antioxidants and cancer. IV. Initiating activity of malonaldehyde as a carcinogen. *J. Natl. Cancer Inst. 53:*1771–1773.
10. Clayton, C. C., and Baumann, C. A. 1949. Diet and azo dye tumors: Effect of diet during a period when the dye is not fed. *Cancer Res. 9:*575–582.
11. Griffin, A. C., and Jacobs, M. M. 1977. Effects of selenium on azo dye hepatocarcinogenesis. *Cancer Lett. 3:*177–181.
12. Daoud, A. H., and Griffin, A. C. 1980. Effect of retinoic acid, butylated hydroxytoluene, selenium and sorbic acid on azo-dye hepatocarcinogenesis. *Cancer Lett. 9:*299–304.
13. Balanski, R. M., and Hadsiolov, D. H. 1979. Influence of sodium selenite on the hepatocarcinogenic action of diethylnitrosamine in rats. *Comptes Rendus Acad. Bulg. Sci. 32:*697–698.
14. Dzhoiev, F. D. 1978. Effect of selenium, phenobarbital, teturam, and carbon tetrachloride on the carcinogenic effect of diethylnitrosamine and 1,2-dimethylhydrazine. in G. O. Loogna (Ed.) *Kantserog N-Nitrozonsoedin: Deistvie, Obraz., Opred., Mater Simp.*, 3rd Tallinn, USSR, pp. 51–53.
15. Harr, J. R., Exon, J. H., Weswig, P. H., and Whanger, P. D. 1973. Relationship of dietary selenium concentration; chemical cancer induction; and tissue concentration of selenium in rats. *Clin. Toxicol. 8:*487–495.

16. Harr, J. R., Exon, J. H., Whanger, P. D., and Weswig, P. H. 1972. Effect of dietary selenium on N-2 fluorenyl-acetamide (FAA)-induced cancer in vitamin E supplemented, selenium depleted rats. *Clin. Toxicol. 5:*187–194.

17. Marshall, M. V., Arnott, M. S., Jacobs, M. M., and Griffin, A. C. 1979. Selenium effects on the carcinogenicity and metabolism of 2-acetylaminofluorene. *Cancer Lett. 7:*331–338.

18. Lotliker, P. D., Enomoto, M., Miller, J. A., and Miller, E. C. 1967. Species variations in the N- and ring-hydroxylation of 2-acetylaminofluorene and effects of 3-methylcholanthrene pretreatment. *Proc. Soc. Exp. Biol. Med. 125:*341–346.

19. Lotliker, P. D., Hong, Y. S., and Baldy, W. L. 1978. Effects of 3-methylcholanthrene pretreatment on 2-acetylaminofluorene N- and ring-hydroxylation by rat and hamster liver microsomes. *Toxicol. Lett. 2:*135–139.

20. Rasco, M. A., Jacobs, M. M., and Griffin, A. C. 1977. Effects of selenium on aryl hydrocarbon hydroxylase activity in cultured human lymphocytes. *Cancer Lett. 3:*295–301.

21. Wortzman, M. S., Besbris, H. J., and Cohen, A. M. 1980. Effect of dietary selenium on the interaction between 2-acetylaminofluorene and rat liver DNA *in vivo. Cancer Res. 40:*2670–2676.

22. Besbris, H. J., Wortzman, M. S., and Cohen, A. M. 1982. Effect of dietary selenium on the metabolism and excretion of 2-acetylaminofluorene in the rat. *J. Toxicol. Environ. Heath 9:*63–76.

23. Chen, J., Goetchius, M. P., Combs, G. F., and Campbell, T. C. 1982. Effects of dietary selenium and vitamin E on covalent binding of aflatoxin to chick liver cell macromolecules. *J. Nutr. 112:*350–355.

24. Lalor, J. H., and Llewellyn, G. C. 1981. Biointeraction of sodium selenite and aflatoxin B_1 in the mongolian gerbil. *J. Toxicol. Environ. Health 8:*387–400.

25. Jacobs, M. M., Jansson, B., and Griffin, A. C., 1977. Inhibitory effects of selenium on 1,2-dimethylhydrazine and methylazoxymethanol acetate induction of colon tumors. *Cancer Lett. 2:*133–138.

26. Jacobs, M. M., Forst, C. F., and Beams, F. A. 1981. Biochemical and clinical effects of selenium on dimethylhydrazine-induced colon cancer in rats. *Cancer Res. 41:*4458–4465.

27. Ankerst, J., and Sjorgren, H. O. 1982. Effect of selenium on the induction of breast fibroadenomas by adenovirus type 9 and 1,2-dimethylhydrazine-induced bowel carcinogenesis in rats. *Int. J. Cancer 29:*707–710.

28. Soullier, B. K., Wilson, P. S., and Nigro, N. D. 1981. Effect of selenium on azoxymethane-induced intestinal cancer in rats fed high fat diet. *Cancer Lett. 12:*343–348.

29. Harbach, P. R., and Swenberg, J. A. 1981. Effects of selenium on 1,2-dimethylhydrazine metabolism and DNA alkylation. *Carcinogenesis 2:*575–580.

30. Banner, W. P., Tan, Q. H., and Zadeck, S. 1981. Studies of the mechanism by which selenium inhibits tumor formation. *Proc. Am. Assoc. Cancer Res. 22:*115.

31. Schrauzer, G. N., and Ishmael, D. 1974. Effects of selenium and of arsenic on the genesis of spontaneous mammary tumors in inbred C_3H mice. *Ann. Clin. Lab. Sci. 4:*411–447.

32. Schrauzer, G. N., White, D. A., and Schneider, C. J. 1976. Inhibition of the genesis of spontaneous mammary tumors in C_3H mice: Effects of selenium and of selenium antagonistic elements and their possible role in human breast cancer, *Bioinorg. Chem. 6:*265–270.

33. Schrauzer, G. N., White, D. A., and Schneider, C. J. 1978. Selenium and cancer: Effects of selenium and of the diet on the genesis of spontaneous mammary tumors in virgin inbred female C_3H/St mice. *Bioinorg. Chem. 8:*387–396.

34. Wester, P. O., Brune, D., and Nordberg, G. 1981. Arsenic and selenium in lung, liver and kidney tissue from dead smelter workers, *Br. J. Indust. Med. 38:*179–184.

35. Shamberger, R. J., and Bratush, C. M. 1980. Cadmium, selenium and zinc levels in kidneys. *Trace Sub. Environ. Health* Hemphill, D. D., (ed.), Univ. Missouri, Columbia XIV:203–210.

36. Schrauzer, G. N., Kuehn, K., and Hamm, D. 1981. Effects of dietary selenium and lead on the genesis of spontaneous mammary tumors in mice. *Biol. Trace Elem. Res. 3:*185–196.

37. Schrauzer, G. N., McGinness, J. E., and Kuehn, K. 1980. The effects of temporary selenium supplementation on the genesis of spontaneous mammary tumors in inbred female $C_3H/St.$ mice. *Carcinogenesis 1:*199–201.

38. Thompson, H. J., and Becci, P. J. 1980. Selenium inhibition of N-methyl-N-nitrosourea-induced mammary carcinogenesis in the rat. *J. Natl. Cancer Inst. 65:*1299–1301.

39. Thompson, H. J., Meeker, L. D., and Becci, P. J. 1981. Effect of combined selenium and retinyl acetate treatment on mammary carcinogenesis. *Cancer Res. 41:*1413–1416

40. Thompson, H. J., and Tagliaferro, A. R. 1980. Effect of selenium on 7,12-dimethylbenzanthracene-induced mammary tumorigenesis. *Fed. Proc. 39:*1117.

41. Thompson, H. J., Meeker, L. D., Becci, P. J., and Kokoska, S. 1982. Effect of short-term feeding of sodium selenite on 7,12-dimethylbenzanthracene-induced mammary carcinogenesis in the rat. *Cancer Res. 42:*4954–4958.

42. Ip, C., and Sinha, D. K. 1981. Enhancement of mammary tumorigenesis by dietary selenium deficiency in rats with a high polyunsaturated diet. *Cancer Res. 41:*31–34.

43. Ip, C. 1981. Factors influencing the anticarcinogenic efficacy of selenium in dimethylbenzanthracene-induced mammary tumorigenesis in rats. *Cancer Res. 41:*2683–2686.

44. Ip, C., 1981, Prophylaxis of mammary neoplasia by selenium supplementation in the initiation and promotion phases of chemical carcinogenesis. *Cancer Res. 41:*4386–4390.

45. Spallholz, J. E., Martin, J. L., Gerlach, M. L., and Heizerling, R. H. 1975. Injectable selenium: Effect on the primary immune response of mice. *Proc. Soc. Exp. Biol. Med. 148:*37–40.

46. Bradley, C. J., Kledzik, G. S., and Meites, J. 1976. Prolactin and estrogen dependency of rat mammary cancers at early and late stages of development. *Cancer Res. 36:*319–324.

47. Ip, C., and Ip, M. M. 1981. Chemoprevention of mammary tumorigenesis by a combined regimen of selenium and vitamin A. *Carcinogenesis 2:*915–918.

48. Young, E. O., and Milner, J. A. 1981. Inhibition of 7,12-dimethylbenzanthracene-induced mammary tumors by selenium. *Fed. Proc. 40:*949.

49. Welsch, C. W., Goodrich-Smith, M., Brown, C. K., Greene, H. D., and Hamel, E. J. 1981. Selenium and the genesis of murine mammary tumors. *Carcinogenesis 2:*519–522.

50. Medina, D., and Shepherd, F. 1981. Selenium-mediated inhibition of 7,12-dimethylbenzanthracene-induced mouse mammary tumorigenesis. *Carcinogenesis 2:*451–455.

51. Birt, D. F., Lawson, T. A., Julius, A. D., Runice, C. E., and Saimasi, S. 1982. Inhibition by dietary selenium of colon cancer induced in the rat by bis(2-oxopropyl)nitrosamine. *Cancer Res. 42:*4455–4459.

52. Thompson, H. J., and Becci, P. J. 1979. Effect of graded dietary levels of selenium on tracheal carcinomas induced by 1-methyl-1-nitrosourea. *Cancer Lett. 7:*215–219.

53. O'Conner, T. P., Youngman, L. D., and Campbell, T. C. 1983. Effect of selenium on development of L-azaserine (Aza) induced preneoplastic abnormal acinar cell nodules (AACN) in rat pancreas. *Fed. Proc. 42:*670.

54. Baldwin, S., Parker, R. S., and Misslbeck, N. 1983. Effect of dietary fat and selenium on the development of preneoplastic lesions in rat liver. *Fed. Proc. 42:*1312.

55. LeBoeuf, R. A., Laishes, B. A., and Hoekstra, W. G. 1983. Effect of dietary selenium concentration on the early post-initiation stages of hepatocarcinogenesis. *Fed. Proc. 42:*669.

56. Chatterjee, M., and Banerjee, M. R. 1982. Selenium mediated dose-inhibition of 7,12-dimethylbenzanthracene-induced transformation of mammary cells in organ culture. *Cancer Lett. 17:*187–195.

57. Witting, C., Witting, U., and Krieg, V. 1982. The tumor-protective effect of selenium in an experimental model. *J. Cancer Res. Clin. Oncol. 104:*109–113.

58. Abdullaev, G. B., Gasanov, G. G., Ragimov, R. N., Teplyakova, G. V., Mekhtiev, M. A., and Dzhafarov, A. I. 1973. Selenium and tumor growth under experimental conditions. *Dokl. Akad. Nauk Azerb. SSR 29*:18–24.

59. Poirier, K. A., and Milner, J. A. 1979. The effect of various seleno-compounds on Ehrlich ascites tumor cells. *Biol. Trace Elem. Res. 1*:25–34.

60. Greeder, G. A., and Milner, J. A. 1980. Factors influencing the inhibitory effect of selenium on mice inoculated with Ehrlich ascites tumor cells. *Science 209*:825–827.

61. Whanger, P. D., and Weswig, P. H. 1975. Effects of selenium, chromium, and anti-oxidants on growth, eye cataracts, plasma cholesterol, and blood glucose in selenium deficient, vitamin A supplemented rats. *Nutr. Rep. Int. 12*:345–357.

62. Mautner, H. G., and Jaffe, J. J. 1958. The activity of 6-selenopurine and related compounds against some experimental mouse tumors. *Cancer Res. 18*:294–298.

63. Milner, J. A., and Hsu, C. Y. 1981. Inhibitory effects of selenium on the growth of L1210 leukemic cells. *Cancer Res. 41*:1652–1656.

64. Medina, D., and Oborn, C. J. 1981. Differential effects of selenium on the growth of mouse mammary cells in vitro. *Cancer Lett. 13*:333–344.

65. Ip, C. 1981. Modification of mammary carcinogenesis and tissue peroxidation by selenium deficiency and dietary fat. *Nutr. Cancer 2*:136–142.

66. Randleman, C. D. 1980. Inhibitory effects of selenium on induced rat ovarian tumors. *BIOS 51*:86–89.

67. Jacobs, M. M., Shubik, P., and Feldman, R. 1980. Influence of selenium on vascularization in the hamster cheek pouch. *Cancer Lett. 9*:353–357.

68. Exon, J. H., Koller, L. D., and Elliott, S. C. 1976. Effect of dietary selenium on tumor induction by an oncogenic virus. *Clin. Toxicol. 9*:273–279.

69. Watson-Williams, E. 1920. The treatment of inoperable cancer with selenium. *Br. J. Surg. 8*:50–58.

70. Prowse, W. B. 1937. Carcinoma of breast with wide-spread metastases. Two cases of recovery. *Br. Med. J. 1*:1021–1023.

71. Gillett, A. S., and Wakeley, C. P. G. 1922. Selenium in the treatment of malignant disease. *Br. J. Surg. 9*:532–539.

72. Shamberger, R. J., and Willis, C. E. 1971. Selenium distribution and human cancer mortality. *CRC Crit. Rev. Clin. Lab. Sci. 2*:211–221.

73. Shamberger, R. J., Tytko, S. A., and Willis, C. E. 1976. Antioxidants and cancer. Part VI. Selenium and age-adjusted human cancer mortality. *Arch. Environ. Health 31*:231–235.

74. Schrauzer, G. N., White, D. A., and Schneider, C. J. 1977. Cancer mortality correlation studies—III: Statistical associations with dietary selenium intakes. *Bioinorg. Chem. 7*:23–24.

75. Schrauzer, G. N., White, D. A., and Schneider, C. J. 1977. Cancer mortality correlation studies—IV: Associations with dietary intakes and blood levels of certain trace elements, notably Se-antagonists. *Bioinorg. Chem. 7*:35–56.

76. Jansson, B., and Jacobs, M. M. 1976. Selenium—a possible inhibitor of colon and rectum cancer. in *Proceedings of the symposium on selenium–tellurium in the environment*. pp. 326–340. Pittsburgh: Industrial Health Foundation.

77. Bogden, J. B., Kemp, F. W., Buse, M., Thind, I. S., Louria, D. B., Forgacs, J., Llanos, G., and Terrones, I. M. 1981. Composition of tobaccos from countries with high and low incidence of lung cancer. I. Selenium, Polonium-210, Alternaria, tar and nicotine. *J. Natl. Cancer Inst. 66*:27–31.

78. Shamberger, R. J., Rukovena, E., Longfield, A. K., Tytko, S. A., Deodhar, S., and Willis, C. E. 1973. Antioxidants and cancer. I. Selenium in the blood of normals and cancer patients. *J. Natl. Cancer Inst. 50*:863–870.

79. Dickson, R. C., and Tomlinson, R. H. 1967. Selenium in blood and human tissues. *Clin. Chem. Acta 16:*311–321.

80. McConnell, K. P., Broghamer, W. L., Blotcky, A. J., and Hurt, O. J. 1975. Selenium levels in human blood and tissues in health and in disease. *J. Nutr. 105:*1026–1031.

81. Broghamer, W. L., McConnell, K. P., and Blotcky, A. J. 1976. Relationship between serum selenium levels and patients with carcinoma. *Cancer 37:*1384–1388.

82. McConnell, K. P., Jagar, R. M., Higgins, P. J., and Blotcky, A. J. 1977. Serum selenium levels in patients with and without breast cancer. in J. Van Eys, M. S. Seelig, and B. L. Nichols (Eds.) *Proceedings of the 18th meeting of the American College of Nutrition. Houston, Texas.* pp. 195–198. New York: S. P. Medical and Scientific Books.

83. McConnell, K. P., Jager, R. M., Bland, K. I., and Blotcky, A. J. 1980. The relationship of dietary selenium and breast cancer. *J. Surg. Oncol. 15:*67–70.

84. Capel, I. D., and Williams, D. C. 1979. Selenium and glutathione peroxidase in breast cancer. *Obstet. Gynecol. 7:*425.

85. Broghamer, W. L., McConnell, K. P., Grimaldi, M., and Blotcky, A. J. 1978. Serum selenium and reticuloendothelial tumors. *Cancer 41:*1462–1466.

86. Calautti, P., Moschini, G., Stievano, B. M., Tomio, L., Calzavara, F., and Perona, G. 1980. Serum selenium levels in malignant lymphoproliferative diseases. *Scand. J. Haematol. 24:*63–66.

87. Goodwin, W. J., Lane, H. W., Bradford, K., Marshall, M. V., Griffin, A. C., Geopfert, H., and Jesse, R. H. 1983. Selenium and glutathione peroxidase levels in patients with epidermoid carcinoma of the oral cavity and oropharynx. *Cancer 51:*110–115.

88. Schrauzer, G. N., and Rhead, W. J. 1971. Interpretation of the methylene blue reduction test of human plasma and the possible protecting effect of selenium. *Experientia 27:*1069–1071.

89. Schrauzer, G. N., Rhead, W. J., and Evans, G. A., 1973, Selenium and cancer: Chemical interpretation of a plasma "cancer test." *Bioinorg. Chem. 2:*329–340.

90. Robinson, M. F., Godfrey, P. J., Thomson, C. D., Rea, H. M., and van Rij, A. M. 1979. Blood selenium and glutathione peroxidase activity in normal subjects and in surgical patients with and without cancer in New Zealand. *Am. J. Clin. Nutr. 32:*1477–1485.

91. Nelson, A. A., Fitzhugh, O. G., and Calvery, H. O. 1943. Liver tumors following cirrhosis caused by selenium in rats. *Cancer Res. 3:*230–236.

92. Shapiro, J. R. 1972. Selenium and carcinogenesis: A review. *Ann. NY Acad. Sci. 192:*215–219.

93. Volgarev, N. N., and Tscherkes, L. A. 1967. Further studies in tissue changes associated with sodium selenate. in O. H. Muth (Ed.) *Symposium: Selenium in biomedicine.* pp. 179–184. Westport, Connecticut: Avi.

94. Schroeder, H. A., and Mitchener, M. 1971. Selenium and tellurium in rats: Effects on growth, survival and tumors. *J. Nutr. 101:1531–1540.*

95. *Schroeder, H. A., and Mitchener, M. 1972. Selenium and tellurium in mice. Arch. Environ. Health 24:66–71.*

96. Harr, J. R., Bone, J. F., Tinsley, I. J., Weswig, P. H., and Yamamoto, R. S. 1967. Selenium toxicity in rats. II. Histopathology. in O. H. Muth (Ed.) *Symposium: Selenium in biomedicine.* pp. 153–178. Westport, Connecticut: Avi.

97. Seifter, J., Ehrlich, W. E., Hudgma, G., and Mueller, G. 1946. Thyroid adenomas in rats receiving selenium. *Science 103:*762.

98. National Cancer Institute Carcinogenesis Test Program. 1980. Bioassay of selenium sulfide (gavage) for possible carcinogenicity. NIH Publ. NIH-80-1750, 130 pp.

99. Walker, G. W. R., and Ting, K. P. 1967. Effect of selenium on recombination in barley. *Can. J. Genet. Cytol. 9:*314–320.

100. Nickerson, W. J., Taber, W. A., and Falcone, G. 1956. Physiological basis of morphogenesis

in fungi. 5. Effect of selenite and tellurite on cellular division of yeastlike fungi. *Can. J. Microbiol.* 2:575–584.

101. Ahmed. Z. U., and Walker, G. W. R. 1975. The effects of urethane, sodium monohydrogen arsenate and selenocystine on crossing-over in Drosophilia melanogaster. *Can. J. Genet. Cytol.* 17:55–66.
102. Jacobs, M. M., Matney, T. S., and Griffin, A. C. 1977. Inhibitory effects of selenium on the mutagenicity of 2-acetylaminofluroene (AAF) and AAF metabolites. *Cancer Lett.* 2:319–322.
103. Shamberger, R. J., Corlett, C. L., Beaman, K. D., and Kasten, B. L. 1979. Antioxidants reduce the mutagenic effect of malonaldehyde and β-propiolactone, Part IX. Antioxidants and cancer. *Mutat. Res.* 66:349–355.
104. Adams, G., Martin, S., and Milner, J. 1980. Effects of selenium on the Salmonella/microsome mutagen test system. *Fed. Proc.* 39:790.
104a. Aherne, W., Piall, E., and Marks, V. 1978. Radioimmunoassay of methotrexate: Use of ^{75}Se-labelled methotrexate. *Ann. Clin. Biochem.* 15:331–334.
105. Martin, S. E., Adams, G. H., Schillaci, M., and Milner, J. A. 1981. Antimutagenic effects of selenium on acridine orange and 7,12-dimethylbenzanthracene in the Ames Salmonella/microsomal system. *Mutat. Res.* 82:41–46.
106. Arciszewska, L. K., Martin, S. E., and Milner, J. A. 1982. The antimutagenic effect of selenium on dimethylbenzanthracene and metabolites in the Ames Salmonella/microsome system. *Biol. Trace Element Res.* 4:259–267.
107. Schillaci, M., Martin, S. E., and Milner, J. A. 1982. The effects of dietary selenium on the biotransformation of 7,12-dimethylbenzanthracene. *Mutat. Res.* 101:31–37.
108. Shamberger, R. J., Baughman, F. F., Kalchert, S. L., Willis, C. E., and Hoffman, G. C. 1973. Carcinogen-induced chromosomal breakage decreased by antioxidants. *Proc. Natl. Acad. Sci. USA* 70:1461–1463.
109. Ray, J. H., Altenburg, L. C., and Jacobs, M. M. 1978. Effects of sodium selenite and methyl methanesulphonate or N-hydroxy-2-acetylaminofluorene co-exposure on sister chromatid exchange production in human whole blood cultures. *Mutat. Res.* 57:359–368.
110. Morimoto, K., Iijima, S., and Koizumi, A. 1982. Selenite prevents the induction of sister–chromatid exchanges by methyl mercury and mercuric chloride in human whole-blood cultures. *Mutat. Res.* 102:183–192.
111. Russell, G. R., Nader, C. J., and Patrick, E. J. 1980. Induction of DNA repair by some selenium compounds. *Cancer Lett.* 10:75–81.
111b. Williams, G. M. 1978. Further improvements in the hepatocyte primary culture DNA repair test for carcinogens: Detection of carcinogenic biphenyl derivatives. *Cancer Lett.* 4:69–75.
112. Lawson, T., and Birt, D. 1981. BOP induced damage of pancreas DNA and its repair in hamsters pretreated with selenium. *Proc. Am. Assoc. Cancer Res.* 22:93.
113. Norppa, H., Westermarck, T., Laasonen, M., Knuutila, L., and Knuutila, S. 1980, Chromosomal effects of sodium selenite *in vivo*. I. Aberrations and sister chromatid exchanges in human lymphocytes. *Hereditas* 93:93–96.
114. Norppa, H., Westermarck, T., Oksanen, A., Rimaila-Parnanen, E., and Knuutila, S. 1980. Chromosomal effects of sodium selenite in vivo. II. Aberrations in mouse bone marrow and primary spermatocytes. *Hereditas* 93:97–99.
115. Kuhnlein, H. V., Levander, O. A., King, J. C., Sutherland, B., and Riskie, L. 1981. Dietary selenium and fecal mutagenicity in young men. *Fed. Proc.* 40:903.
116. Rosin, M. P. 1981. Inhibition of spontaneous mutagenesis in yeast cultures by selenite, selenate, and selenide. *Cancer Lett.* 13:7–14.
117. Nakamuro, K., Yoshikawa, K., Sayato, Y., Kurata, H., Tonomura, M., and Tonomura, A. 1976. Studies on selenium-related compounds. V. Cytogenetic effect and reactivity with DNA. *Mutat. Res.* 40:177–184.

118. Kada, T., Tutikawa, K., and Sadaie, Y. 1972. In vitro and host mediated "rec assay" procedures for screening chemical mutagens, and phloxine, a mutagenic red dye detected. *Mutat. Res. 16:*165–174.

119. Noda, M., Takano, T., and Sakurai, H. 1979. Mutagenic activity of selenium compounds. *Mutat. Res. 66:*175–179.

120. Kanematsu, N., Hara, M., and Kada, T. 1980. Rec assay and mutagenicity studies on metal compounds. *Mutat. Res. 77:*109–116.

121. Ray, J. H., and Altenburg, L. C. 1978. Sister–chromatid exchange induction by sodium selenite: Dependence on the presence of red blood cells or red blood cell lysate. *Mutat. Res. 54:*343–354.

122. Sirianni, S. R., and Huang, C. C. 1983. Inductions of sister chromatid exchange by various selenium compounds in Chinese hamster cells in the presence and absence of S9 mixture. *Cancer Lett. 18:*109–116.

123. Norppa, H., Westermarck, T., and Knuutila, S. 1980. Chromosomal effects of sodium selenite in vivo. III. Aberrations and sister chromatid exchanges in Chinese hamster bone marrow. *Hereditas 93:*101–105.

124. Schwarz, K. 1976. Essentiality and metabolic functions of selenium. *Med. Clin. North Am. 60:*745–758.

125. Lo, L. W., Koropatnick, J., and Stich, H. F. 1978. The mutagenicity and cytotoxicity of selenite, "activated" selenite and selenate for normal and DNA repair-deficient human fibroblasts. *Mutat. Res. 49:*305–312.

126. Lofroth, G., and Ames, B. N. 1978. Mutagenicity of inorganic compounds in Salmonella typhimurium: Arsenic, chromium, and selenium. *Mutat. Res. 53:*65–66.

127. Whiting, R. F., Wei, L., and Stich, H. F. 1980. Unscheduled DNA synthesis and chromosome aberrations induced by inorganic and organic selenium compounds in the presence of glutathione. *Mutat. Res. 78:*159–169.

128. Hsieh, H. S., and Ganther, H. E. 1975. Acid-volatile selenium formation catalyzed by glutathione reductase. *Biochemistry 14:*1632–1636.

129. Schut, H. A. J., and Thorgeirsson, S. S. 1979. Mutagenic activation of N-hydroxy-2-acetylaminofluorene by developing epithelial cells of rat small intestine and effects of antioxidants. *J. Natl. Cancer Inst. 63:*1405–1409.

130. Tkeshelashvili, L. K., Shearman, C. W., Zakour, R. A., Koplitz, R. M., and Loeb, L. A. 1980. Effects of arsenic, selenium, and chromium on the fidelity of DNA. *Cancer Res. 40:*2455–2460.

131. Berenshtein, T. F. 1972. Effect of selenium and vitamin E on antibody formation in rabbits. *Zdrawookhr Boloruss 18:*34–41.

132. Spallholz, J. E., Martin, J. L., Gerlach, M. L., and Heinzerling, R. H. 1973. Immunological responses of mice fed diets supplemented with selenite selenium. *Proc. Soc. Exp. Biol. Med. 143:*685–689.

133. Spallholz, J. E., Martin, J. L., Gerlach, M. L., and Heizerling, R. H. 1973. Enhanced IgM and IgG titers in mice fed selenium. Infect. *Immun. 8:*841–842.

134. Spallholz, J. E., Heinzerling, R. H., Gerlach, M. L., and Martin, J. L. 1974. The effects of selenite, tocopherol acetate and selenite, tocopherol acetate on the primary and secondary immune responses of mice administered tetanus toxoid or sheep red blood cell antigen. *Fed. Proc. 33:*694.

135. Norman, B. B., and Johnson, W. 1976. Selenium responsive disease. *Anim. Nutr. Health 31:*6.

136. Aleksondrovicz, J. 1977. Effects of food enrichment with various doses of sodium selenite on some immune response in laboratory animals. *Rocz. Nauk. Zootech. 4:*113–126.

137. Shakelford, J., and Martin, J. 1980. Antibody response of mature male mice after drinking water supplemented with selenium. *Fed. Proc. 39:*339.

138. Koller, L. D., Issacson-Kerkvliet, N., Exon, J. H., Brauner, J. A., and Patton, N. M. 1979. Synergism of methylmercury and selenium producing enhanced antibody formation in mice. *Arch. Environ. Health 34:*248–251.

139. Marsh, J. A., Dietert, R. R., and Combs, G. F. 1981. Influence of dietary selenium and vitamin E on the humoral immune response of the chick. *Proc. Soc. Exp. Biol. Med. 166:*228–236.

140. Sheffy, B. E., and Schultz, R. D. 1978. Influence of vitamin E and selenium on immune response mechanisms. *Cornell Vet. 68* (Suppl. 7):89–93.

141. Martin, J. L., and Spallholz, J. E. 1977. Selenium in the immune response. pp. 204–225. in *Proceedings of a Symposium on selenium–Tellurium in the environment.* Pittsburgh: Industrial Health Foundation.

142. Serfass, R. E., and Ganther, H. E. 1975. Defective microcidal activity in glutathione peroxidase deficient neutrophils of selenium-deficient rats. *Nature 255:*640.

143. Boyne, R., and Arthur, J. R. 1979. Alterations of neutrophil functions in selenium deficient cattle. *J. Comp. Pathol. 89:*151–158.

144. Berenshtein T. F. 1973. Stimulation of a nonspecific immunity in immunized rabbits by sodium selenite. *Ser. Biyal Navek 1:*87–89.

145. Behrenstein, T. F. 1975. Change in the immunological response of vaccinated rabbits following the administration of selenium and vitamin A. *Selen. Biol. Mater. Nauchen. Konf., 1:*94–96.

146. Berenshtein, T. F., and Zdravoukhi, C. G. 1976. Stimulation of the activity of nonspecific immunity factors by biological bases of molybdenum and selenium. *Belowes 3:*67–68.

147. Desowitz, R. S., and Barnwell, J. W. 1980. Effect of dimethyl dioctadecyl ammonium bromide on the vaccine-induced immunity of Swiss-Webster mice against malaria (Plasmodium berghei). *Infect. Immun. 27:*87–89.

148. Mulhern, S. A., Morris, V. C., Vessey, A. R., and Levander, O. A. 1981. Influence of selenium and chow diets on immune function in first and second generation mice. *Fed. Proc. 40:*935.

149. Golden, M. H. N., Golden, B. E., Harland, P. S. E., and Jackson, A. A. 1978. Zinc and immunocompetence in protein-energy malnutrition. *Lancet 1:*1226–1227.

150. Stocks, P., and Davies, R. I. 1964. Zinc and copper content of soils associated with the incidence of cancer of the stomach and other organs. *Br. J. Cancer 18:*14–24.

151. Schrauzer, G. N., White, D. A., and Schneider, C. J. 1977. Cancer mortality correlation studies. IV. Associations with dietary intakes and blood levels of certain trace elements, notably Se-antagonists. *Bioinorg. Chem. 7:*35–56.

152. Van Rensburg, S. J. 1981. Epidemiologic and dietary evidence for a specific nutritional predisposition to esophageal cancer. *J. Natl. Cancer Inst. 67:*243–251.

153. Issell, B. F., MacFadyen, B. V., Gum, E. T., Valdivieso, M., Dudrick, S. J., and Bodey, G. P. 1981. Serum zinc levels in lung cancer patients. *Cancer 47:*1845–1848.

154. Davies, I. J., Musa, M., and Dormandy, T. L. 1968. Measurements of plasma zinc. I. In health and disease. *J. Clin. Pathol. 21:*359–365.

155. Strain, W. H., Mansour, E. G., Flynn, A., Pories, W. J., Tomaro, A. J., and Hill, O. A. 1972. Plasma-zinc concentrations in patients with bronchogenic cancer. *Lancet 1:*1021–1022.

156. Fisher, G. L., Byers, V. S., Shifrine, M., and Levin, A. S. 1976. Copper and zinc levels in serum from human patients with sarcomas. *Cancer 37:*356–363.

157. Lin, H. J., Chan, W. C., Fong, Y. Y., and Newberne, P. M. 1977. Zinc levels in serum, hair and tumors from patients with esophageal cancer. *Nutr. Rep. Int. 15:*635–643.

158. Gyorkey, F., Min, K. W., Huff, J. A., and Gyorkey, P. 1967. Zinc and magnesium in human prostate gland: Normal, hyperplastic and neoplastic. *Cancer Res.* 27:1348–1353.

159. Griffith, K., Wright, E. B., and Dormandy, T. L. 1973. Tissue zinc in malignant disease. *Nature 241:*60.

160. Mulay, I. L., Roy, R., Knox, B. E., Suhr, N. H., and Delaney, W. E. 1971. Trace metal analysis of cancerous and noncancerous human tissue. *J. Natl. Cancer Inst.* 47:1–11.

161. Kew, M. C., and Mallett, R. C. 1974. Hepatic zinc concentrations in primary cancer of the liver. *Br. J. Cancer 29:*80–83.

162. Janes, J. M., McCall, J. T., and Elveback, I. R. 1972. Trace metals in human osteogenic sarcoma. *Mayo Clin. Proc.* 47:476–478.

163. Olson, K. B., Meggen, G. E., and Edwards, C. F. 1958. Analysis of 5 trace elements in liver of patients dying of cancer and non-cancerous disease. *Cancer 11:*554–561.

164. McBean, L. D., Dove, J. T., Halsted, J. A., and Smith, J. C. 1972. Zinc concentration in human tissues. *Am. J. Clin. Nutr.* 25:672.

165. Shamberger, R. J. 1980. Cadmium, selenium and zinc levels in kidneys. in D. D. Hemphill (Ed.) *Trace substances in environmental health.* Univ. Missouri, Columbia XIV:203–210.

166. Petering, H. G., Buskirk, H. H., and Crim, J. A. 1967. The effect of dietary mineral supplements of the rat on the antitumor activity of 3-ethoxy-2-oxobutyraldehyde bis(thiosemicarbazone). *Cancer Res.* 27:1115–1121.

167. DeWys, W., Pories, W. J., Richter, M. C., and Strain, W. H. 1970. Inhibition of Walker 256 carcinosarcoma growth by dietary zinc deficiency. *Proc. Soc. Exp. Biol. Med.* 135:17–22.

168. Minkel, D. T., Dolhun, P. J., Calhoun, B. L., Saryan, L. A., and Petering, D. H. 1979. Zinc deficiency and growth of Ehrlich ascites tumor. *Cancer Res.* 39:2451–2456.

169. Duncan, J. R., Dreosti, I. E., and Albrecht, C. F. 1974. Zinc intake and growth of a transplanted hepatoma induced by 3-methyl-4-dimethylaminoazobenzene in rats. *J. Natl. Cancer Inst.* 53:277–278.

170. Beach, R. S., Gershwin, M. E., and Hurley, L. S. 1981. Dietary zinc modulation of Moloney sarcoma virus oncogenesis. *Cancer Res.* 41:552–559.

171. Barr, D. H., and Harris, J. W. 1973. Growth of P-388 leukemia as an ascites tumor in zinc deficient mice. *Proc. Soc. Exp. Biol. Med.* 144:284–287.

172. Fenton, M. R., Burke, J. P., Tursi, F. D., and Arena, F. P. 1980. Effect of a zinc-deficient diet on the growth of an IgM-secreting plasmacytoma (TEPC-183). *J. Natl. Cancer Inst.* 65:1271–1272.

173. Fong, L. Y. Y., Sivak, A., and Newberne, P. M. 1978. Zinc deficiency and methylbenzylnitrosamine-induced esophageal cancer in rats. *J. Natl. Cancer Inst.* 61:145–150.

174. DeWys, W., and Pories, W. J. 1972. Inhibition of a spectrum of animal tumors by dietary zinc deficiency. *Cancer Res.* 48:375–381.

175. Woster, A. D., Failla, M. L., Taylor, M. W., and Weinberg, E. D. 1975. Zinc suppression of initiation of sarcoma 180 growth. *J. Natl. Cancer Inst.* 54:1001–1003.

176. Phillips, J. L., and Sheridan, P. J. 1976. Effect of zinc administration on the growth of L 1210 and BW 5147 tumors in mice. *J. Natl. Cancer Inst.* 57:361–363.

177. Poswillo, D. E., and Cohen, B. 1971. Inhibition of carcinogenesis by zinc. *Nature 231:*447–448.

178. Schrauzer, G. N. 1979. Trace elements in carcinogenesis. in H. H. Draper (Ed.) *Advances in nutritional research.* Vol. 2. pp. 219–244. New York: Plenum.

179. Verma, R., Jain, S., Arora, H. L., Sareen, P. M., Kalra, V. B., and Lodha, S. K. 1982. Protective efficacy of zinc supplementation on 20-MCA induced sarcomas: An experimental study in mice. *Ind. J. Cancer 19:*126–130.

180. Beisel, W. R., Edelman, R., Nauss, K., and Suskind, R. M. 1981. Single-nutrient effects on immunologic functions. *JAMA 245:*53–58.

181. Pekarek, R. 1980. Abnormal cellular immune response during acquired zinc deficiency. *Am. J. Clin. Nutr. 32:*1466–1471.

182. Koller, L. D. 1980. Review/commentary—immunotoxicology of heavy metals. *Int. J. Immunopharmacol. 2:*269–279.

183. DePasquale-Jardieu, P., and Fraker, P. J. 1979. The role of corticosterone in the loss in immune function in the zinc deficient A/J mouse. *Fed. Proc. 38:*122.

184. Cunningham-Rundles, C., Cunningham-Rundles, S., Garofalo, J., Dupont, B., and Good, R. A. 1979. The effect of zinc on human B-cell activation. *Fed. Proc. 38:*1222.

185. Duchateau, J., Delesphesse, G., and Vereecke, P. 1981. Influence of oral zinc supplementation on the lymphocyte response to mitogens of normal subjects. *Am. J. Clin. Nutr. 34:*88–93.

186. Good, R. A., Fernandes, G., and West, A. 1979. Nutrition, immunity and cancer—a review (Part 1). *Clin. Bull. 9:*1–12.

187. White, J. R., Yeowell, H. N., and Dearman, H. H. 1981. Role of transition metals in the bactericidal action of streptonigrin. *Bioenergetics IV:*1500–1501.

188. Schrauzer, G. N., White, D. A., and Schneider, G. J. 1977. Cancer mortality correlations studies—IV. Associations with dietary intakes and blood levels of certain trace elements, notably Se-antagonists. *Bioinorg. Chem. 7:*35–56.

189. Hrgovcic, M., Tessner, C. F., Minckler, T. M., Mosler, B., and Taylor, G. H. 1968. Serum copper levels in lymphoma and leukemia: Special reference to Hodgkin's disease. *Cancer 21:*743–755.

190. Hrgovcic, M., Tessmer, C. F., Thomas, F. B., Fuller, L. M., Gamble, J. F., and Shullenberg, C. C. 1973. Significance of serum copper levels in adult patients with Hodgkins's disease. *Cancer 31:*1337–1345.

191. Wilimas, J., Thompson, E., and Smith, K. L. 1978. Value of serum copper levels and erythrocyte sedimentation rates as indicators of disease activity in children with Hodgkin's disease. *Cancer 42:*1929–1935.

192. Schwartz, M. K. 1975. Role of trace elements in cancer. *Cancer Res. 35:*3481–3487.

193. Delves, H., Alexander, F. W., and Lay, H. 1973. Copper and zinc concentrations in the plasma of leukaemic children. *Br. J. Haematol. 24:*525–531.

194. Karcioglu, Z. A., Sarper, R. M., Van Rinsvelt, H. A., Guffey, J. A., and Fink, R. W. 1978. Trace element concentrations in renal cell carcinoma. *Cancer 42:*1330–1340.

195. Fisher, G. L., Spitler, L. E., McNeill, K. L., and Rosenblatt, L. S. 1981. Serum copper and zinc levels in melanoma patients. *Cancer 47:*1838–1844.

196. Roguljic, A., Mikac-Devic, D., and Krusic, J. 1980. Copper, zinc and magnesium levels in healthy tissues and benign and malignant tumors of the uterus. *Periodicum Biologorum 82:*213–216.

197. Lefkowitch, J. H., Muschel, R., Price, J. B., Marboe, C., and Braunhut, S. 1983. Copper and copper-binding protein in fibrolamellar liver cell carcinoma. *Cancer 51:*97–100.

198. Prohaska, J. R., and Lukasewycz, O. A. 1981. Copper deficiency supresses the immune response of mice. *Science 213:*559–561.

199. Kamamoto, Y., Makiura, S., Sugihara, S., Hiasa, Y., Arai, M., and Ito, N. 1973. The inhibitory effect of copper on DL-ethionine carcinogenesis in rats. *Cancer Res. 33:*1129–1135.

200. Yamane, Y., and Sakai, K. 1973. Supressive effect of concurrent administration of metal salts on carcinogenesis by 3-methyl-4-(dimethylamino)azobenzene, and the effect of these metals on aminoazo dye metabolism during carcinogenesis). *Gann 64:*563–573.

201. Larsson, G. G., Sandstrom, A., and Westling, P. 1975. Relationship of Plummer-Vinson disease to cancer of the upper alimentary tract in Sweden. *Cancer Res. 35:*3308–3316.

202. Broitman, S. A., Velez, H., and Vitale, J. J. 1981. A possible role of iron deficiency in gastric cancer in Columbia. *Adv. Exp. Med. Biol. 91:*155–181.

203. Ruddell, W. S. J., Bone, E. S., Hill, M. J., and Walters, C. L. 1978. Pathogenesis of gastric cancer in pernicious anaemia. *Lancet 1:*521–523.

204. Cole, P., and Goldman, M. B. 1975. Occupation. in J. F. Fraumeni (Ed.) *Persons at high risk of cancer: An approach to cancer etiology and control.* pp. 167–183. New York: Academic Press.

205. MacKinnon, A. E., and Bancewicz, J. 1973. Sarcoma after injection of intramuscular iron. *Br. Med. J. 2:*277–279.

206. Armann, R. W., Muller, E., Bansky, J., Schuler, J., and Hacki, W. H. 1980. High incidence of extrahepatic carcinomas in idiopathic hemochromatosis. *Scand. J. Gastroenterol. 15:*733–736.

207. Sweeney, G. D., Jones, K. G., Cole, F. M., Basford, D., and Krestynski, F. 1979. Iron deficiency prevents liver toxicity of 2,3,7,8-tetrachlorodibenzop-dioxin. *Science 204:*332–335.

208. Vitale, J. J., Broitman, S. A., Vavrousek-Jakuba, E., Rodday, P. W., and Gottlieb, L. S. 1978. The effects of iron deficiency and the quality and quantity of fat on chemically induced cancer. *Adv. Exp. Med. Biol. 91:*229–242.

209. Brusick, D., Gletten, F., Jagannath, D. R., and Weeks, U., 1976. The mutagenic activity of ferrous sulfate for Salmonella typhimurium. *Mutat. Res. 38:*386.

210. Joynson, D. H. M., Jacobs, A., Walker, D. M., and Dolby, A. E. 1972. Defect of cell-mediated immunity in patients with iron-deficiency anemia. *Lancet 2:*1058–1059.

211. Yang, C. S. 1980. Research on esophageal cancer in China: A review. *Cancer Res. 40:*2633–2644.

212. Burrell, R. J. W., Roach, W. A., and Shadwell, A. 1966. Esophageal cancer in the Bantu of the Transkei associated with mineral deficiency in garden plants. *J. Natl. Cancer Inst. 36:*201–204.

213. Berg, J. W., Haenszel, W., and Devesa, S. S. 1973. Epidemiology of gastrointestinal cancer. in *Seventh National Cancer Conference proceedings.* pp. 459–464. Philadelphia: J. B. Lippincott.

214. Luo, X. M., Wei, H. J., Hu, G. G., Shang, A. L., Liu, Y. Y., Lu, S. M., and Yang, S. P. 1981. Molybdenum and esophageal cancer in China. *Fed. Proc. 40:*928.

215. Kopf-Maier, P. 1979. Molybdocen-dichlorid als antitumor-Agens. *Z. Naturforsch. 34c:*1174–1176.

216. Wei, H. J., Luo, X. M., Sproat, H. F., and Yang, S. P. 1983. Inhibitory effects of molybdenum on N-methyl-N-nitrosourea-indiced mammary carcinogenesis in female rats. *Fed. Proc. 42:*670.

217. Stoner, G. D., Shimkin, M. B., Troxell, M. C., Thompson, T. L., and Terry, L. S. 1976. Test for carcinogenicity of metallic compounds by the pulmonary tumor response in strain A mice. *Cancer Res. 36:*1744–1747.

218. Nishioka, W. 1975. Mutagenic activities of metal compounds in bacteria. *Mutat. Res. 31:*185–189.

219. Wahner, H. W., Cuello, C., Correa, P., Uribe, L. F., and Gaitan, E. 1966. Thyroid carcinoma in an endemic goiter area, Cali, Columbia. *Am. J. Med. 40:*58–66.

220. Williams, E. D., Doniach, I., Bjarnason, O., and Michie, W. 1977. Thyroid cancer in an iodide rich area. A histopathological study. *Cancer 39:*215–222.

221. Clements, F. W. 1954. The relationship of thyrotoxicosis and carcinoma of the thyroid to endemic goitre. *Med. J. Aust. 2:*894–897.

222. Pendergrast, W. J., Milmore, B. K., and Marcus, S. C. 1961. Thyroid cancer and thyrotoxicosis in the United States: Their relation to endemic goiter. *J. Chron. Dis. 13:*22–28.

223. Bogardus, G. M., and Finley, J. W. 1961. Breast cancer and thyroid disease. *Surgery 49:*461–468.

224. Stadel, B. V. 1976. Dietary idoine and risk of breast, endometrial, and ovarian cancer. *Lancet 1:*890–891.

225. Edington, G. M. 1976. Dietary iodine and risk of breast, endometrial and ovarian cancer. *Lancet 1:*1413–1414.

226. Waterhouse, J., Muir, C., Correa, P., and Powell, J. (Eds.) 1976. *Cancer incidence in five continents.* Vol. 3. IRAC Scientific Publication No. 15. Lyons, France: International Agency for Research on Cancer.

227. Aquino, T. I., and Eskin, B. A. 1972. Rat breast structure in altered iodine metabolism. *Arch. Pathol. Lab. Med. 94:*280–285.

228. Eskin, B. A. 1978. Iodine and mammary cancer. *Adv. Exp. Med. Biol. 91:*293–304.

229. Eskin, B. A., Jacobson, H. I., Bolmarcich, V., and Murray, J. A. 1976. Breast atypia in altered iodine states: Intracellular changes. *Senologia 1:*51.

230. Doniach, I. 1958. Experimental induction of tumors of the thyroid by radiation. *Br. Med. Bull. 14:*181–183.

231. Leach, R. M. 1971. Role of manganese in mycopolysaccharide metabolism. *Fed. Proc. 30:*991–994.

232. Sunderman, F. W., McCully, K. S., Taubman, S. B., Alpass, P. R., Reid, M. C., and Rineheimer, L. A. 1980. Manganese inhibition of sarcoma induction by benzopyrene in rats. *Carcinogenesis 1:*613–620.

233. Sunderman, F. W., Kasprzak, K. S., Law, T. J., Minghetti, P. P., Maeriza, R. M., Becker, N., Onkelinx, C., and Goldblatt, P. J. 1976. Effects of manganese on carcinogenicity and metabolism of nickel subsulfide. *Cancer Res. 36:*1790–1800.

234. Rensburg, S. J., Bruyn, D. B., Schalkwyk, D. J., Sunderman, F. W., McCully, K. S., Trubman, S., Allpass, P., Reid, M., and Rinchimer, L. 1980. Manganese inhibition of carcinoma induction by benzopyrene in rats. *Carcinogenesis 1:*613–620.

235. Yamane, Y., and Sakai, K. 1973. Suppressive effect of concurrent administration of metal salts on carcinogenesis by 3-methyl-4-dimethylaminoazobenzene, and the effect of these metals on aminoazo dye metabolism during carcinogenesis. *Gann 64:*563–573.

236. Yiamouyiannis, J., and Burk, D. 1977. Fluoridation and cancer: Age-dependence of cancer mortality related to artificial fluoridation. *Fluoride 10:*102–123.

237. Doll, R., and Kinlen, L. 1977. Fluoridation of water and cancer mortality in the USA. *Lancet 1:*1300–1302.

238. Hoover, R. N., McKay, F. W., and Fraumeni, J. F. 1976. Fluoridated drinking water and the occurrence of cancer. *J. Natl. Cancer Inst. 57:*757–768.

239. Erickson, J. 1978. Mortality in selected cities with fluroidated and non-fluoridated water supplies. *N. Engl. J. Med. 298:*1112–1116.

240. Oldham, P. D., and Newell, O. J. 1977. Fluoridation of water supplies and cancer—A possible association? *Appl. Stats 26:*125–135.

241. Taves, D. R. 1977. Fluoridation and cancer mortality. *Origins of human cancer.* Book A: *Incidence of cancer in humans.* Vol. 4. pp. 357–366. Cold Spring Harbor, New York: Cold Spring Harbor Laboratory.

242. Bois, P., Sandborn, E. B., and Messier, P. E. 1969. A study of thymic lymphosarcoma developing in magnesium-deficient rats. *Cancer Res. 29:*763–775.

243. Averdunk, R., Bippus, P. H., Gunther, T., and Merker, H. J. 1982. Development and properties of malignant lymphoma induced by magnesium deficiency in rats. *J. Cancer Res. Clin. Oncol. 104:*63–73.

244. Young, G. A., and Parsons, F. M. 1977. The effects of dietary deficiencies of magnesium and potassium on the growth and chemistry of transplanted tumors and the host tissues in the rat. *Eur. J. Cancer 13:*103–113.

245. Mills, B. J., Higgins, P. J., Broghamer, W. L., and Lindeman, R. D. 1983. Magnesium depletion inhibits growth of established tumors. *Fed. Proc. 42:*1312.
246. Yancey, R. S. 1980. Vitamins and trace elements in the etiology and treatment of cancer. *Cancer Bull. 32:*177–179.
247. Merliss, R. R. 1971. Talc-treated rice and Japanese stomach cancer. *Science 173:*1141–1142.
248. Stemmermann, G. N., and Kolonel, L. N. 1978. Talc-coated rice as a risk factor for stomach cancer. *Am. J. Clin. Nutr. 31:*2017–2019.
249. O'Neill, C., Clarke, G., Hodges, G., Jordan, P., Newman, R., Pan, Q. Q., Liu, F. S., Ge, M., Chang, Y. M., and Toulson, E. 1982. Silica fragments from millet bran in mucosa surrounding oesophageal tumours in patients in northern China. *Lancet 1:*1202–1206.
250. O'Neill, C., Hodges, G. M., Riddle, P. N., Jordan, P. W., Newman, R. H., Flood, R. J., and Toulson, E. C. 1980. A fine fibrous silica contaminant of flour in the high esophageal cancer areas of northeast Iran. *Int. J. Cancer 26:*617–628.
251. Cramer, D. W., Welch, W. R., Scully, R. E., and Wojciechowski, C. A. 1982. Ovarian cancer and talc. A case-control study. *Cancer 50:*372–376.

Chapter 6

Mutagens in Food

In recent years there have been many attempts to determine whether carcinogens are present in our foods. A vast number of separate chemical entities are present in our foods: several thousand as additives and several times this number as natural constituents. In addition, some are present because of contamination or are formed during processing. Although most of these chemicals are present in relatively low concentrations, even very low levels of potent carcinogens could be a potential public health problem. It is therefore a problem to test the very large number of chemicals present in the complex mixture called food to see whether they may be contributing to our risk from cancer. To test whether a single chemical may be a carcinogen in the diet of rodents costs as much as $500,000. Clearly, simpler and less expensive tests should be devised as a screen to help decide which chemicals to test in long-term studies.

Initiation of the carcinogenic process seems to involve an alteration in the genetic material of a cell. Chemicals that alter DNA will therefore have a high probability of being mutagens or initiators of carcinogenesis. Because there are chemical similarities of DNA in all organisms, a chemical that is a mutagen in any living system should be suspected as being carcinogenic. However, there are cases in which a mutagen is a noncarcinogen and a carcinogen is a nonmutagen. This uncertainty is related to the class of chemical being investigated. A high degree of correlation exists for some classes of chemical carcinogens, such as aromatic amines, polycyclic hydrocarbons, and direct alkylating agents. There are problems, however, in detecting the mutagenic activity of some types of carcinogens, especially chlorinated compounds. Therefore, caution should be exercised, and the structure and likely metabolites of the chemical being tested should be carefully evaluated.

Mutagenicity tests have helped identify chemical carcinogens and have led to the removal of these compounds from products to which humans are exposed. These compounds include the food preservatives 2-(2-furyl)-3-(5-nitrofuryl)-acrylamide (AF-2), which was extensively used in Japan, the flame-retardant chemical tris(2,3-dibromopropyl)phosphate, which was widely used in children's sleepwear in the United States, and the hair dye ingredient 2,4-diaminoanisole. The fact that simple mutagenic assays correctly predicted the carcinogenic potential of these chemicals adds to our confidence that these tests can assist us in identifying environmental carcinogens.

The most widely used mutagenic assay is the *Salmonella* plate test, commonly known as the Ames test. This assay tests a chemical for its ability to induce mutations in different strains of a bacterium, i.e., *Salmonella typhimurium*. These bacteria do not usually grow on histidine-deficient medium, but when the compound under test mutates the bacteria, they are able to grow on a histidine-deficient medium. Most chemical carcinogens and mutagens do not interact directly with DNA. They require alteration by enzymes in order to become activated. This process of metabolic activation generally cannot be accomplished by enzymes present in bacteria. The enzymes necessary for metabolic activation are usually provided by a microsomal extract of rat liver.

Many other mutagenic test systems, such as chromosomal aberrations in Chinese hamster ovary (CHO) cells and mitotic crossover gene conversion in *Saccharomyces cerevisiae* have been used to test chemicals but, of the mutagenic system tested, the most often used is that of *Salmonella typhimurium*. In addition to the mutagenic testing, mutagenicity assays have been used to study the interactions between chemicals. These interactions have resulted in the discovery of both comutagens or as inhibitors of mutagenesis that may provide helpful tools in investigating the metabolic fate and genetic interactions of chemicals. *In vitro* modification of mutagenic activity may or may not have relevance to *in vivo* effects. Specific *in vitro* effects of modifiers of mutagenesis, such as the inhibition of a particular metabolizing enzyme, may not operate or may have the opposite effect in living organisms. When such modification of mutagenesis is observed, the mechanism should be examined.

MUTAGENS RESULTING FROM COOKING OF FOODS

Beef grilled over a gas or charcoal fire has been found to contain a variety of polycyclic aromatic hydrocarbons (PAH's). Up to 8 μg/kg of benzpyrene has been found in charcoal-broiled steak.[1] The source of the PAH's resulting from charcoal broiling was the smoke generated when pyrolyzed fat was dripped from the meat onto the hot coals. The highest levels of PAH were found in the meats with highest fat content.[2] When meat was cooked in a way that prevented exposure to the smoke generated by the dripping fat, this source of PAH was either reduced or eliminated.

Smoked foods and roasted coffee also contain PAH.[3] PAH's from air, soil, or water can easily contaminate vegetables. In addition, fish and shellfish can assimilate these carcinogens from their marine environment. It is likely the major source of PAH will probably be the smoking or cooking of foods except for vegetable or seafood obtained from highly contaminated environments.

MUTAGENS FROM PYROLIZED PROTEINS AND AMINO ACIDS

Mutagens

Recently, it has become clear that regardless of their source, the PAH's can account for only a small fraction of the mutagenic, and therefore possibly carcinogenic, activity that occurs in foods during cooking. Nagao *et al.* have extracted the charred surfaces of broiled fish and meat with dimethylsulfoxide.[4] The mutagenic activities of these extracts on the histidine-requiring strains of *S. typhimurium* were found to be hundreds of thousands greater than could be accounted for by the benzpyrene contents of these cooked foods. For example, in one experiment the mutagenic activity of charcoal-broiled beefsteak was found to be equivalent to that of 4500 μg benzpyrene per kilogram of steak, in contrast with Lijinsky and Shubik's report of no more than 8 μg of this chemical per kilogram.[1]

The mutagenic activity in both broiled fish and beef could be detected in *S. typhimurium* strain TA 98, suggesting that the agent could induce frame-shift mutations. In order to obtain positive results in these assays, it was necessary to have an *in vitro* metabolic activiation system that utilizes the microsomes from homogenized livers of rats pretreated with polychlorinated biphenyls. There have also been a series of detailed studies on the cooking conditions under which mutagenic activity is produced in several types of fish, meats (including organ meats), as well as eggs, milk, cheese, and tofu. Table 6-1 summarizes the mutagens isolated from cooked foods.

In order to determine which protein constituents of fish and meat contribute to the mutagenic activity produced in the cooking process, the mutagenicity of smoke condensates of various proteins have been examined. The smoke analyzed from pyrolyzed proteins such as lysozyme and histone was found to be highly mutagenic to *S. typhimurium*. In contrast, smoke condensates from pyrolyzed DNA, RNA, starch, or vegetable oil were only slightly mutagenic.[5]

Mutagens from Pyrolyzed Amino Acids

Tryptophan

Tryptophan pyrolysis resulted in more mutagenic activity than any other amino acid, but almost all of the amino acids tested produced some mutagenic

Table 6-1. Mutagenic Activities of the Mutagens Isolated from Cooked Foods[a]

Abbreviation	Chemical name	Mutagenicity (revertants/μm)		Source of mutagen	Concentration of mutagen in heated material (ng/g)
		TA98	TA100		
Trp-P-1	3-Amino-1,4-dimethyl-5*H*-pyrido[4,3-*b*]indole	39,000	1,650	Broiled sun-dried sardine	13.3
				Broiled beef	53 (in raw beef)
Trp-P-2	3-Amino-1-methyl-5*H*-pyrido[4,3-*b*]indole	104,200	1,750	Broiled sun-dried sardine	13.1
Glu-P-2	2-Aminodipyrido-1,2-a-3',2'-*d*-imidazole	1,900	1,200	Broiled sun-dried cuttlefish	280
Phe-P-1	2-Amino-5-phenylpyridine	41	23	Broiled sun-dried sardine	8.6
AαC	2-Amino-9*H*-pyrido[2,3-b]indol	300	20	Grilled beef	650
				Grilled chicken	180
				Grilled onion	1.5
MeAαC	2-Amino-3-methyl-9*H*-pyrido[2,3-]indol	200	120	Grilled beef	64
				Grilled chicken	15
IQ	2-Amino-3-methylimidazo[4,5-*f*]quinoline	433,000	7,000	Broiled sun-dried sardine	158
				Broiled beef	0.59
MeIQ	2-Amino-3,4-dimethylimidazo[4,5-*f*]quinoline	661,000	30,000	Broiled sun-dried sardine	72
MeIQx	2-Amino-3,8-dimethylimidazo[4,5-*f*]quinoxaline	145,000	14,000	Fried beef	No information available

[a]By permission of National Academy Press, Washington, D.C., 1982.

activity when pyrolyzed.[6] Purification of the mutagenic products resulting from pyrolysis of tryptophan resulted in the discovery and isolation of two previously unknown amino-carbolines that are potent mutagens: 3-amino-1,4-dimethyl-5H-pyrido[4,3-b]indole (referred to as Trp-P-1), for tryptophan pyrolysate 1 (Fig. 6-1), and 3-amino-1-methyl-5H-pyrido[4,3-b]indole (Trp-P-2).[7]

Glutamic Acid

The pyrolysis of L-glutamic acid has also been shown to produce mutagenic activity. Two mutagens were formed and, after isolation, were found to be 2-amino-6-methyldipyrido[1,2-a:3,2-d]imidazole (Glu-P-1) and 2-aminodipyrido[1,2-a:3,2-d]imidazole (glu-P-2) (Fig. 6-1).[8] There are apparent structural similarities between these products of glutamic acid pyrolysate and Trp-P-1 and Trp-P-2.

Lysine and Phenylalanine

A different, but structurally related, heterocyclic mutagen has been isolated from pyrolyzed lysine.[9] This compound was 3,4-cyclopentenopyrido[3,2-a]

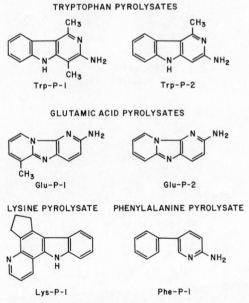

Figure 6-1. Mutagens from amino acid pyrolysates and from cooked foods.

carbazole (Lys-P-1) (Fig. 6-1). Pryolysis of phenylalanine resulted in the formation of the mutagen 2-amino-5-phenylpyridine (Phe-P-1) (Fig. 6-1).

Mutagens from Pyrolyzed Proteins

Globulin

When soybean globulin was pyrolyzed, other mutagenic compounds were formed that were not previously identified as pyrolysis products of any individual amino acid. These compounds 2-amino-gH-pyrido[2,3-b]indole AαC (Fig. 6-2) and 2-amino-3-methyl-9H-pyrido[2,3-b]indole (MeAαC), are quite closely related to the γ-carboline compounds Trp-P-1 and Trp-P-2.[10]

Casein and Gluten

Both Trp-P-1 and Trp-P-2 were found to be present in the pyrolysates of casein and gluten.[11] In addition, Yamaguchi et al. identified Glu-P-2 in the tar

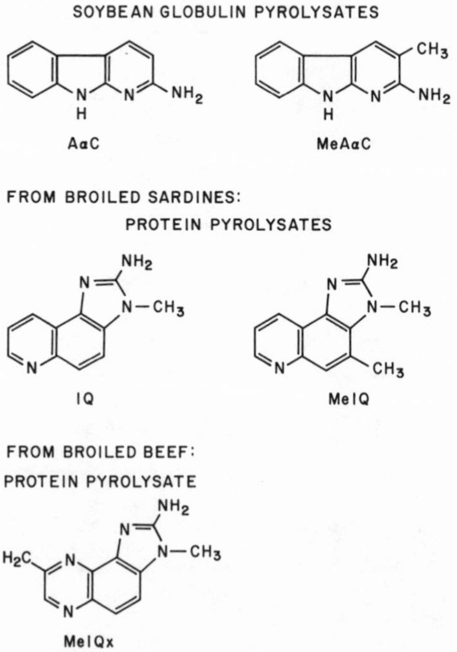

SOYBEAN GLOBULIN PYROLYSATES

AαC

MeAαC

FROM BROILED SARDINES:
PROTEIN PYROLYSATES

IQ

MeIQ

FROM BROILED BEEF:
PROTEIN PYROLYSATE

MeIQx

Figure 6-2. Mutagens from protein pyrolysates and from cooked foods.

resulting from pyrolysis of casein.[12] Glu-P-2 and Glu-P-1 accounted for about 10% of the total mutagenic activity of the pyrolysate.

Cooked Foods

Some of the mutagenic pyrolysis products of amino acids are also present in cooked foods. Trp-P-1 has been found in very well done broiled beef and Glu-P-2 has been found in broiled cuttlefish, although they account for less than 10% of the total mutagenic activity in extracts of these foods.[13,14] When sardines are broiled to a dark brown color, Trp P-1, Trp-P-2, and Phe-P-1 are formed, even though most of the mutagenic activity in these fish was attributable to the presence of other mutagenic compounds[15] (Table 6-1). In pieces of beef or chicken grilled in a high gas flame, AαC and MeαC were found.[16] Similarly, AαC could be identified in grilled onions.

Two previously unknown mutagens were isolated from broiled sardines.[17] These have been identified as 2-amino-3-methylimidazo[4,5-*F*]quinoline (IQ and 2-amino-3,4-dimethylimidazo[4,5-*F*]quinoline (MeIQ), which are unusually potent mutagens to *S. typhimurium* strain TA98.[18] With the exception of the beef containing IQ and possibly MeIQ and 2-amino-3,8-dimethylimidazo[-4,5-*F*]quinoxaline (MeIQx), the foods listed as sources of mutagens in Table 6-1 appear to have been well cooked and even charred on the surfaces to produce the mutagens listed in Table 6-1.

Mutagenicity of Pyrolysates on Mammalian Cells

Four of the mutagenic pyrolysates drived from amino acids or protein-Trp-P-1, Trp-P-2, Glu-P-1, and AαC induce sister chromatid exchanges in a permanent line of human lymphoblastoid cells.[19] In addition, in cultured Chinese hamster lung cells, the basic fraction extracted from pyrolyzed tryptophan caused mutations resulting in resistance to ouabain or 8-azaguanine.[20]

Trp-P-1, Trp-P-2, and Glu-P-1 can transform primary Syrian golden hamster embryo cells.[21] The cells transformed by Trp-P-2 are able to grow in soft agar and result in tumors when inoculated into the cheek pouches of young hamsters with unimpaired immunocompetence.

Carcinogenicity of Pyrolysates

Many of the mutagenic pyrolysates of amino acids or proteins have been tested for *in vivo* carcinogenicity. In Wistar rats given the basic fraction from pyrolyzed tryptophan at 0.2% in the diet, neoplastic nodules, which are thought to be precancerous changes, were found in the livers.[22] Subcutaneous injection of Trp-P-1 (1.5 mg once a week for 20 weeks) induced sarcomas in Syrian golden hamsters and in Fischer rats.[23] Under the same experimental conditions, Trp-P-2 did not induce tumors in either hamsters or rats.[23] When CDF-1 (BALB/ c × DBA) mice were fed a diet containing 0.02% of Trp-P-1 and Trp-P-2, liver tumors were produced.[24] Some of these liver tumors metastasized to the lung. Female mice were more susceptible to these carcinogens than were the males. In addition, six of nine female AC1 rats fed a diet containing Trp-P-2 developed neoplastic nodules of the liver. None of the control animals developed such nodules or tumors.

Glu-P-1, Glu-P-2, AαC, and MeAαC have induced hepatomas in mice.[25] In addition, Glu-P-1 and Glu-P-2 also have induced hemangioendotheliomas between the scapulae of mice fed diets containing 0.5% of either of these two pyrolysate products. It appears that the identification of several of the mutagenic products of pyrolyzed proteins and amino acids was an accurate predictor of carcinogenicity.

Mutagens Formed from Meat at Lower Temperatures

In the experiments studying the mutagenicity pyrolysis products from amino acids and proteins, temperatures of 250°C or greater were used. However, it is now known that simply boiling beef stock at about 100°C results in the formation of bacterial mutagens. In fact, mutagens have formed in beef stock at temperatures as low as 68°C. Frying of fish at 190°C also produces mutagenic activity. When hamburgers are broiled, mutagenic activity also results even though the surface temperature does not exceed 130°C.[26] The mutagenic activity formed from the heated beef extract or from fried beef was found to be due to a chemical with a molecular weight of 198, which has now been shown to be MeIQx (Fig. 6-2). Another heterocyclic mutagenic compound was not identified as an amino acid or protein pyrolysate, but has been found in fried beef. The frying temperature was not specified, but was formed at moderate temperatures. However, this mutagen may result from a browning reaction between sugars and amines rather than from protein pyrolysis.

Mutagen Formation Involving Carbohydrates

The frying of potatoes and the toasting of bread also result in the formation of mutagens, but the chemicals responsible for this activity and its source during the cooking process remain to be determined.[27]

The reaction of amines with sugars may result in the browning of foods. Spingarn and Garvie used a model system for the browning reaction found that mutagenic activity occurred when any of the six different sugars, including glucose, were refluxed with ammonium hydroxide.[28] Heating a mixture of amino acid lysine with glucose at temperatures between 100°C and 121°C in several laboratories results in products that are mutagenic.[29] The increase in mutagenic activity could also be produced by using certain amino acids other than lysine or by replacing glucose with fructose.

Compounds formed by heating mixtures of sugars and amino acids have been identified as pyrazine and four of its alkyl derivatives. These compounds were found to be nonmutagenic to *S. typhimurium,* but capable of inducing chromosomal aberrations in cultured CHO. Chromosome abberations in CHO cells have been shown to be produced by commercial caramel and carmalyzed samples of several sugars prepared by heating sugar solutions. Similarly, furan and six derivatives, which can also be produced in foods by heating carbohydrates, have also been found to cause chromosomal aberrations.[31]

Plant Flavonoids

Among the most widely occurring mutagens that are normal constituents of many foods are the mutagenic flavonoids.

Flavenol Aglycones

Some of the flavonol aglycones that have been shown to be mutagenic to *S. typhimurium* are quercetin, kaempferol, and galangin.[32] Quercetin has also been reported to induce gene conversion in yeast,[33] transformation of both hamster embryo cells,[34] and BALB/c 3T3 mouse cells,[35] as well as mutations and single-stranged DNA breaks in L5178Y mouse cells.[35] In addition, both quercetin and kaempferol have been reported to cause mutations in V79 Chinese hamster cells[36] and heritable mutations (sex-linked recessive lethals) in the fruit fly, *Drosophila melanogaster.*[37]

Mutagenic Plant Products Consumed by Humans

Flavonoids have been identified in some mutagenic plant products consumed by humans. Most of the mutagenic activity of green tea when acid hydrolyzed could be accounted for by three flavenoids: kaempferol, quercetin, and myricetin.[37] In Japanese pickles most of the mutagenic activity comes from the flavonoids kaempferol and isorhamnetin.[39] Quercetin was found to be mutagen in the spice of sumac.[40] The major mutagens in a methanol extract of dill weed were found to be quercetin and isorhamnetin.[41]

Flavonoid Glycosides

The edible portions of most food plants contain flavonoid glycosides, especially quercetin and kaempferol.[32] The average daily intake of flavonoids in the U.S. diet is about 1g and the daily intake of mutagenic flavonoid glycosides may be equivalent to 50 mg quercetin. About 25% of the flavonoid intake comes from tea, coffee, cocoa, fruit jams, red wine, beer, and vinegar.[32] Rutin is a flavonoid which is glycoside of quercetin that can be hydrolyzed to release quercetin by enzymatic or chemical treatment. Hydrolysis by intestinal bacteria can occur when glycosides are consumed in foods. Rutin as well as other glycosides of mutagenic flavonoids were mutagenic to *S. typhimurium* after treatment with glycosidase-containing extracts of the mold *Aspergillus niger*,[41] the snail *Helix. pomatia,*[42] rat cecal contents,[43] or human feces.[44] In addition, mutagenic activity of rutin has been observed in *S. typhimurium* in the absence of glycosidase treatment, but only at doses greater than those needed when glycosidase treatment is used.[45]

Carcinogenicity of Flavonoids

Because of the mutagenicity and widespread distribution of certain flavonoids, especially quercetin. At present, there is contradictory evidence about the carcinogenicity of quercetin. One study added 0.1% quercetin to the diet of albino Norweigan rats for 58 weeks.[46] This treatment resulted in the induction of tumors in the epithelium of the intestine and urinary bladder. In contrast, when Saito *et al.*[47] fed quercetin to ddY mice for their lifetime, there was no significant increase in tumor incidence. In another experiment doses as high as 10% quercetin was fed to rats throughout their lifetime. No significant increases in tumor incidence was observed in AC1 rat[48] or in hamsters.[49] The reason for the differences when the results of Pamukcu *et al.*[46] were compared with the findings of other investigators is not clear, but may relate to sensitivity differences among the species and strain tested.

Mutagenic Activity on Extracts of Food and Beverages

Coffee

Several food substances have been reported to contain mutagenic activity, even though the chemicals responsible for this activity have not been identified. Coffee, for example, whether brewed, instant, or decaffeinated, has been reported to be mutagenic to *Salmonella typhimurium* strain TA 100.[49] Although caffeine has been reported to be mutagenic to bacteria, it is probably not responsible for the mutagenicity of coffee observed in several reports, since decaffeinated coffee was as mutagenic as regular coffee.[49]

Tea

Black tea, green tea, and roasted tea were mutagenic to *S. typhimurium* strain TA without the addition of added enzymes.[50] Tea also became mutagenic to *S. typhimurium* strain TA 98, when extracts of *Aspergillus niger* or human feces containing enzymes capable of hydrolyzing glycosides were added.[50] Acid hydrolysis of green or black tea also caused mutagenic activity to be released. Most of the mutagenic activity of an acid hydrolysate of green tea has recently been shown to be accounted for by the flavonols quercetin, kaempferol, and myricetin.[38] Grape juice was also found to be mutagenic to strain TA 98, but only when tested with fecal extracts containing glycosidases.[44]

Alcoholic Beverages

Mutagenic activity has also been detected in concentrates of 17 of 27 commonly consumed Chinese alcoholic beverages, mostly fermented from rice, barley, and glutinous rice. Mutagens has been found in alcoholic beverages that had been distilled only once or to which herbs or meat had been added. Nagao *et al.* have examined evaporated residues from 12 out of 13 Japanese, Scottish, and North American whiskies and found them to contain mutagenic activity.[52] This activity did not require the addition of mammalian enzymes or glycosidases. This mutagenic activity was found only when using *S. typhimurium* strain TA 100, but not TA 98 indicating that the mutagen was inducing base-pair substitution rather than frameshift mutations. In addition when concentrated or fractionated, some French brandies and apple brandies were also mutagenic.[52]

Food Extracts

Only a few extracts of fruits, vegetables, and beverages have been shown to be mutagenic. When extracts of 28 beverages and 40 fruits vegetables were fractionated, only three beverages and five fruits and vegetables demonstrated mutagenic activity.[53] The mutagenic activity of three of the fruits (strawberries, raspberries, and peaches) was caused by residues of the fungicide Captan. Quercetin was responsible for the mutagenicity of the other fruits and vegetables (raisins and onions) as well as two of the beverages, i.e., red wine and grape juice). The coffee mutagen was not identified. However, 68 other foods did not show any mutagenic activity that had not been previously reported. Bjeldanes *et al.* have found no significant mutagenic activity in extracts of eggs, milk, cheese, or tofu unless these foods were cooked at high temperatures or were darkened during cooking.[54] With the exception of mutagens produced by the cooking of food, it seems unlikely that many new mutagens will be found in common foods. Recently, however, Ceylon cinnamon (the bark of *Cinnamomum Zeylanicum Nees* of the family Lauracease) produces a *rec* mutagenic effect of *Bacillus subtilis*.[55]

Modifiers of Mutagenic Activity

Several substances in food have been reported either to enhance or to decrease the mutagenic activity of other substances. Because most of these effects have been observed in *in vitro* test systems, their importance or relevance to effects in intact mammals is unknown. Modifiers of mutagenicity can be either comutagens or antimutagens. Comutagens are substances that enhance the mutagenic activity of a chemical even though it is not in itself mutagenic. The enhancement of mutagenicity may take one of two forms: (1) it may enhance the mutagenic response of chemicals that are themselves mutagenic, or (2) it may create a mutagenic response from substances that are not normally mutagenic. In contrast, an antimutagen is a substance that reduces or completely eliminates the mutagenic activity of a mutagen.

Harman and Norharman

Harman (1-methyl-β-carboline) and norharman (β-carboline) are among the more interesting comutagens discovered in recent years. Norharman is present in tabacco tar and is also present in toasted bread, broiled beef, and broiled sardines.[56] Harman is also found in these same sources as well as in Japanese sake.[57]

Harman and norharman were identified as comutagens when fractionation of pyrolyzed tryptophan resulted in a significant decrease of mutagenic activity on *S. typhimurium*. However, when Trp-P-1 and Trp-P-1 were added to fractions containing harman and norharman, the mutagenic activity of these mutagens was restored.[58] Norharman is only marginally mutagenic, but has been shown to be comutagenic when mixed with several other chemicals, including 4-dimethylaminoazobenzene, aniline, *o*-toluidine (but not *m*- or *p*-toluidine), nitrosodiphenylamine, 3-aminopyridine, 2-amino-3-methylpyridine, 2-acetylaminofluorene, 2-aminofluorene, and *N*-hydroxy-2-acetylaminofluorene.[59] These chemicals all need an *in vitro* and mammalian metabolic activation system for mutagenic activity. In addition, norharman is comutagenic with *N*-acetoxy-2-acetylaminofluorene, which does not require metabolic activation.[60]

Aniline, which is nonmutagenic in the absence of norharman, was believed for many years to be carcinogenic. Later it was demonstrated to have weak carcinogenic activity. There are also a number of other chemical carcinogens the activity of which has been only observed in the presence of norharman, but data are insufficient to justify the inclusion of norharman in routine testing. There is also a possibility that many false-positives results might be obtained with norharman.

The mechanism of the comutagenic action of harman and norharman is unclear. However, these comutagens are believed to act by metabolically activating the test compounds, but they may act through other mechanisms as well. For example, the mutagenicity of *N*-acetoxy-2-acetylaminofluorene, which is enhanced by harman and norharman, does not require activation.[60]

A number of substances in foods can reduce the activity of certain mutagens in *in vitro* test systems. For example, juices prepared from some common vegetables, fruits, and spices, including cabbage, broccoli, green pepper, eggplant, apple, shallot, ginger, pineapple, and mint leaf, all reduced the mutagenic pyrolysates.[61] Antimutagenic activity has also been found in extracts of wheat sprouts, leaf lettuce, parsley, brussel sprouts, mustard greens, spinach, cabbage, broccoli, and other vegetables.[62] Although they concluded that the antimutagenic substance in these vegetables is chlorophyll, certain food substances that have no chlorophyll, such as apples, also inhibit mutagenic activity, indicating that some factor in foods other than chlorophyll can be antimutagenic.[62]

Hemin

Antimutagenic activity has also been derived from certain pigments derived from animal systems. For example, the activity of a number of polycyclic mutagens, including benzpyrene, 3-methylcholanthrene, 2-acetyaminofluorene, 2-nitrofluorene, and aflatoxin B_1, as well as several mutagenic amino acid pyrolysates, such as Trp-P-1 and Trp-P-2, has been inhibited by hemin.[63] Biliverdin and bilirubin, which are heme metabolites, have also interfered with the mutagenic activity of some of these compounds. The mechanism of these antimutagenic activities is unknown. In addition, hemin has interfered with the mutagenic activity of 2-nitrofluorene and the activated forms of Trp-P-1 and Glu-P-1, all of which are mutagenic to *S. typhimurium* without the addition of a mammalian metabolic activation system. Therefore, at least some of the antimutagenic activity may be unrelated to such activation.

Fatty Acids

Other food chemicals have also been reported to inhibit mutagenic activity. Oleic acid and linoleic acid, which are unsaturated, but not the saturated fatty acids stearic acid and palmitic acid have inhibited the mutagenic activity of a number of chemicals for *S. typhimurium*.[64] The mechanism for this inhibition is unknown.

Nitrite

When pyrolyzed casein, a mutagenic extract of roasted chicken meat, tabacco-smoked condensate, and certain aromatic amines were treated with nitrite under acidic conditions, a decrease was observed in the mutagenic activity of these substances when tested on *Salmonella typhimurium*.[65] Concentrations of sodium nitrite as low as 3 mg/liter were enough to bring about a loss of most of the mutagenic activity of casein pyrolysate. In addition, Tsuda *et al.* have found that acidic treatment with a 2.3-mg/liter solution of sodium nitrite also resulted in the loss of mutagenic activity of Trp-P-1, Trp-P-2, and Glu-P-1.[65]

In regard to the interaction of nitrite with 2-amino-α-carboline, a more complex situation exists. At a pH value of ∼ 4, the reaction results in a loss of mutagenic activity through the conversion of 2-amino-α-carboline to the nonmutagen 2-hydroxy-α-carboline.[67] However, when the pH was below 3.5, a new, direct-acting mutagen was formed, i.e., 2-hydroxy-3-nitroso-α-carboline. Nitrite is thus able to neutralize mutagens or result in the formation of new mutagens. In addition, nitrite has also already been shown to interact with dietary amines to form mutagenic and carcinogenic *N*-nitrosamines, as discussed in Chapter 4.

Antioxidants

Several antioxidants such as butylated hydroxyanisole (BHA), butylated hydroxytoluene (BHT), ascorbic acid vitamin E, sodium bisulfite, and selenium have been shown to inhibit mutagenesis in either mammalian or bacterial mutagenic test systems such as the *S. typhimurium*. In other cases, selenium at higher concentrations and also ascorbic acid have been shown to be mutagenic. These inhibitions or enchancement of mutagenesis are described in either the vitamin (vitamin E, ascorbic acid) (selenium) trace element or the food-additive section (BHA, BHT).

Retinol (vitamin A alcohol) inhibits both the mutagenic activity of 2-aminofluorene and aflatoxin B_1, both of which need metabolic activation, but does not inhibit the mutagenic activity of the direct-acting mutagens adriamycin and diepoxybutane.[68] In a similar manner as the other antioxidants, these results may indicate that retinol inhibits mutagenesis by interfering with metabolic activation rather than by acting as a scavenger of free radicals produced by mutagenic chemicals.

The finding that some constituents of food are able to enhance or inhibit the *in vitro* mutagenicity of other compounds does not necessarily mean that these compounds would produce the similar effects in living animals or humans. If mutagens should be found to cause animal cancer, many factors should be considered before action is taken to reduce exposure. Certainly the cooking of meat and fish can produce mutagens, but cooking also destroys pathogenic microorganisms and parasites.

REFERENCES

1. Lijinsky, W., and Shubik, P. 1964. Benzopyrene and other polynuclear hydrocarbons in charcoal-broiled meat. *Science 145:*53–55.
2. Lijinsky, W., and Ross, A. E. 1967. Production of carcinogenic polynuclear hydrocarbons in the cooking of food. *Food Cosmet. Toxicol. 5:*343–347.
3. Howard, J. W., and Fazio, T. 1980. Analytical methodology and reported findings of polycyclic aromatic hydrocarbons in foods. *J. Assoc. Off. Anal. Chem. 63:*1077–1104.
4. Nagao, M., Honda, M., Seino, Y., Yahagi, T., and Sugimura, T. 1977. Mutagenicities of smoke condensates and the charred surface of fish and meat. *Cancer Lett. 2:*221–226.
5. Nagao, M., Honda, M., Seino, Y., Yahagi, T., Kawachi, T., and Sugimura, T. 1977. Mutagenicities of protein pyrolysates. *Cancer Lett. 2:*335–340.
6. Matsumoto, T., Yoshida, D., Mizusaki, S., and Okamato, H. 1977. Mutagenic activity of amino acid pyrolysates in *Salmonella typhimurium* TA 98. *Mutat. Res. 48:*279–286.
7. Sugimura, T., Kawachi, T., Nagao, M., Yahagi, T., Seino, Y., Okamoto, T., Shudo, K., Kosuge, T., Tsuji, K., Wakabayashi, K., Itaka, Y., and Itai, A. 1977. Mutagenic principle(s) in tryptophan and phenylalanine pyrolysis products. *Proc. Jpn. Acad. 53:*58–61.
8. Yamamoto, T., Sutji, K., Kosuge, T., Okamoto, T., Shudo, K., Takeda, K., Iitaka, Y., Yamaguchi, K., Seino, Y., Yahagi, T., Nagao, M., and Sugimura, T. 1978. Isolation and structure determination of mutagenic substances in L-glutamic acid pyrolysate. *Proc. Jpn. Acad. 54:*248–250.
9. Wakabayashi, K., Tsuji, K., Kosuge, T., Takeda, K., Yamaguchi, K., Shudo, K., Iitaka, Y., Okamoto, T., Yahagi, T., Nagao, M., and Sugimura, T. 1978. Isolation and structure determination of a mutagenic substance in L-lysine pyrolsate. *Proc. Jpn. Acad. 54(B):*569–571.
10. Yoshida, D., and Matsumoto, T. 1978. Changes in mutagenicity of protein pyrolyzates by reaction with nitrite. *Mutat. Res. 58:*35–40.
11. Uyeta, M., Kanada, T., Mazaki, M., Taue, S., and Takahashi, S. 1979. Assaying mutagenicity of food pyrolysis products using the Ames test. in E. C. Miller, J. A. Miller, I. Hirono, T. Sugimura, and S. Takayama (Eds.) *Naturally occurring carcinogens—mutagens and modulators of carcinogenesis.* pp. 169–176. Baltimore: University Park Press.
12. Yamaguchi, K., Zenda, H., Shudo, K., Kosuge, T., Okamoto, T., and Sugimura, T. 1979. Presence of 2-aminodipyrido[1,2-a:3,2-d]imidazole in casein pyrolysate. *Gann 70:*849–850.
13. Yamaguchi, K., Shudo, K., Okamoto, T., Sugimura, T., and Kosuge, T. 1980. Presence of 3-amino-1,4-dimethyl-5*H*-pyrido[4,3-*b*]indole in broiled beef. *Gann 71:*745–746.
14. Yamaguchi, K., Shudo, K., Okamoto, T., Sugimura, T., and Kosuge, T. 1980. Presence of 2-aminodipyrido[1,2-*a*:3,2-*d*]imidoazole in broiled cuttlefish. *Gann 71:*743–744.
15. Yamaizumi, Z., Shiomi, T., Kasai, H., Nishimura, S., Takahashi, Y., Nagao, M., and Sugimura, T. 1980. Detection of potent mutagens, Trp-P-1 and Trp-P-2, in broiled fish. *Cancer Lett. 9:*75–83.
16. Matsumoto, T., Yoshida, D., and Tomita, H. 1981. Determination of mutagens, amino-α-carbolines in grilled foods and cigarette smoke condensate. *Cancer Lett. 12:*105–110.

17. Kasai, H., Nishimura, S., Wakabayashi, K., Nagao, M., and Sugimura, T. 1980. Chemical synthesis of 2-amino-3-methylimidazo[4,5-*f*]quinoline (IQ), a potent mutagen isolated from broiled fish. *Proc. Jpn. Acad. 56(B):*382–384.

18. Kasai, H., Yamaizumi, Z., Shiomi, T., Yokoyama, S., Miyazawa, K., Wakabayashi, M., Nagao, M., Sugimura, T., and Nishimura, S. 1981. Structure of a potent mutagen isolated from fried beef. *Chem. Lett. 4:*485–488.

19. Tohda, H., Oikawa, A., Kawachi, T., and Sugimura, T. 1980. Introduction of sister–chromatid exchanges by mutagens from amino acid and protein pyrolysates. *Mutat. Res. 77:*65–69.

20. Inui, N., Nishi, Y., Hasegawa, M. M., and Kawachi, T. 1980. Introduction of 8-azaguanine or ouabain resistant somatic mutation of Chinese hamster lung cells by treatment with tryptophan pyrolysis products. *Cancer Lett. 9:*185–189.

21. Takayama, S., Hirakawa, T., Tanaka, M., Kawachi, T., and Sugimura, T. 1979. *In vitro* transformation of hamster embryo cells with a glutamic acid pyrolysis product. *Toxicol. Lett. 4:*281–284.

22. Matsukura, N., Kawachi, T., Wakabayashi, K., Ohgaki, H., Morino, K., Sugimura, T., Nukaya, H., and Kosuge, T. 1981. Liver cancer and precancerous changes in rats induced by the basic fraction of tryptophan pyrolysate. *Cancer Lett. 13:*181–186.

23. Ishikawa, T., Takayama, S., Kitagawa, T., Kawachi, T., Kinebuchi, M., Matsukura, N., Uchida, E., and Sugimura, T. 1979. *In vivo* experiments on tryptophan pyrolysis products. in E. C. Miller, J. A. Miller, I. Hirono, T. Sugimura, and S. Takayama (Eds.) *Naturally occurring carcinogens— mutagens and modulators of carcinogenesis.* pp. 169–167. Baltimore: University Park Press.

24. Matsukura, N., Kawachi, T., Morino, K., Ohgaki, H., Sugimura, T., and Takayama, S. 1981. Carcinogenicity in mice of mutagenic compounds from a tryptophan pyrolyzate. *Science 213:*346–347.

25. Hosaka, S., Matsushima, T., Hirono, I., and Sugimura, T. Carcinogenic activity of 3-amino-1-methyl-5*H*-pyrido[4,3-b]indole (TRP-P-2), a pyrolysis product of tryptophan. *Cancer Lett. 13:*23–28.

26. Weisburger, J. H., and Spingarn, N. E. 1979. Mutagens as a function of mode of cooking meats. in E. C. Miller, J. A. Miller, I. Hirono, T. Sugimura, and S. Takayama (Eds.) *Naturally occurring carcinogens—mutagens and modulators of carcinogenesis.* pp. 177–184. Baltimore: University Park Press.

27. Spingarn, N. E., and Garvie, C. T. 1979. Formation of mutagens in sugar-ammonia model systems. *J. Agric. Food Chem. 27:*1319–1321.

28. Powrie, W. D., Wu, C. H., Rosin, M. P., and Stich, H. F. 1981. Clastogenic and mutagenic activities of Maillard reaction model systems. *J. Food. Sci. 46:*1433–1438.

29. Stich, H. F., Stich, W., Rosin, M. P., and Powrie, W. D. 1980. Mutagenic activity of pyrazine derivatives: A comparative study with *Salmonella typhimurium, Saccharomyes cerevisiae,* Chinese hamster ovary cells. *Food Cosmet. Toxicol. 18:*581–584.

30. Stich, H. F., Stich, W., Rosin, M. P., and Powrie, W. D. 1981. Clastogenic activity of carmel and carmelized sugars. *Mutat. Res. 91:*129–136.

31. Stich, H. F., Rosin, M. P., Wu, C. H., and Powrie, W. D. 1981. Clastogenicity of furans found in food. *Cancer Lett. 13:*89–95.

32. Brown, J. P. 1980. A review of the genetic effects of naturally occurring flavonoids, anthraquinones and related compounds. *Mutat. Res. 75:*243–277.

33. Hardigree, A. A., and Epler, J. L. 1978. Comparative mutagenesis of plant flavonoids in microbial systems. *Mutat. Res. 58:*231–239.

34. Umezawa, K., Shirai, A., Matsushima, T., and Sugimura, T. 1978. Comutagenic effect of norharman and harman with 2-acetylaminofluorene derivatives. *Proc. Natl. Acad. Sci. (USA) 75:*928–930.

35. Meltz, M. L., and MacGregor, J. T. 1981. Activity of the plant flavanol quercetin in the mouse lymphoma L5178Y TK +/− mutation, DNA single-strand break, and Balb/C 3T3 chemical transformation assays. *Mutat. Res. 88:*317–324.

36. Maruta, A., Enaka, K., and Umeda, M. 1979. Mutagenicity of quercetin and kaempferol on cultured mamalian cells. *Gann 70:*273–276.

37. Watson, W. A. F. 1982. The mutagenic activity of quercetin and kaempferol in Drosophilia melanogaster. *Mutat Res. 103:*145–147.

38. Uyeta, M., Taue, S., and Mazaki, M. 1981. Mutagenicity of hydrolysates of tea infusions. *Mutat. Res. 88:*233–240.

39. Takahashi, Y., Magao, M., Fujino, T., Yamaizumi, Z., and Sugimura, T. 1979. Mutagens in Japanese pickles identified as flavonoids. *Mutat. Res. 68:*117–123.

40. Seino, Y., Nagao, M., Yahagi, T., Sugimura, T., Yasuda, T., and Nishimura, S. 1978. Identification of a mutagenic substance in a spice, sumac, as quercetin. Mutat. Res. 58:225–229.

41. Fukouka, M., Yoshihira, K., Natori, S., Sakamoto, K., Iwahara, S., Hosaka, S., and Hirono, I. 1980. Characterization of mutagenic principles and carcinogenicity test of dill weed and seeds. *J. Pharmacobio-Dyn. 3:*236–244.

42. Nagao, M., Takahashi, Y., Wakabayashi, K., and Sugimura, T. 1981. Mutagenicity of alcoholic beverages. *Mutat. Res. 88:*147–154.

43. Brown, J. P., and Dietrich, P. S. 1979. Mutagenicity of plant flavonols in the Salmonella/mamalian microsome test. Activation of flavonol glycosides by mixed glycosidases from rat cecal bacteria and other sources. *Mutat. Res. 66:*223–240.

44. Tamura, G., Gold, C., Ferro-Luzzi, A., and Ames, B. N. 1980. Fecalase: A model for activation of dietary glycosides to mutagens by intestinal flora. *Proc. Natl. Acad. Sci. (USA) 77:*4961–4965.

45. Hardigree, A. A., and Epler, J. L. 1978. Comparative mutagenesis of plant flavonoids in microbial systems. *Mutat. Res. 58:*231–239.

46. Pamukcu, A. M., Yalciner, S., Hatcher, J. F., and Bryan, G. T. 1980. Quercetin, a rat intestinal and bladder carcinogen present in bracken fern (*Pteridium aquilinum.*) *Cancer Res. 40:*3468–3472.

47. Saito, D., Shirai, A., Matsushima, T., and Hirono, I. 1980. Test of carcinogenicity of quercetin, a widely distributed mutagen in food. *Teratog. Carcinogen. Mutagen. 1:*213–221.

48. Hirono, I., Ueno, I., Hosaka, S., Takanashi, H., Matsushima, T., Sugimura, T., and Natori, S. 1981. Carcinogenicity examination of quercetin and rutin in AC1 rats. *Cancer Lett. 13:*15–21.

49. Aeschbacher, H. U., Chappuis, C., and Wurzner, H. P. 1980. Mutagenicity of testing of coffee: A study of problems encountered with the Ames Salmonella test system. *Food Cosmet. Toxicol. 18:*605–613.

50. Nagao, M., Takahashi, Y., Yamanaka, H., Sugimura, T. 1979. Mutagens in coffee and tea. *Mutat. Res. 68:*101–106.

51. Lee, J. S. K., and Fong, L. Y. Y. 1979. Mutagenicity of Chinese alcohol spirits. *Food Cosmet. Toxicol. 17:*575–578.

52. Nagao, M., Takahashi, Y., Wakabayashi, K., and Sugimura, T. 1981. Mutagenicity of alcoholic beverages. *Mutat. Res. 88:*147–154.

53. Stoltz, D. R., Stavric, B., Krewski, D., Klassen, R., Bendall, R., and Junkins, B. 1982. Mutagenicity screening of foods. I. Results with beverages. *Environ. Mutagen. 4:*447–492.

54. Bjeldanes, L. J., Morris, M. M., Felton, J. S., Healys, S., Stuermer, D., Berry, P., Timourian, H., and Hatch, F. T. 1982. Mutagens from the cooking of food. II. Survey by Ames/*Salmonella* test of mutagen formation in the major protein-rich foods of the American diet. *Food Chem. Toxicol. 20:*357–363.

55. Ungsurungsie, M., Suthienkul, O., and Paovalo, C. 1983. Mutagenicity screening of popular Thai spices. *Food Chem. Toxicol. 20:*527–530.

56. Yasuda, T., Yamaizumi, Z., Nishimura, S., Nagao, M., Takahashi, Y., Fujiki, H., Sugimura, T., and Tsuji, K. 1978. Detection of comutagenic compounds, harman and norharman in pyrolysis product of proteins and food by gas chromatography-mass spectrometry. *Nippon Gan Gakkai Sokai Kiju 37:*6. (Abst. 41.)

57. Takeuchi, T., Ogawa, K., Linuma, H., Suda, H., Ukita, K., Nagatsu, T., Kato, M., and Omezawa, H. 1973. Monoamine oxidase inhibitors isolated from fermented broths. *J. Antibiot. 26:*162–167.

58. Nagao, ., Yahagi, T., Sugimura, T., Kosuge, T., Tsuji, K., Wakabayashi, K., Mizusakai, S., and Matsumoto, T. 1977. Comutagenic action of northarman and harman. *Proc. Jpn. Acad. 53(B):*34–37.

59. Sugimura, T., Nagao, M., and Wakabayashi, K. 1982. The metabolic aspects of the comutagenic action of norharman. in R. Synder, D. Park, J. T. Kocsis, D. T. Jollow, C. G. Gibson, and C. M. Witmer (Eds.) *Biological Reactive Intermediates 2.* Part B, pp. 1011–1025.

60. Umezawa, K., Shirai, A., Matsushima, T., and Sugimura, T. 1978. Comutagenic effect of norharman and harman with 2-acetyl aminofluorene derivatives. *Proc. Natl. Acad. Sci. (USA) 75:*928–930.

61. Morita, K., Hara, M., and Kada, T. 1978. Studies on natural desmutagens: Screening for vegetable and fruit factors active in inactivation of mutagenic pyrolysis products from amino acids. *Agric. Biol. Chem. 42:*1235–1238.

62. Lai, C., Butler, M. A., and Matney, T. S. 1980. Antimutagenic activities of common vegetables and their chlorophyll content. *Mutat. Res. 77:*245–250.

63. Arimoto, S., O'Hara, Y., Namba, T., Negishi, T., and Hayatsu, H. 1980. Inhibition of the mutagenicity of amino acid pyrolysis products by hemin other biological pyrrole pigments. *Biochem. Biophys. Res. Commun. 92:*662–668.

64. Hayatsu, H., Inoue, K., Ohta, H., Namba, T., Togawa, K., Hayatsu, T., Makita, M., and Wataya, Y. 1981. Inhibition of the mutagenicity of cooked-beef basic fraction. *Mutat. Res. 91:*437–442.

65. Yoshida, D., and Matsumoto, T. 1978. Changes in mutagenicity of protein pyrolyzates by reaction with nitrite. *Mutat. Res. 58:*35–40.

66. Tsuda, M., Takahashi, Y., Nagao, M., Hirayama, T., and Sugimura, T. 1980. Inactivation of mutagens from pyrolysates of tryptophan and glutamic acid by nitrite in acidic solution. *Mutat. Res. 78:*331–339.

67. Hirayama, T., and Sugimura, T. 1981. Nitrite converts a non-mutagen, and 2-hydroxy-3-nitroso-α-carboline, a direct mutagen. *Mutat. Res. 83:*61–68.

68. Busk, L., and Ahlborg, U. C. 1980. Retinol (vitamin A) as an inhibitor of the mutagenicity of aflatoxin B_1. *Toxicol. Lett. 6:*243–249.

Chapter 7

Naturally Occurring Carcinogens

Some toxic chemicals, especially those produced by microbes and plant cells, exhibit carcinogenic activity. Even though some of these compounds are integral components of foods relatively common in the diet of humans, many of these carcinogens have also been found in unusual food sources or in foods contaminated by microorganisms or unwanted plant materials. Sometimes the potential hazards to human health by these components or contaminants of foods range from small to very large. Very low levels of exposure to chemicals with weak carcinogenic activity in laboratory animals may be of little risk to human populations. However, the presence of aflatoxin B_1 in foods is a matter of considerable concern, because aflatoxin B_1 is a potent carcinogen for a number of species, and epidemiological data suggest that this carcinogen may play a role in the development of cancer in humans living in some parts of Africa and the Far East.[1,2]

MYCOTOXINS

Mycotoxins have been defined as toxic secondary products resulting from mold metabolism. About 45 mycotoxins have been identified as being either carcinogenic or mutagenic, but only 17 have been reported to occur naturally in food or feed. However, only 13 mycotoxins are involved if one considers the aflatoxin group as a single compound.

The selection of the mycotoxins discussed was made on the basis of their occurrence in food and the data demonstrating their carcinogenicity. These include aflatoxin, sterigmatocystin, ochratoxin A, zearalenone, T-2 toxin, patulin, penicillic acid, griseofuvin, luteoskyrin, cyclochlorotine, and ergot.

Aflatoxins

The molds that produce aflatoxin are ubiquitous. They are frequently encountered as outgrowths of *Aspergillus flavus* and *A. parasiticus* on stored commodities, especially under conditions prevailing in many tropical areas. Aflatoxin contamination in the United States is generally restricted to those crops invaded by the aflatoxin-producing molds before harvest, most frequently peanuts, corn, and cottonseed, and to a much lesser degree, tree nuts, including almonds, walnuts, pecans, and pistachios. Aflatoxin contamination is greater in the southeastern United States.

The most important source of human exposure in the United States is corn and peanuts. Other direct dietary sources, such as tree nuts, are of minor significance, because either contamination is infrequent or because only small quantities are eaten.

It is not likely that secondary exposures results from the ingestion of aflatoxin residues in tissues of animals fed aflatoxin-contaminated feed, except possibly for aflatoxin M_1, a metabolite that sometimes appears in the milk of lactating mammals exposed to aflatoxins. Even though large amounts of milk are consumed, this exposure is probably negligible compared with the direct exposure from peanuts and corn. In addition, aflatoxins are cleared from tissues of the pig within 2–4 days after removal from a contaminated diet.

Aflatoxins are classified as unavoidable contaminents. According to the U.S. Food and Drug guidelines, the maximum allowable limit of total aflatoxin in consumer peanut products is currently 20 μg/kg.[3]

Epidemiological Evidence

Liver Cancer. Oettle first suggested that aflatoxin ingestion might cause liver cancer. He postulated that the geographic distribution of liver cancer in Africa might be explained by differing levels of exposure to aflatoxin in the diet.[4] An apparent association has been observed between the consumption of ground nuts contaminated with aflatoxin and the occurrence of liver cancer in different regions of Swaziland[5] and Uganda.[6] In a later study in Swaziland, Peers *et al.* measured aflatoxin levels in foods consumed by a representative sample of the population in 11 geographic areas.[7] A significant correlation was found between the aflatoxin contamination and the incidence of primary liver cancer among adult males. In the Murang's district of Kenya, there was a similar correlation found between aflatoxin levels in dietary staples of three district subdivisions and liver cancer incidence.[8] In addition, high rates of liver cancer as well as a high daily intake of aflatoxin have been reported in Mozambique. One problem with these studies is the inadequacy of the liver cancer incidence data, since cancer registration is not well established in these areas.

Aflatoxin contamination of ingested foodstuffs have also been conducted in Thailand, where there was an overall correlation between aflatoxin intakes in two regions and liver cancer incidence.[9] Correlations have also been made between the frequency with which aflatoxin was detected in foods and liver cancer mortality in Guangxi province in China.[10] Where the liver cancer mortality rates are high in Taiwan, dietary staples (e.g., peanuts and peanut oil, which are widely used in cooking) are frequently contaminated with aflatoxin.[11]

Linsell and Peers have observed a strong correlation between estimated levels of aflatoxin ingested and liver cancer incidence from studies conducted in Africa.[12] They also observed that there were no areas where high levels of aflatoxin ingestion have been associated with low rates of liver cancer.

Even though the studies suggest a correlation between aflatoxin and primary hepatocellular carcinoma (PHC), several other reports have also documented a high correlation between PHC and hepatitis B virus exposure.[13] These studies do not differentiate whether present or past exposure to this virus is more closely associated with the development of PHC. Kew et al. have observed that active hepatitis B viral infection is present in about 80% to 90% of the patients with PHC.[14] In addition, about 5–10% of the vitamins of hepatitis with persistent liver damage. The liver cells of these affected individuals are believed to regenerate more quickly, thereby increasing the likelihood that a biochemical lesion that initiates neoplasia will become fixed in the genes of the subsequent cell population. There is a possibility that the influences of aflatoxin and hepatitis B virus on the risk for PHC are not completely independent.

Esophageal Cancer. Aflatoxin may also be involved in the etiology of esophageal cancer. Correlations have been observed between mortality from esophageal cancer and the consumption of large amounts of pickled vegetables and other fermented or moldy food in Linxian county of Henan province in northern China.[15] It is difficult to determine the role of aflatoxin in the etiology of this disease, even though *Aspergillus flavus* has been isolated from some products, because these foods also contain other fungal species, mutagens, and carcinogens, including *N*-nitroso compounds.

In Western countries epidemiological studies have not been undertaken, but there have been studies indicating the presence of aflatoxin B_1 in autopsy samples in liver cancer patients in Czechoslovakia,[16] New Zealand,[17] and the United States.[18] Aflatoxin B_1 has been detected in four of six liver samples obtained from patients with PHC in the United States. The significance of these results is not yet known.

Experimental Evidence: Carcinogenicity

Liver Cancer. One of the most potent hepatocarcinogens known is aflatoxin B_1, being about 1000 times more powerful than butter yellow (*p*-dimethylaminoazobenzene) in rats. There have been a great number of studies on the carcinogenicity of aflatoxins in a variety of species and strains of laboratory animals, including mice, marmosets, tree shrews, trout, ducks, rhesus monkeys, hamsters, and several strains of rats. Out of all the various species tested, the male Fischer 344 rat was found to be the most sensitive to aflatoxin-induced carcinogenesis.[19]

Other Cancers. Even though aflatoxin B_1 induced mainly hepatocellular carcinomas in rats, other studies in rats have indicated that aflatoxin B_1 may also induce a very low incidence of carcinomas of the glandular stomach,[20] cancers of the colon,[21] renal epithelial neoplasia,[22] and lung adenomas.[23] Usually males are much more sensitive to aflatoxin than females within a susceptible species and strain.[24]

Species Resistance. However, mice are more resistant to aflatoxin-induced carcinogenesis using conditions that result in 100% tumor incidence in Fischer rats. In one experiment, however, hepatomas were induced in 82 of 105 inbreed (C57BL × C3H)F_1 mice injected intraperitoneally during the first 7 days after birth with low doses of aflatoxin B_1.

Other Animals. When nonhuman primates (170 animals in 12 different investigations) were compared with Fischer rats, they were relatively resistant to aflatoxin-induced carcinogenesis.[25] In monkeys liver tumors do not occur spontaneously, but a female rhesus monkey developed a primary liver carcinoma after ingesting ~ 500 mg aflatoxin over a 6-year period.[26] One of nine marmosets developed liver tumors in another study after 50 weeks on a diet (5 days a week) containing aflatoxin B_1 at 2 μg/gm.[27] These workers also observed liver cirrhosis, which is not an usual symptom of aflatoxicosis in rats. When tree shrews were intermittently fed a 2-μg/gm diet of aflatoxin B_1, 9 of 18 developed liver cancers after 74–172 weeks of treatment.[28]

Experimental Evidence: Mutagenicity

Ueno *et al.* observed that aflatoxin B_1 was mutagenic to *Salmonella typhimurium* strains TA98 and TA100 with and without S9 fractions.[29] In addition, aflatoxin B_1 was mutagenic in the *Bacillus subtilis rec* assay.[30] Mutants that were 8-azaguanine resistant and chromosomal aberations induced by aflatoxin have been observed in FM3A mouse cells.[31] Aflatoxin M_1, the metabolite of aflatoxin B_1, was mutagenic in the Ames assay,[32] but was found to be inactive in *B. subtilis rec* assay.[30]

OTHER MYCOTOXINS

Myotoxins other than aflatoxins may be found in food. Even though most of these mycotoxins are mutagenic in bacterial systems as well as other short-term tests and/or are carcinogenic in laboratory animals, there is no epidemiological evidence that they are carcinogenic in humans.

Sterigmatocystin

Occurrence

Sterigmatocystin is occasionally found in feed that is obviously moldy, as well as in moldy cheese rind, but this mycotoxin is less often in green coffee beans. Sterigmatocystin is mainly a product of *Aspergillus* or *Penicillium*.

Carcinogenicity and Epidemiological Evidence

Oral administration of sterigmatocystin has induced liver tumors in rats.[33] There are no epidemiological data available that sterigmatocystin affects humans.

Mutagenicity

Sterigmatocystin has been shown to be positive in the Ames test,[29] as well as in the *B. subtilis rec* assay.[30] Sterigmatocystin has also been demonstrated to be mutagenic and clastogenic in mouse cells.[31]

Ochratoxin A

Occurrence

Ochratoxin A is frequently found in grains and related foods and is found less often in wheat seeds and green coffee beans.

Carcinogenicity and Epidemiological Evidence

Oral administration to mice has induced both liver and kidney tumors.[33] There is some circumstantial evidence that it may play a role in kidney tumors in the Balkans, but no epidemiological studies have been conducted.

Mutagenicity

Ochtratoxin A has not been found to be mutagenic in the Ames assay.[34]

Zearalenone

Occurrence

Zearalenone is frequently found in food grains, maize, and soybeans. Its occurrence is related to periodic *Fusarium roseum* infection of the grains.

Carcinogenicity and Epidemiological Evidence

Oral administration was not carcinogenic to rats, but was found to be carcinogenic to B6C3F$_1$ mice. This mycotoxin might be involved in cervical cancer in South Africa; however, no epidemiological studies have been conducted.

Mutagenicity

This mycotoxin is not mutagenic in the Ames test,[29] but is positive in the *B. subtilis rec* assay.[30]

T-2 Toxin

Occurrence

There is limited information about the occurrence of T-2 toxin due to inadequate analytical methods. T-2 toxin has been found in maize, barley, safflower seeds, and sorghum invaded by *Fusarium tricinctum*.

Carcinogenicity and Epidemiological Evidence

The gastric administration of T-2 toxin in a LD$_{50}$ dose to rats induced cancer of the digestive tract and the brain.[35] There is circumstantial evidence that T-2 toxin may be involved in esophageal cancer in China and South Africa; however, no epidemiological studies have been conducted.

Mutagenicity

T-2 toxin was not mutagenic in the Ames test[39] and in the *B. subtilis rec* assay.[30]

Patulin

Occurrence

Patulin occurs frequently in apple juice and also in some other fruits subject to soft rot by *Penicillium expansum.*

Carcinogenicity and Epidemiological Evidence

Subcutaneous injection of patulin has produced sarcomas in rats.[36] However, chronic oral administration of patulin to rats was not carcinogenic.[37] There is no epidemiological evidence that patulin is carcinogenic in humans.

Mutagenicity

Patulin was negative in the Ames assay,[34] but was positive in the *B. subtilis rec* assay.[30] In addition, mutations were induced in mouse cells.[31]

Penicillic Acid

Occurrence

Limited studies indicate that penicillic acid occurs in dried beans and in corn with mold damage known as "blue eye."

Carcinogenicity and Epidemiological Evidence

When injected under the skin of rats, local sarcomas were produced.[36] There is no epidemiological evidence that penicillic acid is carcinogenic in humans.

Mutagenicity

Penicillic acid is negative in the Ames test[34] and in the *B. subtilis rec* assay.[30] However, penicillic acid induced DNA breaks in HeLa cells.[38]

Griseofulvin

Occurrence

Griseofulvin and several of its ring-substituted derivatives are produced by certain *Penicillium* species. Griseofulvin is used as a fungicide in the treatment of mycoses. There is no information available on its natural occurrence.

Carcinogenicity and Epidemiological Evidence

Liver tumors have been induced by mice in dietary administration of griseofulvin.[39] There is no epidemiological evidence that griseofulvin is carcinogenic in humans.

Mutagenicity

Griseofulvin is negative in the Ames test[34] and also in the *B. subtilis rec* assay.[30]

Luteoskyrin, Cyclochlorotine: *Penicillium islandicum*

Occurrence

These substances produce three toxins in laboratory cultures and are a common component of grain mycoflora. There is no evidence of the natural occurrence of these toxins in the grains.[39] Stored rice is quite susceptible to contamination by many fungi, especially *Penicillium* and *Aspergillus,* resulting in yellow rice, which also contain toxins largely due to luteoskyrin and cyclochlorotine.

Carcinogenicity and Epidemiological Evidence

Dietary luteoskyrin has induced hepatic tumors in mice.[39] Few liver tumors developed in mice fed cyclochlorotine.[39] There is no epidemiological evidence that these substances are carcinogenic in humans.

Mutagenicity

Luteoskyrin is negative in the Ames test[29] but is positive positive in *S. typhimurium* TM 677.[40]

Ergot

Occurrence

The dried sclerotium of the fungus *Claviceps purpurea* that grows on rye and certain other grasses contains many alkaloids such as ergot and other physiologically active substances.[41]

Carcinogenicity and Epidemiological Evidence

Five percent ergot fed in the diet to rats for 2 years induced neurofibromas of the ears. These tumors regressed when feeding of the ergot was stopped, but reappared when ergot feeding was resumed.[42] There is no epidemiological evidence that ergot is carcinogenic in humans.

Mutagenicity

There is no known evidence that ergot is mutagenic.

HYDRAZINES

Epidemiological Evidence

No epidemiological studies have been conducted to determine the effects of hydrazines on carcinogenesis in humans. Hydrazines are found primarily in mushrooms, which are consumed widely throughout the world. The main types of mushrooms consumed include *Agaricus bisporus* and *Gyromitra esculenta* (false morel).

Agaricus bisporous is a commonly eaten cultivated mushroom found in Europe, North America, as well as other parts of the world. The exact amount of *Agaricus bisporus* consumed is not known, but it has been estimated that about 213 million kilograms of this mushroom were available for consumption (production and imports) in the United States in 1980.

Agaricus bisporous contains agarithine or *N*-glutamyl-4-hydroxymethyl-phenylhydrazine at levels up to 0.04%[43]; 4-hydroxymethylbenzenediazoniumion,[44] 4-hydroxymethylphenylhydrazine, and 4-methylphenylhydrazine, which are breakdown products of agaritine have been found in *A. bisporous*.[45]

Each year, about 1 million people throughout the world eat the mushroom *Gyromitra esculenta*, about 100,000 living in the United States. There have been more than 500 reports of poisonings resulting from the ingestion of this mushroom. Some of these poisonings have been fatal. There are no studies relating the ingestion of this mushroom to human cancer mortality. Gyromitrium (acetaldehyde N-methyl-N-formylhydrazone and its acid decomposition product, N-methyl-N-formylhydrazine have been identified as major poisonous constituents (up to 0.3% and 0.5% of the dry weight).

Experimental Evidence: *Agaricus bisporous*

Carcinogenicity

When N-acetyl-4-(hydroxymethyl)phenylhydrazine was administered in the drinking water to Swiss mice from 6 weeks of age to the end of their lives, lung and blood vessel tumors were induced.[43] An increased incidence of the subcutis and skin tumors were induced when 4-(hydroxymethyl)benzenediazonium tetrafluoroborate was administered to Swiss mice in weekly subcutaneous injections.[46] When 4-methylphenylhydrazine hydrochloride was administered to Swiss mice in seven weekly intragastric instillations, lung and blood vessel tumors were induced.[47]

Mutagenicity

N-Acetyl-4-(hydroxymethyl)-phenylhydrazine was found to be mutagenic when *S. typhimurium* TA1537 was tested without metabolic activation; it also showed some marginal DNA-modifying activity only when the S9 fraction was included.[48] 4-(Hydroxymethyl)benzenediazonium tetrafluoroborate was weakly mutagenic in TA1535 and strongly mutagenic to TA1537, showing toxicity in both strains.[48]

Agaritine itself has produced equivocal results in two *in vitro* assays. There was a slight enhancement of mutagenicity in *S. typhimurium* TA1537 without metabolic activation, as well as marginal DNA-modifying activity in the presence of S9 fraction.[48] In addition, 4-methylphenylhydrazine S9 fraction in *S. typhimurium* TA98 and TA100.[49]

Experimental Evidence: *Gyromitra esculenta*

Carcinogenicity

Eleven hydrazines and hydrazones have been found in *G. esculenta*. Many of these compounds have been studied to determine their carcinogenicity. When N-methyl-N-formylhydrazine (MFH) was continuously administered in the drinking water to 6-week-old outbred Swiss mice for life, tumors of the liver, lung, gallbladder, and bile duct were produced. Under identical conditions, a higher dose had no tumorigenic effect, since it was too toxic for the mice.[43] Later the carcinogenicity of MFH was confirmed in mice[50] and in Syrian golden hamsters.[51] Acetaldehyde methylformylhydrazone, the main ingredient of *G. esculenta,* was administered to Swiss mice in propylene glycol in 52 weekly intragastric instillations, induced tumors of the lungs, preputial glands, forestomach, and clitoral glands.[51] When hydrazine sulfate and methylhydrazine sulfate were administered in drinking water to 6-week-old randomly bred Swiss mice for their lifetime, the incidence of lung tumors increased in Swiss mice. Methylhydrazine also enhanced the development of this neoplasm by shortening their latent period.

A solution of methylhydrazine was administered daily in the drinking water of 2-week-old randomly bred Syrian golden hamsters for the rest of their lifetime. This treatment caused malignant histiocytomas of the liver and tumors of the cecum.

Mutagenicity

N-Methyl-*N*-formylhydrazine, which is present in *G. esculenta,* was mutagenic in *S. typhimurium* TA1537 without activation, but had no DNA-modifying activity.[48]

Methylhydrazine was mutagenic in *S. typhimurium* TA1535 and TA1537. When the S9 fraction activating system was added, the mutagenicity in both strains was increased.[48] The DNA-modifying activity of methylhydrazine was observed previously by von Wright *et al.*[52]

PLANT CONSTITUENTS AND METABOLITES

Pyrrolizidine Alkaloids

Pyrrolizidine alkaloids occur in many nonedible plant species, including the genera *Senecio* (ragworts), *Crotalaria* (rattleboxes), and *Heliotropium* (heliotropes). These alkaloids occur in amounts ranging from trace amounts to as much as 5% of the dry weight. The members of this group that contain a nuclear double bond alpha to an esterified carbinol are very potent toxins in the liver and lung of rodents and certain farm livestock. Plants containing the pyrrolizidine alkaloids may contaminate forages and food grains.

Carcinogenicity

Monocrotaline, retrorsine, lasiocarpine, heliotrine, senkirkine, symphytine, and petasitenine, are all α,β-unsaturated esters that are carcinogenic when administered to rats orally or parenterally when administered to rats orally or parenterally under conditions that permit long-term survival. In most cases tumor induction involved multiple doses of moderate levels of the alkaloids, but low tumor incidence after long latent periods has resulted from only one or a few doses. Tumors have also been induced in rats after the administration of plants, such as coltsfoot (*Tussilago, Farfars*) or comfrey (*Symphytum* sp.), which contain high levels of pyrrolizidine alkaloids. Liver tumors occur most frequently, but some tumors have developed in other tissues, including the skin and lungs.

In addition, plants containing pyrrolizidine alkaloids may also contaminate forages and food grains. Occasionally acute and chronic contamination of livestock have resulted in some parts of the world. Humans may also be exposed by consuming such alkaloid-containing plants as drugs or foods. One species of comfrey (*Symphtum officinale*) is consumed as a green vegetable in Japan.[53] Because of the widespread occurrence of some pyrrolizidine alkaloids and their carcinogenic potency, these α,β-unsaturated esters may play a role in the induction of hepatic cancer in humans in some parts of the world. There are no reliable data, however, to support this hypothesis.

Mutagenicity

In the *Salmonella*/microsome assay, retrorsine, lasiocarpine, heliotrine, senkirkine, symphytine, and petasitenine, but not monocrotaline, have been shown to be mutagenic.

Allylic and Propenylic Benzene Derivatives

In the essential oils of a wide variety of plants there are numerous allylic and propenylic benzene derivatives. Some of these plants or their extracts are used as flavoring agents for human foods or as medicines consumed by humans. The most extensively studied of the naturally occurring allylic benzene derivatives is safrole, (1-allyl-3,4-methylenedioxybenzene), which is a major component of oil of sassafras, estragole (1-allyl-4-methoxybenzene), which is present in tarragon and anise; and myristicin which is a component of nutmeg, carrots, parsnips, and bananas.

Carcinogenicity

Low to moderate incidences of hepatic tumors have been induced in adult rats fed safrole at levels of 0.5% of the diet for as long as 2 years.[39] Within 18 months after adult female CD-1 mice were fed safrole for about 1 year, both safrole and estragole induced hepatic tumors and subcutaneous angiosarcomas. When less than 1 mg of either compound or of methyl eugenol was fed to CD-1 or (C57BL/6 × C3H/He) F_1 male mice before weaning, a high incidence of hepatomas resulted by the age of 12 months.

Mutagenicity

Safrole has been shown to be mutagenic *in vitro* and in the host-mediated assay.[55] However, it did not prove mutagenic in the Ames test.[56] Safrole has also been shown to be positive in the *Bacillus subtrilis rec* assay[57] and in Saccharomyces *cerevisiae* D3.[58]

Estragole was mutagenic to *S. typhimurium* TA100.[56] However, eugenol was not mutagenic to Ames *Salmonella* strains *in vitro* and in the host-mediated assay.[56]

Bracken Fern Toxin(s)

Bracken fern (*Pteridium aquilinum*) occurs widely in nature and is consumed by humans in several parts of the world, especially in Japan.[59] For about 30 years, it has been known that consumption of this plant damages the bone marrow and the intestinal mucosa of cattle, but the chemical compound(s) responsible for these toxic effects have not been identified.

Epidemiological Evidence

Hirayama found in a prospective cohort study in Japan, a significantly higher risk of esophageal carcinoma associated with the daily intake of hot gruel or bracken fern every day, especially in people who ate both foods daily.[60] In contrast, in a case-control study in Canada, there was no association found between bladder cancer and consumption of fiddlehead greens.[61]

Carcinogenicity

The carcinogenicity of bracken fern was first observed in the early 1960s, when polyps were found in the urinary bladder mucosa of cattle fed large amounts of bracken fern (25–40% of the diet). The formation of urinary bladder carcinomas in cattle, urinary bladder carcinomas and intestinal adenocarcinomas in rats, urinary bladder tumors in guinea pigs, pulmonary adenomas in mice, and intestinal adenocarcinomas in Japanese quail as also observed when these animals were fed bracken fern.[63]

The greatest concentration of the toxin(s) is present in young plants before the fronds have uncurled, and the rhizome has greater carcinogenic activity than that of the stalk or fronds. The toxicity of the fern is reduced by cooking, but not eliminated.[59]

Several studies have attempted to identify the carcinogenic agent(s) in bracken fern,[59,62,63] Quercetin (3,3,4,5,7-pentahydroxyflavone) occurs as a conjugate in bracken fern and in numerous other plants. In culture, quercetin has induced morphological transformations of cryopreserved golden hamster embryo cells[64] and has also produced mutations in *S. typhimurium*,[65] but its carcinogenicity continues to be disputed. Addition of quercetin to the diet of rats for as long as one year resulted in an 80% incidence of intestinal tumors and a 20% incidence of urinary bladder tumors.[66] In contrast, in another study, Hirono, *et al.* fed ACI rats 1–10% quercetin in the diet. No significant increase of tumors were observed.

Indirect evidence for the carcinogenicity of bracken fern may also be derived from observations that milk from cows fed high levels of bracken fern contained compounds that were shown to be carcinogenic in rats. When rats were fed high levels of fresh or powdered milk from cows that had consumed 1g of bracken fern per k. of body weight for about 2 years, carcinomas of the intestine, urinary bladder, and the kidney/pelvis were observed.[68] No tumors were observed in the rats fed milk from control cows.

Estrogenic Compounds

There are several known plant estrogens. These include estrone (from palm kernels), genistein (from soybean and clover), coumestrol (from alfalfa and other forage crops), and mirestrol (from certain legumes). Zearalenone, a product of *Fusarium* molds that sometimes infects grains, also possesses estrogenic activity.

Plant estrogens are usually very weak estrogens compared with the hormones from animals; however, they sometimes occur in relatively large amounts. Fat-free soybeans, for example, may contain as much as 0.1% genistein.

Carcinogenicity

There are almost no data pertaining to the carcinogenicity of plant estrogens, other than one report on zearalenone, already discussed in the mycotoxin section. Certain of the nonsteroidal phytoestrogens, which are natural components of some foods, compete for estrogen receptors in rat uterine cytosol in tissue sections from 7,12-dimethylibenzanthracene-induced mammary tumors as well as in mammary tumor tissue from humans. The significance of these findings in the etiology of neoplasia in humans unknown.

Mutagenicity

Genistein and coumestrol were tested and found not to be mutagenic in the *Salmonella* microsome assay.[65]

Coffee

Epidemiological Evidence

Bladder Cancer. Coffee drinking has been associated with an elevated risk of bladder cancer in several case-control studies.[69-71] However, no evidence of a dose–response relationship has been demonstrated, with only two possible exceptions in males,[69,70] and it appears that the association is not causal.

Pancreatic Cancer. A direct dose–response relationship was reported between coffee consumption and the risk of pancreatic cancer.[72] In another study, an association was observed between pancreatic cancer and the use of decaffeinated coffee.[73]

Other Cancer. Other associations have been reported between coffee drinking and caner, but they have been scattered and inconsistent. Martinez has found an association between oral and esophageal cancers combined and consumption of hot beverages, mostly coffee.[74] In contrast, Stocks did not find a significant correlation between coffee consumption and esophageal cancer, but did observe a significant association between coffee drinking and pancreatic cancer or prostatic cancer.[75] Shennan has reported a direct correlation between per capital coffee intake and mortality from renal cancer ($r = 0.8$).[76] This association, even though less strong, also appeared in the correlational data of Armstrong and Doll.[77] Other case-control studies of renal cancer did not confirm this association.[78]

Carcinogenicity

In Sprague-Dawley rats fed a diet containing 5% instant coffee for 2 years, no bladder tumors were observed in the rats, even though the animals had received an equivalent of 85 cups of coffee per day.[79] In Sprague-Dawley rats fed the maximum tolerated dose of regular and decaffeinated instant coffees (6% of the diet) for 2 years, there was no evidence of carcinogenesis.[80] In these experiments it was also observed that high levels of caffeine led to a lower incidence of tumors. However, Challis and Bartlett have reported that readily oxidized phenolic compounds, which are constituents of coffee, are able to catalyze nitrosamine formation from nitrite and secondary amines at gastric pH. It is likely that 4-methylcatechol and the phenolic components of chlorogenic acid that constitute 13% of the dry weight of the soluble constituents of coffee also catalyzed nitrosamine formation. These results might indicate that several foodstuffs and beverages have carcinogenic properties.

Mutagenicity

Whether coffee is brewed, instant, or decaffeinated, it is mutagenic to *Salmonella typhimurium* strain TA100.[82] Even though caffeine has been reported to be mutagenic to bacteria,[83] it is not likely responsible for the mutagenicity of coffee, because decaffeinated coffee was found to be as mutagenic as regular coffee, and caffeine itself was not detected as a mutagen under the test conditions used.[82]

Methylxanthines

Carcinogenicity

Methylxanthines, which include caffeine, are another widely consumed class of compounds. Oral administration of caffeine has been tested in Wistar rats.[84] Caffeine was placed in their drinking water for 18 months starting at the age of 8 weeks. There was no significant increase in the incidence of any type of tumor in caffeine-treated animals, as compared with that in control animals.

Mutagenicity

Three of the methylxanthines present in tea and coffee are mutagenic in at least some test systems. Caffeine, theophylline, and theobromine have been found to be mutagenic to bacteria and also to cause abnormalities in the chromosomes of plant cells.[85] However, similar mutagenic effects of these compounds in mammals have not been clearly demonstrated *in vivo*. Nevertheless, caffeine can enhance the genetic effects of other chemicals, even *in vivo*.[86] This activity is presumably due to the ability of caffeine to inhibit repair of DNA damage caused by chemical mutagens.

Cycasin

Cycasin (methylazoxymethanol-β-glucoside) is one of the most potent carcinogens found in plants. This compound and at least one related glucoside (macrozamin) were isolated from the palmlike cycad trees of the family Cycadacease. In tropical and subtropical regions, these trees have provided food for natives and their livestock. Generally, the sliced nuts are extracted with water before use, but acute poisonings have been observed.

The ingestion of cycasid and cycad nuts has been proposed as an etiological factor in Guam and Okinawa. However, in one study conducted in the Miyako Islands of Okinawa, no correlation was found between mortality from hepatoma and the ingestion of cycad nuts.[87]

Carcinogenicity

When cycasin is administered orally, tumors have been induced in the liver, kidney, and colon of rats, but tumors have also been induced in other species.[88] Hydrolysis of cycasin generally depends on the action of intestinal bacteria, but the tissues of rats contain low levels of β-glucosidase, which hydrolyzes cycasin. The product of hydrolysis, methylazoxymethanol (MAM), decomposes at neutral pH to form an electrophilic intermediate capable of methylating nucleic acids and proteins both *in vitro* and *in vivo*. These results and the carcinogenic activity of MAM have suggested that MAM is a proximate carcinogenic metabolite of cycasin.[88]

Mutagenicity

Cycasin was not mutagenic in the standard Ames test, but it became mutagenic when preincubated with β-glucosidase from almonds.[89]

Thiourea

Thiourea occurs naturally in laburnum shrubs and in certain fungi (e.g., *Verticillium albo-atrum* and *Bortrylio cinerea*).

Carcinogenicity

When administered to rats in the drinking water or diet for as long as 2 years, thiourea has been shown to cause thyroid tumors, hepatic adenomas, and epidermoid carcinomas.[90]

Mutagenicity

In the standard Ames *Salmonella*/microsome assay, thiourea was negative, but positive in the host-mediated assay.[91] Thiourea has also induced transformations in hamster embryo cells.[92]

Tannic Acid and Tannins

Tannins, which are found in many plants, may be divided into two groups—the nonhydrolyzable condensed tannins and the hydrolyzable tannins—which are subdivided into ellagitannins or gallotannins. The term tannic acid usually applies to hydrolyzable gallotannins, including taratannic acid. Tannins are widely distributed in plants, but are also naturally present in small amounts in coffee and tea. U.S. food processors also use tannic acid as a clarifying agent in the brewing and wine industries, and it is also used as a flavoring agent in such products as butter, caramel, fruit, brandy, maple, syrup, and nuts.

Carcinogenicity

Subcutaneous administration of tannic acid have produced skin necrosis, ulcers and hepatic tumors in rats.[91] No adequate studies have been conducted to test the carcinogenicity of orally administered tannins. In mice, repeated subcutaneous injections of three condensed nonhydrolyzable tannins produced liver tumors and sarcomas.[92]

Mutagenicity

When *Saccharomyces cerevisiae* D4 and Ames *Salmonella typhimurium* were used with and without metabolic activation, tannic acid was not found to be mutagenic.[93] Tannins from apple juice, grape juice, wine, and betel nuts were found to be strongly clastogenic for CHO cells, but they do not produce mutations in the Ames test.

Coumarin

Coumarin is also present in a number of plants, including tonka beans, cassia, and woodruff, as well as their essential oils.[39]

Carcinogenesis

In rats fed coumarin in the diet for 18 months, bile duct carcinomas were induced.

Mutagenicity

The *Escherichia coli* pol A assay found coumarin to be negative.[94] Coumarin interferes with excision repair processes in ultraviolet-damaged DNA and with host cell reactivation of ultraviolet-damaged DNA and ultraviolet-irradiated phage T1 in *E. coli* WP2.[95]

Parasorbic Acid

Parasorbic acid is found in ripe berries of the Moravian mountain ash *Sorbus aucuparia*. It has not been found in a number of common fruits, such as pears, apples, lemons, cranberries, grapes, oranges, or tomatoes.[39]

Carcinogenicity

Sarcomas resulted within 2 years in rats that had received repeated subcutaneous injections of parasorbic acid.[39]

Mutagenicity

No studies concerning the mutagenicity of parasorbic acid could be identified.

METABOLITES OF ANIMAL ORIGIN

Tryptophan and Its Metabolites

Carcinogenicity

Hyperplasia of the urinary bladder developed in dogs fed high levels of tryptophan.[96] When tryptophan was given to rats that had received subcarcinogenic doses of a nitrofuran, a prompting effect was observed on the formation of tumors in the urinary bladder.[97] In another study, four metabolites of tryptophan (3-hydroxykynurenine, 3-hydroxyanthranilic acid, 2-amino-3-hydroxyacetophenone, and xanthurenic acid-8-methyl ether) each induced bladder tumors when these substances were implanted as pellets in the urinary bladders of mice.[98] Attempts to relate the development of tumors in the urinary bladder of humans to abnormal tryptophan metabolism have not been definitive.

Mutagenicity

In the *Salmonella*/microsome assay, tryptophan and its metabolites were not mutagenic.[99]

Hormones

Carcinogenicity

Several endogenous peptide and steroid hormones facilitate the development of tumors of the endocrine glands of laboratory animals.[100] However, humans consume only a very small amount of hormones from the tissues of animals. There is also no indication that hormones from food sources are significant factors in the development of human cancer. One exception, of course, is diethylstilbestrol (DES), which is discussed in Chapter 9.

Fermentation Product: Ethyl Carbamate

Ethyl carbamate, or urethan, is a fermentation product. Low levels of ethyl carbamate have been detected in wines treated with the synthetic sterilant diethyl pyrocarbonate. In addition, naturally fermented foods and beverages (e.g., wines, bread, beers, and yogurt) contain detectable but very low levels of ethyl carbamate. Ethyl carbamate may result from the reaction of ethanol and carbamoylphosphate, which are both normal metabolic products in the yeast.

Carcinogenicity

Ethyl carbamate has been studied for several years as a synthetic carcinogen in the rat, mouse, and hamster. Tumors are induced by administering the compound during the prenatal and preweanling periods as well as adult animals. Carcinogenicity is observed when ethyl carbamate is administered orally, by inhalation, or by subcutaneous or intraperitoneal injection. The susceptible tissues include the lungs, lymphoid tissues, skin, liver, mammary gland, and the Zymbal's gland.[90] The significance of naturally occuring ethyl carbamate in the development of human cancer is unknown, but the levels are very low in comparison to the dose used to induce tumors in laboratory enzymes.

Mutagenicity

Urethan was not mutagenic in the Ames *Salmonella* strains or in the host-mediated assay.[59] However, ethyl carbamate did induce transformation in hamster embryo cells.[101]

REFERENCES

1. Peers, F. G., Gilman, G. A., and Linsell, C. A. 1976. Dietary aflatoxins and human liver cancer. A study in Swaziland. *Int. J. Cancer 17:*167–176.
2. van Rensberg, S. J., van der Watt, J. J., Purchase, I. F. H., Coutinho, L. P., and Markham, R. 1974. Primary liver cancer rate and aflatoxin intake in the high cancer area. *South Afr. Med. J.* 48:2508a–2508d.
3. U.S. Food and Drug Administration. 1980. Nuts. in *Compliance policy guidelines*. Washington, D.C.: Division of Field Regulatory Guidance, Bureau of Foods, Food and Drug Administration.
4. Oettle, A. G. 1965. The aetiology of primary carcinoma of the liver in Africa: A critical appraisal of previous ideas with an outline of the mycotoxin hypothesis. *South Afr. Med. J.* 39:917–925.
5. Keen, P., and Martin, P. 1971. The toxicity and fungal infestation of foodstuffs in Swaziland in relation to harvesting and storage. *Trop. Geogr. Med. 23:*35–43.
6. Alpert, M. E., Hutt, M. S. R., Wogan, G. N., and Davidson, C. S. 1971. Association between aflatoxin content of food and hepatoma frequency in Uganda. *Cancer 28:*253–260.
7. Peers, F. G., Gilman, G. A., and Linsel, C. A. 1976. Dietary aflatoxins and human liver cancer. A study in Swaziland. *Int. J. Cancer 17:*167–176.
8. Peers, F. G., and Linsell, C. A. 1973. Dietary Aflatoxins and liver cancer—A population based in Kenya. *Br. J. Cancer 27:*473–484.
9. Wogan, G. N. 1975. Dietary factors and special epidemiological situations of liver cancer in Thailand and Africa. *Cancer Res. 35:*3499–3502.
10. Armstrong, B. 1980. The epidemiology of cancer in the People's Republic of China. *Int. J. Epidemiol. 9:*305–315.
11. Tung, T. C., and Ling, K. H. 1968. Study on aflatoxin of foodstuffs in Taiwan. *J. Vitaminol.* 14(Suppl.):48–52.
12. Linsell, C. A., and Peer, F. G. 1977. Aflatoxin and liver cell cancer. *Trans. R. Soc. Trop. Med. Hyg. 71:*471–473.
13. Chien, M. C., Tong, M. J., Lo, K. J., Lee, J. K., Milich, D. R., Voyas, G. N., and Murphy, B. L. 1981. Hepatitis B viral markers in patients with primary hepatocellular carcinoma in Taiwan. *J. Natl. Cancer Inst. 66:*475–479.
14. Kew, M. C., Desmyter, J. Bradfurne, A. F., and Macnab, G. M. 1979. Hepatitis B virus infection in southern African blocks with hepatocellular cancer. *J. Natl. Cancer Inst. 62:*517–520.
15. Yang, C. S. 1980. Research on esophageal cancer in China: A review. *Cancer Res. 68:*211–216.
16. Dvorackova, I., Kusak, V., Vesely, D., Vesela, J., and Nesnidal, P. 1977. Aflatoxin and encephalopathy with fatty degeneration of viscera (Reye). *Ann. Nutr. Aliment. 31:*977–989.
17. Becroft, D. M. D., and Webster, D. R. 1972. Aflatoxin and Reye's disease. *Br. Med. J.* 4:117.
18. Siraj, M. Y., Hayes, A. W., Unger, P. D., Hogan, G. R., Ryan, N. J., and Wray, B. B. 1981.

Analysis of Aflatoxin B_1 in human tissues with high-pressure liquid chromatography. *Toxicol. Appl. Pharmacol. 58:*422–430.

19. Wogan, G. N. 1973. Aflatoxin carcinogenesis. in H. Busch (Ed.) *Methods in cancer research.* Vol. 7. pp. 309–344. New York: Academic Press.

20. Butler, W. H., and Barnes, J. M. 1966. Carcinoma of the glandular stomach in rats given diets containing aflatoxin. *Nature 209:*90.

21. Newberne, P. M., and Rogers, A. E. 1973. Rat colon carcinomas associated with aflatoxin and marginal vitamin A. *J. Natl. Cancer Inst. 50:*439–448.

22. Epstein, S. M., Bartus, B., and Farber, E. 1969. Renal epithelial neoplasms in male Wistar rats by oral aflatoxin B_1. *Cancer Res. 29:*1045–1050.

23. Newberne, P. M., Hunt, C. E., and Wogan, G. N. 1967. Neoplasms in the rat associated with administration of urethan and aflatoxin. *Exp. Mol. Pathol. 6:*285–299.

24. Vesselinovitch, S. D., Mihailovich, N., Wogan, G. N., Lombard, L. S., and Rao, K. V. N. 1972. Aflatoxin B_1, a hepatocarcinogen in the infant mouse. *Cancer Res. 32:*2289–2291.

25. Stoloff, L., and Friedman, L. 1976. Information bearing on the evaluation of the hazard to man from aflatoxin ingestion. *PAG Bull. 6:*21–32.

26. Adamson, R. H., Correa, P., and Dalgard, D. W. 1973. Occurrence of a primary liver carcinoma in a rhesus monkey fed aflatoxin B_1. *J. Natl. Cancer Inst. 50:*549–553.

27. Lin, J. J., Liu, C., and Svoboda, D. J. 1974. Long-term effects of aflatoxin B_1 and viral hepatitis on marmoset liver. *Lab. Invest. 30:*267–278.

28. Reddy, J. K., Svoboda, D. J., and Rao, M. S. 1976. Induction of liver tumors by aflatoxin B_1 in the tree shrews (*tupaiaglis*), a non-human primate. *Cancer Res. 36:*151–160.

29. Ueno, Y., Kubota, K., Ito, T., and Nakamura, Y. 1978. Mutagenicity of carcinogenic mycotoxins in *Salmonella typhimurium*. *Cancer Res. 38:*536–542.

30. Ueno, Y., and Kubota, K. 1976. DNA-attacking ability of carcinogenic mycotoxins in recombination-deficient mutant cells of *Bacillus subtilis*. *Cancer Res. 36:*445–451.

31. Umeda, M., Tsutsui, T., and Saito, M. 1977. Mutagenicity and inducibility of DNA single-strand breaks and chromosome aberrations by various mycotoxins. *Gann 68:*619–625.

32. Wong, J. J., and Hsieh, D. P. H. 1976. Mutagenicity of aflatoxins related to their metabolism and carcinogenic potential. *Proc. Natl. Acad. Sci. (USA) 73:*2241–2244.

33. Kanisawa, M., and Suzuki, S. 1978. Induction of renal and hepatic tumors in mice by ochratoxin A, a mycotoxin. *Gann 69:*599–600.

34. Wehner, F. C., Thiel, P. G., van Rensburg, S. J., and Demasius, I. P. C. 1978. Mutagenicity to *Salmonella typhimurium* of some Aspergillus and Penicillium mycotoxins. *Mutat. Res. 58:*193–203.

35. Schoental, R., Joffe, A. Z., and Yagen, B. 1979. Cardiovascular lesions and various tumors found in rats given T-2 toxin, a trichothecene metabolite of Fusarium. *Cancer Res. 39:*2179–2189.

36. Dickens, F., and Jones, H. E. H. 1965. Further studies on the carcinogenic action of certain lactones and related substances in the rat and mouse. *Br. J. Cancer 19:*392–403.

37. Becci, P. J., Hess, F. G., Johnson, W. D., Gallo, M. A., Babish, J. G., Cox, G. E., Daily, R. E., and Parent, R. A. 1981. Long-term carcinogenicity and toxicology studies of patulin in the rat. *J. Appl. Toxicol. 1:*256–261.

38. Umeda, M., Yamamoto, T., and Saito, M. 1972. DNA-strand breakage of Hela cells induced by several mycotoxins. *Jpn. J. Exp. Med. 42:*527–537.

39. International Agency for Research on Cancer. 1976. *LARC monographs on the evolution of the carcinogenic risk of chemicals in man*. Vol. 10: *Some naturally occurring substances*. Lyons, France: International Agency for Research on Cancer.

40. Stark, A. A., Townsend, J. M., Wogan, G. N., Demain, A. L., Manmade, A., and Ghosh, A.

C. 1978. Mutagenicity and antibacterial activity of mycotoxins produced by Penicillium islandicum Sopp and Penicillium regulosum. *J. Environ. Pathol. Toxicol. 2:*313–324.

41. Miller, J. A. 1973. Naturally occurring substances that can induce tumors. in *Toxicants occurring naturally in foods.* 2nd ed. pp. 508–549. Washington, D.C.: Food and Nutrition Board, National Academy of Sciences.

42. Nelson, A. A., Fitzhugh, O. G., Morris, H. J., and Calvery, H. O. Neurofibromas of rat ears produced by prolonged feeding of crude ergot. *Cancer Res. 2:*11–15.

43. Toth, B., Nagel, D., Patil, K., Erickson, J., and Antonson, K. 1978. Tumor induction with the *N'*-acetyl derivative of 4-hydroxymethylphenylhydrazine, a metabolite of agaritine of *Agaricus bisporus.*

44. Levenberg, B. 1962. An aromatic diazoneium compound in the mushroom Agaricus bisporus. *Biochim. Biophys. Acta 63:*212–214.

45. Levenberg, B. 1964. Isolation and structure of agaritine, a glutamylsubstituted arylhydrazine derivative from Agaricaceae. *J. Biol. Chem. 239:*2267–2273.

46. Toth, B., Smith, J., and Patil, K. 1981. Cancer incidence in mice with acetaldehyde methylformylhydrazone of the false morel mushroom. *J. Natl. Cancer Inst. 67:*881–887.

47. Toth, B., Tompa, A., and Patil, K. 1977. Tumorigenic effect of 4-methylphenylhydrazine hydrochloride in Swiss mice. *Z. Krebsforsch. Klin. Onkol. 89:*245–252.

48. Rogan, E. G., Walker, B. A., Gingell, R., Nagel, D., and Toth, B. 1982. Microbial mutagenicity of selected hydrazines. *Mutat Res. 102:*447–455.

49. Shimizu, H., Hayashi, K., and Takemura, N. 1978. Relationships between the mutagenic and carcinogenic effects of hydrazine derivatives. *Nippon Eiseigaku Zasshi 33:*474–485.

50. Toth, B., and Patil, K. 1981. Cyromitrin as a tumor inducer. *Neoplasma 28:*559–564.

51. Toth, B., and Patil, K. 1979. Carcinogenic effects in the Syrian golden hamster of N-methyl-N-formylhydrazine of the false morel mushroom *Gyromitra esculenta. J. Cancer Res. Clin. Oncol. 93:*109–121.

52. von Wright, A., Niskanen, A., and Physalo, H. 1977. The toxicities and mutagenic properties of ethyliden gyromitrin and N-methylhydrazine with *Escherichia Coli* as test organism. *Mutat. Res. 56:*105–110.

53. Hirono, I., Mori, H., Haga, M., Fujii, M., Yamada, K., Hirata, Y., Takanashi, H., Uchida, E., Hosaka, S., Ueno, I., Matsushima, T., Umezawa, K., and Shirai, A. 1979. Edible plants containing carcinogenic pyrrolizidine alkaloids in Japan. in E. C. Miller, J. A. Miller, I. Hirono, T. Sugimura, and S. Takayama (Eds.) *Naturally occurring carcinogens—mutagens and modulators of carcinogenesis.* pp. 79–87. Baltimore: University Park Press.

55. Green, N. R., and Savage, J. R. 1978. Screening of safrole, eugenol, their ninhydrin positive metabolites and selected secondary amines for potental mutagenicity. *Mutat. Res. 57:*115–121.

56. Swanson, A. B., Chambliss, D. D., Blomquist, J. C., Miller, E. C., and Miller, J. A. 1979. The mutagenicities of safrole, estragole, eugenol, trans.-anethole, and some of their known or possible metabolites for *Salmonella typhimurium* mutants. *Mutat. Res. 60:*143–153.

57. Rosenkranz, H. S., and Poirier, L. A. 1979. Evaluation of the mutagenicity and DNA-modifying activity of carcinogens and noncarcinogens in microbial systems. *J. Natl. Cancer Inst. 62:*873–891.

58. Simmon, V. F. 1979. In vitro assays for recombinogenic activity of chemical carcinogens and related compounds with *Saccharomyces cerevisiae* D3. *J. Natl. Cancer Inst. 62:*901–909.

59. Hirono, I. 1981. Natural carcinogenic products of plant origin. *CRC Crit. Rev. Toxicol. 8:*235–277.

60. Hirayama, T. 1979. Epidemiological evaluation of the role of naturally occurring carcinogens and modulators of carcinogenesis. in E. C. Miller, J. A. Miller, I. Hirono, T. Sugimura, and S. Takayama (Eds.) *Naturally occurring carcinogens—mutagens and modulators of carcinogenesis.* pp. 359–380. Baltimore: University Park Press.

61. Howe, G. R., Burch, J. D., Miller, A. B., Cook, G. M., Esteve, J., Morrison, P., Gordon, P., Chambers, L. W., Fodor, G., and Winsor, G. M. 1980. Tobacco use, occupation, coffee; various nutrients and bladder cancer. *J. Natl. Cancer Inst.* *64:*701–713.

62. Pamukcu, A. M., and Bryan, G. T. 1979. Bracken fern, a natural urinary bladder and intestinal carcinogen. in E. C. Miller, J. A. Miller, I. Hirono, T. Sugimura, and E. Takayama (Eds.) *Naturally occurring carcinogens—mutagens and modulators of carcinogenesis.* pp. 89–99. Baltimore: University Park Press.

63. Evans, I. A. 1976. The bracken carcinogen. in C. E. Searle (Ed.) *Chemical carcinogens.* ACS Monograph 173. pp. 690–700. Washington, D.C.: American Chemical Society.

64. Umezawa, K., Matsushima, T., Sugimura, T., Hirakawa, T., Tanaka, M., Katoh, Y., and Takayama, S. 1977. In vitro transformation of hamster embryo cells by quercetin. *Toxicol. Lett.* *1:*175–178.

65. Bartholomew, R. M., and Ryan, D. S. 1980. Lack of mutagenicity of some phytoestrogens in the Salmonella/mammalian microsome assay. *Mutat. Res.* *78:*317–321.

66. Pamukcu, A. M., Yalciner, S., Hatcher, J. F., and Bryan, G. T. 1980. Quercetin, a rat intestinal and bladder carcinogen present in bracken fern (*Pteridium aquilinum*). *Cancer Res.* *40:*3468–3472.

67. Hirono, I., Ueno, I., Hosaka, S., Takanashi, H., Matsushima, T., Sugimura, T., and Natori, S. 1981. Carcinogenicity examination of quercetin and rutin in ACI rats. *Cancer Lett.* *13:*15–21.

68. Pamukcu, A. M., Erturk, E., Yalciner, S., Milli, U., and Bryan, G. T. 1978. Carcinogenic and mutagenic activities of milk from cows fed bracken fern (*Pteridium aquilinum*). *Cancer Res.* *38:*1556–1560.

69. Bross, I. D. J., and Tidings, J. 1973. Another look at coffee drinking and cancer of the urinary bladder. *Prev. Med.* *2:*445–451.

70. Wynder, E. L., and Goldsmith, R. 1977. The epidemiology of bladder cancer. A second look. *Cancer* *40:*1246–1268.

71. Howe, G. R., Burch, J. D., Miller, A. B., Cook, G. M., Esteve, J., Morrison, B., Gordon, P., Chambers, L. W., Fodor, G., and Winsor, G. M. 1980. Tobacco use, occupation, coffee, various nutrients and bladder cancer. *J. Natl. Cancer Inst.* *64:*701–713.

72. MacMahon, B., Yen, S., Trichopoulous, D., Warren, K., and Nardi, G. 1981. Coffee and cancer of the pancreas. *N. Engl. J. Med.* *304:*630–633.

73. Lin, R. S., and Kessler, I. I. 1981. A multifactorial model for pancreatic cancer in man: Epidemiological evidence. *JAMA* *245:*147–152.

74. Martinez, I. 1969. Factors associated with cancer of the esophagus, mouth, and pharynx in Puerto Rico. *J. Natl. Cancer Inst.* *42:*1069–1094.

75. Stocks, P. 1970. Cancer mortality in relation to national consumption of cigarettes, solid fuel, tea and coffee. *Br. J. Cancer* *24:*215–225.

76. Shennan, D. H. 1973. Renal carcinoma and coffee consumption in 16 countries. *Br. J. Cancer* *28:*473–474.

77. Armstrong, B., and Doll, R. 1975. Environmental factors and cancer incidence and mortality in different countries with special reference to dietary practices. *Int. J. Cancer* *15:*617–631.

78. Armstrong, B., Garrod, A., and Doll, R. 1976. A retrospective study of renal cancer with special reference to coffee and animal protein consumption. *Br. J. Cancer* *33:*127–136.

79. Zeitlin, B. R. 1972. Coffee and bladder cancer. *Lancet* *1:*1066.

80. Wurzner, H. P., Lindstrom, E., Vuatz, L., and Luginbuhl, H. 1977. A 2-year feeding study of instant coffees in rats. II. Incidence and types of neoplasms. *Food Cosmet. Toxicol.* *15:*289–296.

81. Challis, B. C., and Bartlett, C. D. 1975. Possible cocarcinogenic effects of coffee constituents. *Nature* *254:*532–533.

82. Aeschbocher, H. U., and Wurzner, H. P. 1980. An evaluation of instant and regular coffee in the Ames mutagenicity test. *Toxicol. Lett. 5:*139–145.

83. Clarke, C. H., and Wade, M. J. 1975. Evidence that caffeine, 8-methoxypsoralen and steroidal diamines are frameshift mutagens for *E. coli* K-12. *Mutat. Res. 28:*123–125.

84. Takayama, S., and Kuwabara, N. 1982. Long-term study on the effect of caffeine in Wistar rats. *Gann 73:*365–371.

85. Kihlman, B. A. 1977. *Caffeine and chromosomes.* New York: Elsevier.

86. Jenssen, D., and Ramel, C. 1978. Factors affecting the induction of micronuclei at low doses of x-rays, MMS and dimethylnitrosamine in mouse erythroblasts. *Mutat. Res. 58:*51–65.

87. Hirono, I., Kachi, H., and Kato, T. 1970. A survey of acute toxicity of cycads and mortality rate from cancer in the Miyako Islands, Okinawa. *Acta Pathol. Jpn. 20:*327–337.

88. Laquer, G. L., and Spatz, M. 1968. Toxicology of cycasin. *Cancer Res. 28:*2262–2267.

89. Matsushima, T., Matsumoto, H., Shirai, A., Sawamura, M., and Sugimura, T. 1979. Mutagenicity of the naturally occurring carcinogens cycasin and synthetic methylazoxymethanol conjugates in *Salmonella typhimurium. Cancer Res. 39:*3780–3782.

90. International Agency for Research on Cancer. 1974. Thiourea. in IARC Monographs on the Evaluation of the Carcinogenic Risk of Chemicals to Man. Vol. 7: *Some anti-thyroid and related substances, nitrofurans and industrial chemicals.* Lyons, France: International Agency for Research on Cancer.

91. Korpassy, B. 1961. Tannins as hepatic carcinogens. *Prog. Exp. Tumor Res. 2:*245–290.

92. Kirby, K. S. 1960. Induction of tumors by tannin extracts. *Br. J. Cancer 14:*147–150.

93. Litton Bionetics. 1975. Mutagenic evaluation of compound 001401554 tannic acid. Prepared for the Bureau of Foods, Food and Drug Administration under Contract No. 73-56. Kensington, Maryland: Litton Bionetics.

94. Rosenkranz, H. S., and Leifer, Z. 1981. Determining the DNA-modifying activity of chemicals using DNA-polymerase deficient *Escherichia coli. Chem. Mutagens 6:*109–147.

95. Grigg, C. W. 1972. Effects of coumarin, pyronin y, 6, 9-dimethyl 2-methyliopurine and caffeine or excision repair and recombination repair in *Escherichia coli. J. Gen. Microbiol. 70:*221–230.

96. Radomski, J. L., Greenwald, D., Hearn, W. L., Block, N. L., and Woods, F. M. 1978. Nitrosamine formation in bladder infections and its role in the etiology of bladder cancer. *J. Urol. 120:*48–58.

97. Cohen, S. M., Arai, M., Jacobs, J. B., and Friedell, G. M. 1979. Promoting effect of saccharin and DL-tryptophan in urinary bladder carcinogenesis. *Cancer Res. 39:*1207–1217.

98. Clayson, D. B., and Garner, R. C. 1976. Carcinogenic aromatic amines and related compounds. in C. E. Searle (Ed.) *Chemical carcinogens.* ACS Monograph 173. pp. 366–461. Washington, D.C.: American Chemical Society.

99. Bowden, J. P., Chung, K. T., and Andrews, A. W. 1976. Mutagenic activity of tryptophan metabolites produced by rat intestinal microflora. *J. Natl. Cancer Inst. 57:*921–924.

100. Clifton, K. N., and Sridharan, B. N. 1975. Endocrine factors and tumor growth. in F. F. Becker (Ed.) *Cancer: a comprehensive treatise. Biology of tumors.* Vol. 3: *Cellular biology and growth.* pp. 249–285. New York: Plenum.

101. Pienta, R. J. 1981. Transformation of Syrian hamster embryo cells by diverse chemicals and correlation with their reported carcinogenic and mutagenic activities. *Chem. Mutagens 6:*175–202.

Chapter 8

Additives and Contaminants

ADDITIVES

This chapter presents data on a few selected compounds that are added directly to foods, as well as processing aids and some compounds that may migrate into foods in small amounts during packaging.

Saccharin

Saccharin is a nonnutritive sweetener that has been used since 1907. In 1977, an estimated 2.2 million kg saccharin and sodium saccharin was produced in the United States and an additional 1.3 million kg was imported. During 1977, about 2.9 million kg (about 83% of the domestic and imported saccharin) was added to foods.

Epidemiological Studies

Population Studies. Nonnutritive sweeteners have been studied mainly to determine their association with bladder cancer. When diabetics were studied, no direct association was found between saccharin use and bladder cancer.[1] However-er, diabetics may not be representative of the general population in epidemiological studies of cancer incidence and mortality, since they differ from the general population in several important respects. Diabetics as a group smoke less and, since smoking has been related to bladder cancer, less cancer of the bladder could be anticipated among these subjects.[2]

In addition, Burbank and Fraumeni found no mortality increase from bladder cancer mortality in the United States after the widespread use of nonnutritive sweeteners.[3] These workers examined mortality rates for this cancer after saccharin was introduced early in this century and also after a 10:1 mixture of cyclamate : saccharin came into use in 1962. From 1911 to 1970 in England and Wales analysis of bladder cancer mortality showed no major change in mortality trends for either males or females.[4] However, time-trend studies may not detect weak effects and can pick up no effects for diseases with long latency periods, if only a short time has elapsed between exposure to the substances and the observation.

Case-Control Studies

Bladder Cancer/Several case-control studies have compared the consumption of saccharin by bladder cancer patients and by healthy controls. Most of these studies were not originally designed to investigate the relationship between nonnutritive sweeteners and bladder cancer. In a case-control study based on responses to questionnaires from 74 female cases, 158 male cases and an equal number of matched controls, Morgan and Jain were unable to find an increased cancer risk in males or females.[5] In another study based on mailed questionnaires to women only, there were no differences found between the cases and controls in either saccharin or cyclamate use.[6] In contrast, Howe *et al.* conducted a case-control study of 480 male and 152 female sex-matched pairs. Males who used nonnutritive sweeteners had a 60% increase in bladder cancer risk and showed evidence of a dose–response relationship. However, women showed no significant increase. In a later study, these preliminary findings were confirmed even when confounding factors such as smoking were controlled.[8]

In case-control studies of 519 bladder cancer patients and 1038 controls,[9] of 265 bladder cancer patients and 530 controls,[10] of 13 bladder cancer cases and 10,784 controls,[11] and of 302 men and 65 women with bladder cancer and an equal number of controls,[12] there was no significant risk associated with the regular use of nonnutritive sweeteners.

In another case-control study, of 592 patients and 596 controls, there was no increase in risk for urinary tract cancer among users of nonnutritive sweeteners.[13] However, in a subgroup of nonsmoking women, there were elevated risks of 2.1 for use of sugar substitutes and 2.6 for use of dietetic beverages.

The National Cancer Institute and the Food and Drug Administration have designed a study to evaluate the relationship between nonnutritive sweetener consumption and bladder cancer.[14] Subjects who had never used either nonnutritive sweeteners or artificially sweetened foods or beverages were not found to have an increased risk of bladder cancer. However, White nonsmoking women who had not been exposed to known bladder carcinogens such as azo dyes were found to have a relative risk of 2.7 to 3.0 in heavy users of nonnutritive sweeteners for at least 10 years and a suggested dose–response relationship. Users of both table-top sweeteners and diet drinks, with a heavy use of at least one of the two, showed a relative risk of 1.5.[14]

Morrison *et al.* evaluated case-control studies in Manchester, United Kingdom, and Nagoya, Japan, where extensive use of saccharin occurred 30–40 years ago. A broad-based series of cases (555 in Manchester, 293 in Nagoya) were interviewed and compared with a series of controls (735 in Manchester, 589 in Nagoya).[15] Use of saccharin was not associated with an elevated risk of bladder cancer in either study area.

In a case-control study conducted in 1978 in Detroit, Michigan, based on interviews with 305 hospital controls, 440 population controls as well as 391 patients with transitional or squamous cell carcinoma of the lower urinary tract, there was a relative risk of 1.1 for males but not females when artificial sweetener users were compared with the general population.[16] Jensen and Kamby have studied the risk of bladder tumors in humans in Denmark after *in utero* exposure to saccharin.[17] When the risk of bladder cancer at ages 20–34 (born 1941–1945) was compared with the risk in men or women born 1931–1940, the relative risk for men was 1.0 and for women 0.3. There was no evidence of an increased risk of human bladder cancer during the first 30–35 years of life associated with *in utero* saccharin exposure.

*Pancreatic Cancer/*An increase of deaths from pancreatic cancer was found in diabetics who consumed saccharin.[1] A direct correlation was also found between pancreatic cancer mortality and diabetes mellitus in women, but not in men, who consumed saccharin in a study done by county in the United States.[18] Wynder *et al.,* in a case-control study, found a direct association of pancreatic cancer with early-onset diabetes in women who used saccharin.[19]

Carcinogenicity

In a number of single-generation studies in which various doses of saccharin were fed to several strains of mice and rats and to hamsters and rhesus monkeys, there was no evidence of saccharin-induced carcinogenesis. In a single-generation study, Wistar specific-pathogen-free rats were fed saccharin or saccharin and *o*-toluenesulfonamide (OTS) in the drinking water daily for 2 years.[20] Treated males in both groups developed more tumors than did the untreated controls, but there was no significant difference in the females. Charles River CD rats fed sodium saccharin (free of OTS) for their lifetime had a greater incidence of benign and malignant bladder tumors than was observed in the untreated controls.[21]

Saccharin has also been tested in two-generation carcinogenicity bioassays in which parent animals, baby animals *in utero,* and their offspring are given the same diet as their parents. In one such study, there was no difference in the incidence of tumors in treated or control Swiss SPF mice in either generation.[22] In three two-generation studies with Charles River and Sprague-Dawley rats, the incidence of bladder tumors in the second-generation male rats was greater than in the control rats.[21]

Saccharin has increased the incidence of and decreased the latent period for tumor development in animals treated with N-nitroso-N-methylurea (NMU)[17] or with N-[4(5-nitro-2-furyl)-2-thiazolyl]formamide (FANFT).[20] In several *in vitro* cell culture systems, saccharin also exhibited an activity similar to the tumor-promoting activity exhibited by tetradecanoylphorbol acetate.[21]

Mutagenicity

Conflicting results have resulted from efforts to test saccharin for mutagenicity. No mutagenicity was observed in several studies,[25] but Batzinger *et al.* reported that saccharin was weakly mutagenic to *S. typhimurium* TA98 and TA100 strains in a modified plate assay and that the urine of animals fed saccharin contained mutagens for TA98 and TA100 strains.[26] In the mouse lymphoma assay, weak mutagenic effects were observed.[27] Dominant lethal mutations have been found in animals fed sodium saccharin in the diet,[28] and Ochi and Tonomura have reported a dose-dependent increase in unscheduled DNA synthesis.[29]

Continuous exposure to saccharin after treatment of C3H/10T1/2 cells with 3-methylcholanthrene has led to a significant increase in the number of transformed colonies.[30] Saccharin also induces chromosomal aberrations in mammalian cells,[31] as well as sister chromatid exchanges in cells from humans.[32]

Cyclamate

Cyclamic acid, sodium cyclamate, and calcium cyclamate were used as nonnutritive sweeteners, in carbonated beverages, in dry beverage bases, in diet foods, and in sweetener formulations until 1970, when cyclamates were banned from use in the United States.

Epidemiological Evidence

Because cyclamates were rarely used without saccharin, epidemiological data on cyclamates alone are inadequate. Studies were not generally able to distinguish the consumption of cyclamate-containing mixtures from the consumption of saccharin.

Carcinogenicity

There was no evidence of the carcinogenicity of cyclamates in a study performed on Swiss and Charles River CD mice that received up to 5% sodium cyclamate for 18 or 24 months.[33] When 0.6% sodium cyclamate was administered in drinking water to mice for their lifetime, there was no evidence of carcinogenesis in male and female C3H mice, but there was an increased incidence of lung tumors in RIII male and XVIII female mice and of hepatocellular carcinomas in (C3H × RIII)F$_1$ male mice.[34] In female SPF mice fed diets containing up to 7% sodium cyclamate for 80 weeks, a higher but statistically insignificant increase was observed in the incidence of lymphosarcomas as compared with the controls.[35]

Cyclamates fed to Sprague-Dawley rats for 2 years led to a slight increase in the incidence of bladder tumors.[36] When Osborne Mendel rats were fed cyclamate in their diet for 101 weeks, there was an increased incidence of transitional cell papillomas of the urinary bladder; however, in this study only a small number of animals were examined histopathologically.[37]

Lifetime studies in one generation of Syrian golden hamsters and rhesus monkeys and a six-generation study of Swiss SPF mice produced no evidence that sodium cyclamate is carcinogenic.[38]

Female Wistar SPF rats treated with NMU and cyclamate in their diets for their lifetime or up to 2 years had a significantly greater incidence of bladder cancer and a significant decrease in the latent period as compared with both animals treated with NMU only and the untreated controls.[39]

In another study, NMU was instilled into the urinary bladder of female Wistar rats before the animals were started on a diet containing sodium cyclamate that would continue for the rest of their lives.[40] The overall incidence of urinary tract tumors was 70% in those given NMU and sodium cyclamate, 57% in animals receiving NMU alone, and 65% in another control group given NMU and calcium carbonate.[40]

Mutagenicity

There are no data available on the ability of cyclamates alone to induce mutations in either microbial or mammalian cells. However, two studies found cyclamates to induce chromosomal breaks in human leukocytes.[41,42]

No increases in chromosomal aberrations were observed in hamsters given oral doses of either sodium cyclamate or cyclohexylamine sulfate.[43]

Aspartame

Aspartame, the methyl ester of the amino acid phenylalanine and aspartic acid, is about 180 times sweeter than sugar; it was approved in 1981 by the FDA for use as a sweetener or flavoring agent in certain foods. However, aspartame cannot be used in soft drinks because of its instability in liquids during storage.

Epidemiological Evidence

Because aspartame has only been on the market since 1981 and in only a few countries (e.g., Belgium, France, and Canada), there have been no epidemiological studies regarding its association with cancer in humans.

Carcinogenicity

The G. D. Searle Company has been feeding aspartame to Charles River mice for the past 2 years. No tumors attributable to aspartame ingestion have been reported to date.[44] Another study demonstrated no statistically significant differences in the incidence of neoplasms in the urinary bladders of control and in treated mice 26 weeks after implantation of cholesterol pellets or its breakdown product diketopiperazine (DKP).

These findings are possible in contrast to those of another study, in which male and female Sprague-Dawley rats were fed various levels of aspartame for up to 2 years. An independent review board of the FDA examined the data and concluded that aspartame was a possible carcinogen on the basis of three of the study's findings: (1) a greater incidence of brain neoplasms in aspartame-fed rats than that of the controls; (2) a possible dose–response relationship as demonstrated by tumor incidence in the two lower doses as compared with the two higher-dose treatment groups combined; and (3) a decrease in the latent period for gliomas.[45] Investigators at the G. D. Searle Company did not agree with the FDA's statistical interpretation of the results. However, in a follow-up study by the Searle group, rats were exposed *in utero* to three levels of aspartame for the duration of their lives. There was no statistical difference between the control and treated groups.

In another study by Searle, groups of five male and female beagle dogs were fed aspartame at four dietary levels for more than 106 weeks. No evidence of neoplasia was observed in any of the treated or control groups.

Mutagenicity

Aspartame and DKP were negative in the Ames test with and without using the S9 fractions from rats, in the host-mediated assay in rats and mice, and was also negative in the *in vivo* dominant lethal assay in rats.[46] The additional carcinogenic and mutagenicity studies have led the FDA to conclude that aspartame is not carcinogenic in animals.

Food Colorings

Food colors have received special attention over the years. At one time they were tested by subcutaneous injection; several food colors resulted in the induction of sarcomas. It was generally accepted, however, that such tests for food additives were not appropriate and that the resultant sarcomas might be a result of physical rather than chemical properties of the test materials. The general principle that food additives should be tested orally is probably more reliable.

One of the first carcinogens to be used extensively in the laboratory was p-dimethylaminobenzene known previously as a food color, butter yellow. Butter yellow is mainly known for its ability to induce hepatomas in the rat, but does not seem to be active in other species.

The presence of residues of the well-known carcinogen, 2-naphthylamine in yellow OB and yellow AB resulted in control of these compounds. Red 2 or amaranth still remains controversial not only as a possible carcinogen but as a teratogen. In one experiment the ratio of malignant to benign tumors did increase in females given diets containing 3% amaranth (the highest dose). The FDA did not claim amaranth to be a carcinogen but that safety had not been demonstrated. There was also no evidence of a public health hazard.

Eight food dyes or commercial color mixtures certified for use in the United States have been tested for their ability to transform *in vitro* a serial line of Fischer rat embryo cells which have been reported to be a sensitive indicator of chemicals having carcinogenic potential.[47] Malignant cell transformation was induced by a commercial mixture (G2024) of two of these dyes (Blue 1 and Yellow 5) and by Blue 2, Green 3 (one of two experiments), and Red 4. However, food dyes Blue 1, Red 3, Yellow 5, and Yellow 6 did not induce cell transformation.

Auramine is a compound whose manufacture causes cancer in man which seems to result from an as yet unidentified impurity.

Butylated Hydroxytoluene (BHT) and Butylated Hydroxyanisole (BHA)

Butylated hydroxytoluene (BHT) and butylated hydroxyanisole (BHA) are widely used as food additives mainly because of their preservative and antioxidant properties. Both BHA and BHT are included in the FDA list of substances generally accepted as safe (GRAS) and many acute and chronic toxic tests have been done on them. Based on the evidence from these studies, the FDA in 1977 recommended that BHT be removed from the GRAS list and proposed interim regulations pending future studies.

Epidemiological Evidence

There are no epidemiological studies in regard to the effects of BHT and BHA on human health.

Carcinogenicity of BHT

BHT was fed in the diet to male and female mice for 107 to 108 weeks.[48] In the female mice receiving the low dose, the incidence of alveolar/bronchiolar adenomas or carcinoma was significantly higher than the controls, but there was no dose response. When male and female Fischer 344 rats were studied in a similar study, the incidence of tumors in treated animals was not statistically different from that in controls.

Promoting Effect of BHT

Three groups of A/J mice were injected with urethan, 3-methylcholanthrene, or nitrosodimethylamine and then given repeated injections of BHT. BHT treatment significantly increased the multiplicity of lung tumors induced by all three carcinogens.[48] In addition, BHT administered orally increased the multiplicity of lung tumors induced by all three carcinogens.[48] An increase of lung tumor incidence was still observed even if urethan injections were started as late as 5 months after the urethan was administered. These results suggest that BHT was a tumor promotor.[49] BHT also appeared to have promoting activity in BALB/c mice and in male Sprague-Dawley rats treated with 2-aminoacetylfluorene (2-AAF).

Mutagenicity of BHT

BHT has inhibited the cell-to-cell communication of mammalian cells *in vitro*—an indication of promoting activity.[50] When BHT was added to phytohemagglutinin-stimulated cultures of human leukocytes, it resulted in a dose-dependent decrease in cell survival as well as in an uncoiling of the chromosomes.[51] However, in the sister chromatid exchange assay, BHT was negative and did not increase chromosomal aberrations.[52]

Carcinogenicity of BHA

In contrast to BHT, when BHA was administered there was no significant effect on the tumor yield or the number of tumors in Swiss Webster mice injected with urethan and then given BHA in the diet.[49]

Mutagenicity of BHA

BHA was positive in the sister chromatid exchange assay with Chinese hamster cells as indicator organisms; however, no chromosomal aberrations were induced in these cells.

Inhibition of Carcinogen-Induced Neoplasia by BHA

Anticarcinogenicity. BHA has proven to be a important inhibitor of carcinogenesis and has been extensively studied for its capacity to inhibit carcinogen-induced neoplasia.[53] Table 8-1 lists experiments in which BHA has been shown to have inhibitory effects. In these studies, BHA was administered before and/or during exposure to the carcinogen.

Mechanism. Studies of the mechanism by which BHA inhibits chemically induced carcinogenesis have shown that this phenolic compound produces a coordinated enzyme response that may be interpreted as causing a greater rate of detoxification.[54] Increases in both glutathione *S*-transferase and tissue glutathione levels have been observed in mice that have been fed BHA for 1–2 weeks in carcinogen inhibition experiments.[55] Glutathione *S*-transferase is an important enzyme for detoxifying chemical carcinogens.[54,55]

Uridine diphosphate (UDP)-glucuronyl transferase, which is another important conjugated enzyme in the detoxification system, is also increased.[56] The feeding of BHA has also been reported to increase epoxide hydrolase activity[57] and also altered the microsomal monoxygenase system.[58]

Table 8-1. Inhibition of Carcinogen-Induced Neoplasia by BHA[a]

Carcinogen inhibited	Species	Site of neoplasm
Benzo[*a*]pyrene	Mouse	Lung
Benzo[*a*]pyrene	Mouse	Forestomach
Benzo[*a*]pyrene-7,8-dehydrodiol	Mouse	Forestomach, lung, and lymphoid tissue
7,12-Dimethylbenz[*a*]anthracene	Mouse	Lung
7,12-Dimethylbenz[*a*]anthracene	Mouse	Forestomach
7,12-Dimethylbenz[*a*]anthracene	Mouse	Skin
7,12-Dimethylbenz[*a*]anthracene	Rat	Breast
7-Hydroxymethyl-12-methyl-benz[*a*]anthracene	Mouse	Lung
Dibenz[*a,h*]anthracene	Mouse	Lung
Nitrosodiethylamine	Mouse	Lung
4-Nitroquinoline-*N*-oxide	Mouse	Lung
Uracil mustard	Mouse	Lung
Urethan	Mouse	Lung
Methylazoxymethanol acetate	Mouse	Large intestine
trans-5-Amino-3-[2-(5-nitro-2-furyl)vinyl]-1,2,4-oxadiazole	Mouse	Forestomach, lung, and lymphoid tissue

[a]By permission of National Academy Press, Washington, D.C., *Diet, nutrition and cancer*, 1982.

Antimutagenicity. BHA has also been shown to inhibit host-mediated muta-genesis resulting from exposure to hycanthone, metrifonate, praziquantel, and metronidazole.[59]

Other phenolics. Several naturally occurring phenolic compounds inhibit carcinogenesis in mice.[60] These phenols are cinnamic acid derivatives that are common constituents of plants. These include *o*-hydroxycinnamic acid, *p*-hydroxycinnamic acid, 3,4-dihydroxycinnamic acid (caffeic acid), and 4-hydroxy-3-methoxycinnamic acid (ferulic acid). Preliminary data on these derivatives indicate that their inhibition of benzopyrene-induced neoplasia in the mouse is considerably weaker than that of BHA.[60] Many other phenols are present in plants, including plants consumed by humans, but their inhibitory activity is unknown.

Indoles

Indole-3-acetonitrile, 3,3[1]-diindolymethane and indole-3-carbinol are found in edible cruciferous vegetables such as brussels sprouts, cabbage, cauliflower, and broccoli. Of these three, indole-3-acetonitrile is the most abundant. These indoles have been studied for their effects on neoplasia induced by benzpyrene (BaP) and 7,12-dimethylbenzanthracene (DMBA) in rodents.[61] If these indoles were added to the diet of mice before and after administration of BaP, all three indoles inhibited BaP-induced neoplasia of the forestomach and pulmonary adenoma formation. In addition, in other experiments, indole-3-carbinol and 3,3[1]-diindolylmethane inhibited DMBA-induced mammary tumor formation in female Sprague-Dawley rats. However, indole-3-acetonitrile was inactive in the rat. All three indoles are able to alter the microsomal monoxygenase oxidase activity.[62] All three compounds increased the activity of this enzyme system with indole-3-carbinol and 3,3-diindolylmethane more strongly than indole-3-acetonitrile. All three indoles have also increased glutathione *S*-transferase activity.

Aromatic Isothiocyanates

Both benzyl isothiocyanates and phenethyl isothiocyanate are also constituents of cruciferous plants. These aromatic isothiocyanates have been shown to inhibit neoplasia induced by polycyclic aromatic hydrocarbons (PAH's) when they were administered during the initiation phase under several different experimental conditions. These results were obtined when the aromatic isothiocyanate was fed before and during administration of the PAH's.[63] The mechanism of inhibition is not known, but it is known that benzyl isothiocyanate is a potent inducer of glutathione S-transferase activity. This compound has also inhibited 1,2-dimethylhydrazine-induced neoplasia of the large intestine when the exposures were begun 1 week after administration of the carcinogen.[64] The mechanism of these inhibitory effects is unknown.

Flavones

The study of flavones (found in fruits and vegetables) as possible inhibitors was started after it was shown that several inducers of increased microsomal mixed function oxidase activity were shown to inhibit chemically induced carcinogenesis. Three flavones have been studied to see if they inhibit BaP-induced carcinogenesis. Of the three flavones, two were synthetic—β-naphthoflavone (5,6-benzoflavone) and quercetin pentamethyl ether—and one naturally occurring compound—rutin-(3,3,4,5,7-pentahydroxyflavone-3-rutinoside).

Induction of Aryl Hydrocarbon Hydroxylase

All three flavones induce aryl hydrocarbon hydroxylase (AHH) activity. Of the three, β-naphthoflavone is the most potent inducer, quercetin pentamethyl ether is a moderate inducer, and rutin has the weakest inducing capacity.

When added to the diet of A/HeJ mice subsequently given orally administered BaP, β-naphthoflavone caused almost total inhibition of pulmonary adenoma formation, and quercetin pentamethyl ether reduced the number of these neoplasms by one-half. In both the animals fed rutin as well as the controls, the number of adenomas was the same. Thus, the potency of the three flavones in inducing increased AHH activity parallels the inhibitory effects of BaP-induced neoplasia.[65] In addition, β-naphthoflavone has been shown to induce activity of conjugating enzymes, including glutathione S-transferase. This is a major detoxification system that catalyzes the finding of a vast variety of electrophiles to the sulfhydryl group of glutathione. Since the reactive ultimate carcinogenic forms of chemicals are electrophiles, the glutathione S-transferase system is likely very important for carcinogen detoxification. *In vitro* enhancement of the enzyme activity has been shown to be associated with the decreased response of tissues to chemical carcinogens.[66]

Induction of Glutathione S-Transferase

Diets containing large quantities of cruciferous vegetables induce increased glutathione S-transferase.[67] Green coffee beans induce such activity to a remarkable extent. Two potent inducers of glutathione S-transferase activity have been isolated from green coffee beans. These compounds are kahweol palmitate and cafestol palmitate.[68] When diets containing large amounts of cabbage and brussels sprouts were fed to healthy volunteers between 21 and 32 years of age, they metabolized antipyrine and phenacetin more rapidly than did subjects on a control diet.[69]

Structure of Flavones and Mutagenicity

The mitogenic flavones have multiple hydroxyl groups. In general, flavones having protective effects do not have free polar groups; they either contain methoxy substituents or are unsubstituted.[70]

Protease Inhibitors

Protease inhibitors are widely distributed in plants, and are especially abundant in seeds. Soybeans are major source of protein in many vegetarian diets, and lima beans contain a number of these compounds. Protease inhibitors are able to inhibit protease enzymes as well as tumor promotion.[71] When rats were fed a diet rich in protease inhibitors after exposure to radiation, there was a reduced incidence of breast cancer.[71] Protease inhibitors also block the transformation of C3H10T1/2 cells by X-rays followed by incubation with 12-*O*-tetradecanoyl-pharbol-13-acetate (TPA).[72] Troll has suggested that protease inhibitors prevent formation of free radicals by tumor promotors. Since BHA and some related antioxidants inhibit promotion, there could be a common mechanism among inhibitors that would lead to synergistic effects.

β-Sitosterol

β-Sitosterol is a common plant sterol that is present in many different vegetables and vegetable oils. β-Sitosterol has shown protective effects in an experimental system with *N*-nitrosomethylurea-a direct-acting carcinogen. β-Sitosterol, when fed in the diet through the entire course of the experiment or only during the promotion phase of carcinogenesis, reduced the incidence of large bowel cancer from 54 to 33%.[73] Other plant sterols of similar structure have not been studied for possible inhibitory effects.

CONTAMINANTS

Vinyl Chloride

Containers made from polyvinyl chloride (PVC) are widely used packaging and storing foods. Because of reports linking several fatal cases of a rare form of liver tumor with prolonged industrial exposure to vinyl chloride, considerable attention has been paid to the possible carcinogenicity and other toxic effects of the monomer vinyl chloride, of which PVC is composed.

Vinyl chloride has been detected in a variety of alcoholic drinks (0.2 to 1 mg/liter), in vinegars (9.4 mg/liter), in edible oils (0.05–14.8 mg/kg), (0.05 mg/kg) has been detected in margarine and butter, and 10.0 μg/liter is the highest concentration found in finished drinking water in the United States.

Epidemiological Evidence

There have been no epidemiological studies on exposure to vinyl chloride as a food contaminant. Creech and Johnson were the first investigators to report an association between inhalation exposure to vinyl chloride and hepatic angiosarcomas.[74] In males who had been occupationally exposed to vinyl chloride for at least 1 year, Tabershaw and Goffey observed an excess of cancer of the digestive system, liver (mainly angiosarcoma) respiratory tract, and brain, as well as lymphomas.[75] A 50% excess of deaths due to all cancers in workers producing and polymerizing vinyl chloride.[76] Other studies have indicated an association between exposure to vinyl chloride and increased mortality from cancer at various sites.[77]

Carcinogenicity

When male and female Sprague-Dawley rats received gastric intubations of vinyl chloride in doses up to 50 mg/kg body weight, angiosarcomas and cancers of the Zymbal's gland mainly developed.[78]

When vinyl chloride monomer was fed to Wistar rats throughout their lifetime, hepatocellular carcinomas, hepatic angiosarcomas, pulmonary angiosarcoma, extraphetic abdominal angiosarcomas, Zymbal gland tumors, abdominal mesotheliomas, and adenocarcinomas of the mammary glands developed.[79]

Inhalation exposures to vinyl chloride have produced cancers of the lung, mammary gland, and liver in mice; cancers of Zymbal's gland, the liver, kidney, and brain in Sprague-Dawley rats; and cancers of the liver, skin, and stomach in hamsters.[78]

Mutagenicity

Vinyl chloride vapors have induced mutations in the Ames *Salmonella* strains,[80] *Escherichia coli, Schizosaccharomyces pombe, Drosophila melanogaster* and mammalian cells. Vinyl chloride also induce gene conversions in yeast.[81] In addition, male workers occupationally exposed to vinyl chloride have been reported to have more chromosomal aberrations than were observed in unexposed workers.[82]

Acrylonitrile

Acrylonitrile is produced on a large scale in industry. Its use in food packaging and the migratory quality of the monomer, which is present in small amounts in the polymer, has led to its being an "indirect" additive or contaminant. Three foods, which have been wrapped in acrylonitrile-based packaging materials (margarine, olive oil, and bologna), contain acrylonitrile in concentrations ranging from 13 to 49 ng/kg.

Epidemiological Studies

The significance of such exposure of the general public to acrylonitrile has not been evaluated. A retrospective cohort study of 1345 male employees exposed to acrylonitrile in a textile plant indicated a trend toward an increased risk at all sites, especially the lung. As the duration and amount of exposure increased, the risk increased.[83]

Carcinogenicity

After rats received acrylonitrile in their drinking water for 1 year, they developed stomach papillomas, tumors of the central nervous system and carcinomas's of the Zymbal's gland. Rats developed tumors of the central nervous system and ear duct, as well as masses in the mammary region.[84]

Mutagenicity

In the Ames test[85] and in *Escherichia coli,* acrylonitrile induced mutations.[86] In contrast, chromosome aberrations in workers exposed to acrylonitrile for an average of 15.3 years did not exceed those in unexposed controls.[87]

Diethylstilbestrol

Among the approximately 20 growth hormones commonly used in animal feed, attention has mainly focused on diethylstilbestrol (DES), whose residues have been monitored for many years following reports that DES was carcinogenic in animals.[88] Until June 1978, DES was permitted for use by humans as a control for functional menstrual disorders; for prevention of postpartum breast engorgement; as chemotherapy for prostate cancer and for breast cancer in postmenopausal women; as a "morning-after pill;" and as therapy for estrogen deficiencies related to the climateric and other hormone-related conditions.

Until 1979, when the use of DES was terminated, it was also permitted as a growth promotor for cattle and sheep under certain conditions outlined by the FDA. In 1972 and 1973, the U.S. Department of Agriculture detected low levels of DES residues in beef. Since 1973 no residues of DES have been detected in beef at these low levels.

Epidemiological Studies

There have been no reports of epidemiological studies in regard to the health effects of DES residues in food. Herbst and Cole have reported that therapeutic doses of DES during pregnancy have been associated with an increase in vaginal and cervical adenocarcinoma among the daughters of DES users, especially in those between the ages of 10 and 30 years.[89]

Men treated with DES for prostate cancer sometimes will develop breast cancer after the start of the treatment.[90] Of 24 female patients treated with DES for five years or more with gonadal dysgenesis (Turner's syndrome),[91] two developed endometrial carcinoma, but the risk of endometrial carcinoma in untreated patients is not known.

Carcinogenicity

When DES was fed to C3H male or female mice, mammary carcinomas were produced in increasing incidence with increased doses.[92] At the highest doses of DES, the latent period was reduced from 49 weeks to 31 weeks. In addition, when C3H/An were fed DES, the incidence of mammary cancers was significantly greater than the controls.[93] In another study Sprague-Dawley rats were fed DES daily in the diet for 2 years. Male rats developed pituitary tumors, some hepatomas (females only), and mammary tumors (males and females)[94] In the progeny of pregnant Syrian golden hamsters which were administered DES by intragastric tube, a high incidence of metaplastic, dyplastic and neoplastic lesions were observed in the genital tract.[95]

Mutagenicity

Diethylstilbestrol was not mutagenic in the Ames test with and without metabolic activation,[96] and in *E. coli*.[97] DES has induced chromosome aberrations in Chinese hamster fibroblast,[98] and in murine bone marrow cells *in vivo*.[99] Other studies have demonstrated that DES induced mutations in mouse lymphoma cells,[100] unscheduled DNA synthesis in HeLa cells,[101] and aneuploidy *in vivo* in several mouse strains.[102]

Pesticides

Environmental contaminants in food can be loosely divided into three categories: some trace metals and organometallic compounds, some natural and synthetic radioactive substances, and some natural and synthetic organic compounds such as pesticides.

Agricultural commodities will sometimes contain residues of pesticides after they have been harvested and prepared for consumer purchase. Processed foods derived from these commodities are also sometimes found in processed foods. Even though the general population has been exposed to low levels of pesticides from numerous sources, especially foods and drinking water, little is known about their effect on human health. Because many of the pesticides which are present in food, are known or suspected carcinogens in some animal species, there is a basis for concern about their potential effects on human health.

Levels of pesticides in food are very low and they vary only slightly from region to region. The organo-chlorine compound tend to accumulate in fat-containing foods such as meat, fish, poultry, and dairy products, whereas the organoposphates are generally more common in cereal products.

Residues of a few organochlorine, organophosphate, and carbamate pesticides are commonly detected in the diet at levels which are usually one to two orders of magnitude below their generally acceptable daily intake (ADI). In contrast to the organophosphates and carbamates, most of the organophosphates have the potential to alter the activity of microsomal enzymes and to engage in synergistic interactions.

Epidemiological Studies

Data from the few epidemiological studies that have been conducted allow no conclusion to be drawn about the carcinogenic risk to humans exposed to pesticides.

Carcinogenicity

Organochlorine Pesticides. The evidence for carcinogenicity is based on the production of parenchymal liver cell tumors in mice for most organochlorine pesticides.[103] With the exception of methoxychlor, which has not been found to be mutagenic or carcinogenic, several other organochlorine pesticides were mutagens or carcinogens. These include dieldrin, DDT, captan, heptachlor, heptachlor epoxide, pentachloronitrobenzene, hexachlorobenzene, toxaphene, lindane, chlordane, and kepone.

Rat tests results indicate that toxaphene and kepone are carcinogenic and that heptachlor, hexachlorobenzene, and lindane may be carcinogenic. Hexachlorobenzene also causes cancer in hamsters.

Organophosphates. In bioassays conducted by the National Cancer Institute, the organophosphates malathion, methyl parathion, and diazinon did not increase tumor incidence in rats or mice. Parathion, however, resulted in an increased incidence of cortical tumors of the adrenal gland in Osborne Mendel rats. In bacterial tests parathion and diazinon were not mutagenic, but studies have indicated that parathion induces chromosome abnormalities in guinea pigs[104] and that diazinon induces chromosome abnormalities in the lymphocytes of humans.[105] Aldicarb is a very toxic compound, but does not appear to be carcinogenic in rats and mice.

Carbamate Pesticides. The carbaryl data are inconclusive and do not permit carcinogenicity assessment. Carbaryl is able to react with nitrite under mildly acidic conditions to produce *N*-nitrosocarbaryl, which is a known carcinogen in rats.[106]

The results of mutagenicity and other short-term tests for some organochlorine pesticides did not coincide with data from experiments to study carcinogenicity in animals. This difference may indicate the limited value of mutagenicity tests for screening organochlorine compounds for possible adverse effects.

Polychlorinated Biphenyls

Polychlorinated biphenyls (PCB's), which are complex mixtures of chlorinated hydrocarbons, have been used for industrial purposes the last fifty years. Initial concern about the adverse health effects of various commercial PCB mixtures started when chloracne and hepatic changes were observed among workers engaged in the production of these compounds.[107] When the Environmental Protection Agency realized that PCB's are highly toxic and persistant to the environment, they suspended their manufacture and commercial use.

The major source of human exposure to low levels of PCB's is the diet. Generally, PCB's have been found only in the flesh or products of animals (e.g., fish, milk, eggs, and cheese) and in animal feed derived from animal products (e.g., fish meal).[108] Between 1969 and 1975 the levels of PCB's decreased in all foods examined, except fish. Daily dietary intakes measured between 1974 and 1977 showed that PCB's had dropped to levels well below the tolerance levels in individual foods.[109] PCB's also tend to accumulate in the adipose tissue of humans, in milk and in blood.[110]

Epidemicological Studies

Because of the lack of data from epidemiological studies, it is difficult to determine the significance of these findings for human health.

Carcinogenicity Studies

On the basis of several experiments, it appears that Kanechlor 500 and Aroclor 1254 induce cancer in mice and that Aroclor 1260 is carcinogenic in rats. All three of these compounds have induced benign and malignant liver cell tumors in laboratory animals.[103] When PCB's were tested as promoting agents, it appears that Kanechlor 400 and 500 enhance the hepatocarcinogencity of 3-methyl-4-aminoazobenzene (3^1-DMAB) and N-nitrosodiethylamine (NDEA) in rats and of lindane in mice. In contrast, when Kanechlor 500 was administered to rats at the same time as the carcinogen, the hepatocarcinogenicity of 3^1-DMAB, 2-AAF, and NDEA.[111]

Mutagenicity Studies

Aroclor 1221 and 1268 are mutagenic,[112] but a number of other PCB's, e.g., Aroclor 1254 are negative in the dominant lethal assay in rats and do not induce chromosomal aberrations in cultures of lymphocytes from humans. These results are difficult to interpret for Aroclor 1254, which induces dose-related hepatocellular carcinoma in female rats and also enhances NDEA-induced hepatocellular carcinoma in rats.

Polybrominated Biphenyls

Polybrominated biphenyl's (PBB's), which are chemically related to the PCB's, have been used in industrial processes as flame retardants. Like the PCB's, PBB's persist in the environment and also can accumulate in body fat.

Epidemiological Evidence

Even though exposure to PBB's in Michigan in 1973 indicated that the exposure was associated with a number of adverse health effects, because of the relatively short interval between the time of exposure and the measurement of effects, there was no definitive information about the relationship between PBB's and cancer.

Experimental Evidence

A high incidence of hepatocellular carcinomas have resulted from giving Sherman rats PBB's by gavage.[113] In addition, PBB has been shown to be a tumor promotor in rats.[103]

Mutagenicity

No mutations were induced in the Ames test and in Chinese hamster uterine cells.[103] When administered orally to mice, PBB's did not induce chromosomal aberrations in bone marrow cells.[113]

Polycyclic Aromatic Hydrocarbons

Polycyclic aromatic hydrocarbons are organic compounds containing two or more benzene rings. More than 100 of these compounds have been identified in the environment and in foods. Fewer than 20 of these have been shown to cause cancer in laboratory animals, but only five of these have induced cancer after oral administration : benzpyrene (BaP), dibenzanthracene (DBA), benzanthracene, 3-methylcholanthrene, 7,12-dimethylbenzanthracene. Of these PAH's, 3MCA and 7,12-DMBA are synthetic chemicals that do not normally occur in the diet.

Sources of PAH Contamination

The major sources of the PAH contamination of food are curing smokes, contaminated soils, polluted air and water, and endogenous biosynthesis by plants and microorganisms. The methods with which foods are cooked or processed will also affect their PAH content.

There is widespread contamination of foods by PAH's. These compounds have been detected in fresh meats, smoked fish and meats, grilled and roasted foods, leafy and root vegetables, vegetable oils, grains, plants, fruits, seafoods, and whiskies.

The total PAH burden is increased by the smoking of meat.[114] In addition, hot air drying and roasting are potential sources of contamination of grain and coffee.[115] Most foods contain low levels of PAH's but shellfish seem to concentrate these compounds and are unable to metabolize them. Extremely low levels of various PAH's including BaP, benzanthracene, and chrysene, have been detected in scotch whiskey and Japanese whiskies.[116] Spinach, kale, and tobacco are leafy plants that contain greater levels of BaP, but only a small fraction appears to be removed by washing.[117]

Even though BaP constitutes only 1–20% of the total amount of carcinogenic PAH's in the environment, the levels of BaP in various foods have been studied extensively,[118] but the levels of other carcinogenic PAH's are still fragmentary. In the German Democratic Republic, the average annual intake of BaP ranged from 340 to 1200 μg per person annually,[119] and in Hungary estimations were calculated to be 290 to 612 micrograms/per person annually.[120] In these studies the main sources of ingested BaP were fruits and vegetables, however, the smoked foods contributed only a minor fraction of the total BaP intake. Even though there is information about specific foods, such as oils and smoked meats, the total intake of BaP from all sources has not been reported in the United States.

Epidemiological Studies

The association between cancer in humans (mainly cancer of the skin and lung) and exposure to PAH's is derived from studies of humans exposed occupationally to PAH's in soot from chimneys, coal tar, creasote oil, and other petroleum products.[121] However, in spite of this association, there is little information concerning the relationship between ingestion of PAH-contaminated food and cancer in humans. Some investigators have speculated that a high incidence of stomach cancer in Hungary and Iceland may be associated with consumption of smoked meat and fish, which are potential sources of PAH's and/or nitrosamines and their precursors, but this has not been conclusively demonstrated.

Carcinogenicity

The toxic, carcinogenic, and mutagenic effects of PAH's are exerted only after being metabolized by the mixed-function oxidases of various tissues.[122] The carcinogenic activity of PAH's varies from being weak to being potent. Some of the PAH's have been shown to be carcinogenic to mice, rats,hamsters, rabbits, and monkeys when administered topically, orally, or parenterally.[122] Many PAH's have also been found to be mutagenic. Some of those PAH's detected in foods and found to be carcinogenic when administered orally include benzopyrene, dibenzanthracene and benzanthracene.[102] Since studies in animals have shown that PAH's are carcinogenic when administered orally, and occupational exposure to substances containing PAH's have been associated with skin and lung cancer, it would be desirable to minimize exposure to PAH's.

REFERENCES

1. Armstrong, B. A., Lea, A. J., Adelstein, A. M., Donovan, J. W., White, G. C., & Ruttle, S. 1976. Cancer mortality and saccharin consumption in diabetics. *Br. J. Prev. Soc. Med. 30:*151–157.

2. Christiansen, J. S. 1978. Cigarette smoking and prevalence of microangiopathy in juvenile-onset insulin-independent diabetes mellitus. *Diabetes Care 1:*146–149.

3. Burbank, F., and Fraumeni, J. F. 1970. Synthetic sweetener consumption and bladder cancer trends in the United States. *Nature 227:*296–297.

4. Armstrong, B., and Doll, R. 1974. Bladder cancer mortality in England and Wales in relation to cigarette smoking and saccharin consumption. *Br. J. Prev. Soc. Med. 28:*233–240.

5. Morgan, R. W., and Jain, M. G. 1974. Bladder cancer: Smoking, beverages and artificial sweeteners. *Can. Med. Assoc. J. 111:*1067–1070.

6. Simon, D., Yen, S., and Cole, P. 1975. Coffee drinking and cancer of the lower urinary tract. *J. Natl. Cancer Inst. 54:*587–591.

7. Howe, G. R., Burch, J. D., Miller, A. B., Morrison, B., Gordon, P., Weldon, L., Champbers, L. W., Fodor, G., and Winsor, G. M. 1977. Artificial sweeteners and human bladder cancer. *Lancet 2:*578–581.

8. Howe, G. R., Burch, J. D., Miller, A. B., Cook, G. M., Esteve, J., Morrison, G., Gordon, P., Chambers, L. W., Fodor, G., and Winsor, G. M. 1980. Tobacco use, occupation, coffee, various nutrients, and bladder cancer. *J. Natl. Cancer Inst. 64:*701–713.

9. Kessler, I. I., and Clark, J. P. 1978. Saccharin, cyclamate and human bladder cancer. No evidence of an association. *JAMA 240:*349–355.

10. Miller, C. T., Neutel, C. I., Nair, R. C., Marrett, L. D., Last, J. M., and Collins, W. E. 1978. Relative importance of risk factors in bladder carcinogenesis. *J. Chron. Dis. 31:*51–56.

11. Morrison, A. S. 1979. Use of artificial sweeteners by cancer patients. *J. Natl. Cancer Inst. 62:*1397–1399.

12. Wynder, E. L., and Stellman, S. D. 1980. Artificial sweetener use and bladder cancer: A case control study. *Science 207:*1214–1216.

13. Morrison, A. S., and Burling, J. E. 1980. Artificial sweeteners and cancer of the lower urinary tract. *N. Engl. J. Med. 302:*537–541.

14. Hoover, R. N., and Strassner, P. H. 1980. Saccharin: A bitter aftertaste? (Editorial.) *N. Engl. J. Med. 302:*573–575.

15. Morrison, A. S., Verhoek, W. G., Leck, I., Aoki, K., Ohno, Y., and Obata, K. 1982. Artificial sweeteners and bladder cancer in Manchester, U.K., and Nagoya, Japan. *Br. J. Cancer 45:*332–336, 1982.

16. Silverman, D. T., Hoover, R. N., and Swanson, G. M. 1983. Artificial sweeteners and lower urinary tract cancer: Hospital vs. population controls. *Am. J. Epidemiol. 117:*326–334.

17. Jensen, O. M., and Kamby, C. 1982. Intra-uterine exposure to saccharin and risk of bladder cancer in man. *Int. J. Cancer 29:*507–509.

18. Blot, W. J., Fraumeni, J. F., and Stone, B. J. 1978. Geographic correlates of pancreas cancer in the United States. *Cancer 42:*373–380.

19. Wynder, E. L., Mabuchi, K., Maruchi, N., and Fortner, J. G. 1973. Epidemiology of cancer of the pancreas. *J. Natl. Cancer Inst. 50:*645–667.

20. Chowaniec, J., and Hicks, R. M. 1979. Response of the rat to saccharin with particular reference to the urinary bladder. *Br. J. Cancer 39:*355–375.

21. Arnold, D. L., Moodie, C. A., Grice, H. C., Charbonneau, S. M., Stavric, B., Collins, B. T., McGuire, P. F., Zawidzka, Z. Z., and Munro, I. C. 1980. Long-term toxicity of *ortho*-toluenesulfonamide and sodium saccharin in the rat. *Toxicol. Appl. Pharmacol. 52:*113–152.

22. Kroes, R., Peters, P. W. J., Berkrens, J. M., Verschuuren, H. G., de Vries, T., and Van Esch, G. J. 1977. Long term toxicity and reproduction study (including a teratogenicity study) with cyclamate, saccharin and cyclohexylamine. *Toxicology 8:*285–300.

23. Cohen, S. M., Arai, M., Jacobs, J. B., and Friedell, G. H. 1979. Promoting effect of saccharin and DL-tryptophan in urinary bladder carcinogenesis. *Cancer Res. 39:*1207–1217.

24. Trosko, J. E., Yotti, L. P., Warren, S., Tsushimoto, G., and Chang, C. C. 1982. Inhibition of cell–cell communication by tumor promotors. In E. Hecker, W. Kunz, S. Marx, N. E. Fusenig, and H. W. Phielmann (Eds.) *Carcinogenesis: A comprehensive survey.* Vol. 7: *Carcinogenesis and biological effects of tumor promotors.* pp. 565–585. New York: Raven Press.

25. Poncelot, F., Roberfroid, M., Mercier, M., and Lederer, J. 1979. Absence of mutagenic activity in *Salmonella typhimurium* of some impurities found in saccharin. *Food Cosmet. Toxicol. 17:*229–231.

26. Batzinger, R. P., Ou, S. Y. L., and Bueding, E. 1977. Saccharin and other sweeteners: Mutagenic properties. *Science 198:*944–946.

27. Clive, D., Johnson, K. O., Spector, J. F. S., Batson, A. G., and Brown, M. M. M. Validation and characterization of the L5178Y/TK$^{+/-}$ mouse lymphoma mutagen assay system. *Mutat. Res. 59:*61–108.

28. Rao, M. S., and Qureshi, A. B. 1972. Induction of dominant lethals in mice by sodium saccharin. *Indian J. Med. Res. 60:*599–603.

29. Ochi, H., and Tonomura, A. 1978. Presence of unscheduled DNA synthesis in cultured human cells after treatment with sodium saccharin. *Mutat. Res. 54:*224.

30. Mondel, S., Brankow, D. W., and Heidelberger, C. 1978. Enhancement of oncogenesis in C3H/10T1/2 mouse embryo cell cultures by saccharin. *Science 201:*1141–1142.

31. Yoshida, S., Masubuchi, M., and Hiraga, K. 1978. Induced chromosome aberrations by artificial sweeteners in CHO-K1 cells. *Mutat. Res. 54:*262.

32. Wolff, S., and Rodin, B. 1978. Saccharin-induced sister chromatid exchanges in Chinese hamster and human cells. *Science 200:*543–545.

33. Homburger, F. 1978. Negative lifetime carcinogen studies in rats and mice fed 50,000 ppm saccharin. in C. L. Galli, R. Paoletti, and G. Vettorazzi (Eds.) *Chemical toxicology of food.* pp. 359–373. New York: Elsevier/North-Holland Biomedical Press.

34. Rudali, G., Coezy, E., and Muranyi-Kovacs, I. 1969. Recherches sur l'action cancerigène du cyclamate de soude chez les souris. *C.R. Hebd. Seances Acad. Sci. Ser. D 269:*1910–1912.

35. Brantom, P. B., Gaunt, I. F., and Grasso, P. 1973. Long-term toxicity of sodium cyclamate in mice. *Food Cosmet. Toxicol. 11:*735–746.

36. Hicks, R. M., Chowaniec, J., and Wakefield, J. St. J. 1978. Experimental induction of bladder tumors in a two-stage system. in T. J. Slaga, A. Sivak, and R. K. Boutwell (Eds.) *Carcinogenesis: A comprehensive survey.* Vol. 2: *Mechanisms of tumor promotion and cocarcinogenesis.* pp. 475–489. New York: Raven Press.

37. Friedman, L., Richardson, H. L., Richardson, M. E., Lethco, E. J., Wallace, W. C., and Sauro, F. M. 1972. Toxic response of rats to cyclamates in chow and semisynthetic diets. *J. Natl. Cancer Inst. 49:*751–764.

38. Kroes, R., Peters, P. W. J., Berkvans, J. M., Verschuuren, H. G., de Vries, T., and van Esch, G. J. 1977. Long term toxicity and reproduction study (including a teratogenicity study) with cyclamate, saccharin, and cyclohexylamine. *Toxicology 8:*285–300.

39. Hicks, R. M., Chowaniec, J., and Wakefield, J. St. J. 1978. Experimental induction of bladder tumors by a two-stage system. in T. J. Slaga, A. Sivak, and R. K. Boutwell (Eds.) *Carcinogenesis—A comprehensive survey.* Vol. 2: *Mechanisms of tumor promotion and cocarcinogenesis.* pp. 475–489. New York: Raven Press.

40. Mohr, U., Green, U., Althoff, J., and Schneider, P. 1978. Syncarcinogenic action of saccharin

and sodium-cyclamate in the induction of bladder tumours in MNU-pretreated rats. in B. Guggenheim (Ed.) *Health and sugar substitutes*. pp. 64–69. New York: S. Kargar.

41. Ebenezer, L. N., and Sadasivan, G. 1970. *In vitro* effect of cyclamates on human chromosomes. *Q. J. Surg. Sci. 6:*116–118.

42. Tokumitsu, T. 1971. Some aspects of cytogenetic effects of sodium cyclamate on human leucocytes in vitro. *Proc. Jpn. Acad. 47:*635–639.

43. Machemer, L., and Lorke, D. 1976. Evaluation of the mutagenic potential of cyclohexylamine on spermatogonia of the Chinese hamster. *Mutat. Res. 40:*243–250.

44. Searle, G. D., and Co. 1974. An evaluation of mutagenic potential employing the host-mediated assay in the mouse. P-T No. 1095S73. Skokie, Illinois: G. D. Searle and Co.

45. U.S. Food and Drug Administration. 1981. Aspartame; commissioner's final decision. *Fed. Regist. 46:*38283–38308.

46. Searle, G. D. and Co. 1978. An evaluation of the mutagenic potential employing the Ames Salmonella/microsome assay. Final report. S.A. 13-85. Skokie, Illinois: G. D. Searle and Co.

47. Price, P. J., Suk, W. A., Freeman, A. E., Lane, W. T., Peters, R. L., Vernon, M. L., and Huebner, R. J. 1978. In vitro and in vivo indications of the carcinogenicity and toxicity of food dyes. *Br. J. Cancer 21:*361–367.

48. National Cancer Institute. 1979. Bioassay of butylated hydroxytoluene (BHT) for possible carcinogenicity. NCI carcinogenesis techical report series no. 150. NIH Publ. No. 79-1706. Bethesda, Maryland: Carcinogenesis Testing Program, National Cancer Institute.

49. Witschi, H. P. 1981. Enhancement of tumor formation in mouse lung by dietary butylated hydroxytoluene. *Toxicology 21:*95–104.

50. Trosko, J. E., Yotti, L. P., Warren, S., Tsushimoto, G., and Chang, C. C. 1982. Inhibition of cell–cell communication by tumor promotors. in E. Hecker, W. Kunz, S. Marx, N. E. Fusenig, and H. W. Phielmann (Eds.) *Carcinogenesis: A comprehensive survey*. Vol. 7: *Carcinogenesis and biological effects of tumor promotors*. New York: Raven Press.

51. Sciorra, L. J., Kaufmann, B. N., and Maier, R. 1974. The effects of butylated hydroxytoluene on the cell cycle and chromosome morphology of phytohaemagglutinin-stimulated leucocyte cultures. *Food Cosmet. Toxicol. 12:*33–44.

52. Abe, S., and Sasaki, M. 1977. Chromosome aberrations and sister chromatid exchanges in Chinese hamster cells exposed to various chemicals. *J. Natl. Cancer Inst. 58:*1635–1641.

53. Wattenberg, L. W. 1979. Inhibitors of chemical carcinogens. in P. Emmelot and E. Kriek (Eds.) *Environmental carcinogenesis*. pp. 241–263. Amsterdam: Elsevier/North-Holland Biomedical Press.

54. Wattenberg, L. W. 1981. Inhibitions of chemical carcinogens. in J. H. Burchenol and H. F. Oettgen (Eds.) *Cancer: Achievements, challenges and prospects for the 1980's*. Vol. 1. pp. 517–539. New York: Grune & Stratton.

55. Benson, S. M., Cha, Y. N., Bueding, E., Heine, H. S., and Talalay, P. 1979. Elevation of extrahepatic glutathione 5-transferase and epoxide hydratase activities by 2(3)-*tert*-butyl-4-hydroxyanisole. *Cancer Res. 39:*2971–2977.

56. Cha, Y. N., and Bueding, E. 1979. Effect of 2(3)-*tert*-butyl-4-hydroxyanisole administration on the activities of several hepatic microsomal and cytoplasmic enzymes in mice. *Biochem. Pharmacol. 28:*1917–1921.

57. Cha, Y. N., Martz, F., and Bueding, E. 1978. Enhancement of liver microsome epoxide hydratase activity in rodents by treatment with 2(3)-*tert*-butyl-4-hydroxyanisole. *Cancer Res. 38:*4496–4498.

58. Lam, L. K. T., Fladmoe, A. V., Hochalter, J. B., and Wattenberg, L. W. 1980. Short time interval effects of butylated hydroxyaninsole on the metabolism of benzopyrene. *Cancer Res. 40:*2824–2828.

59. Batzinger, R. P., Ou, S. Y. L., and Bueding, E. 1978. Antimutagenic effects of 2(3)-*tert*-butyl-4-hydroxyanisole and of antimicrobial agents. *Cancer Res. 38:*4478–4485.
60. Wattenberg, L. W., Coccia, J. B., and Lam, L. K. T. 1980. Inhibitory effects of phenolic compounds on benzopyrene-induced neoplasia. *Cancer Res. 40:*2820–2823.
61. Wattenberg, L. W., and Loub, W. D. 1978. Inhibition of polycyclic hydrocarbon-induced neoplasia by naturally occurring indoles. *Cancer Res. 38:*1410–1413.
62. Pantuck, E. J., Hsiao, K. C., Loub, W. D., Wattenberg, L. W., Kuntzman, R., and Conney, A. H. 1976. Stimulatory effect of vegetables on intestinal drug metabolism in the rat. *J. Pharmacol. Exp. Ther. 198:*278–283.
63. Wattenberg, L. W. 1979. Naturally occurring inhibitors of chemical carcinogenesis. in E. C. Miller, J. A. Miller, I. Hirono, T. Sugimura, and S. Takayama (Eds.) *Naturally occurring carcinogens—mutagens and modulators of carcinogenesis.* pp. 315–329. Baltimore: University Park Press.
64. Wattenberg, L. W. 1981. Inhibition of carcinogen-induced neoplasia by sodium cyanate, tert-butyl isocyanate and benzyl isothiocyanate administered subsequent to carcinogen exposure. *Cancer Res. 41:*2991–2994.
65. Wattenberg, L. W., and Leong, J. L. 1970. Inhibition of the carcinogenic action of benzopyrene by flavones. *Cancer Res. 30:*1922–1925.
66. Sparnins, V. L., and Wattenberg, L. W. 1981. Enhancement of glutathione S-transferase activity of the mouse forestomach by inhibitors of benzopyrene-induced neoplasia of forestomach. *J. Natl. Cancer Inst. 66:*769–771.
67. Sparnins, V. L. 1980. Effects of dietary constituents on glutathione S-transferase (GST) activity. *Proc. Am. Assoc. Cancer Res. 21:*80.
68. Lam, L. K. T., Sparnins, V. L., and Wattenberg, L. 1982. Isolation and identification of kahweol palmitate and cafestol palmitate as active constituents of green coffee beans that enhance glutathione S-transferase activity in the mouse. *Cancer Res. 42:*1193–1198.
69. Pantuck, E. J., Pantuck, C. B., Garland, W. A., Min, B. H., Wattenberg, L. W., Anderson, K. E., Kappas, A., and Conneg, A. H. 1979. Stimulatory effect of brussels sprouts and cabbage on human drug metabolism. *Clin. Pharmacol. Ther. 25:*88–95.
70. MacGregor, J. T., and Jurd, L. 1978. Mutagenicity of plant flavonoids: Structural requirements for mutagenic activity in *Salmonella typhimurium. Mutat. Res. 54:*297–309.
71. Troll, W. 1981. Blocking of tumor promotion by protease inhibitors. in J. H. Burchenol and H. F. Oettgen (Eds.) *Cancer: Achievements, challenges, and prospects for the 1980's.* Vol. 1. pp. 549–555. New York: Grune & Stratton.
72. Kennedy, A. R., and Little, J. B. 1981. Effects of protease inhibitors on radiation transformation *in vitro. Cancer Res. 41:*2103–2108.
73. Cohen, B. I., and Raicht, R. F. 1981. Plant sterols: Protective role in chemical carcinogenesis. in M. S. Zedeck and M. Lipkin (Eds.) *Inhibition of tumor induction and development.* pp. 189–201. New York: Plenum.
74. Creech, J. L., and Johnson, M. N. 1974. Angiosarcoma of liver in the manufacture of polyvinyl chloride. *J. Occup. Med. 16:*150–151.
75. Tabershaw, I. R., and Goffey, W. R. 1974. Mortality study of workers in the manufacture of vinyl chloride and its polymers. *J. Occup. Med. 16:*509–518.
76. Monson, R. R., Peters, J. M., and Johnson, M. N. 1974. Proportional mortality among vinyl-chloride workers. *Lancet 2:*397–398.
77. Fox, A. J., and Collier, P. F. 1977. Mortality experience of workers to vinyl chloride monomer in the manufacture of polyvinyl chloride in Great Britain. *Br. J. Indust. Med. 34:*1–10.
78. Maltoni, C. 1977. Vinyl chloride carcinogenicity: An experimental model for carcinogenesis studies. in H. H. Hiatt, J. D. Watson, and J. A. Winsten (Eds.) *Origins of human cancer.* Book

A: *Incidence of cancer in humans*. pp. 119–146. Cold Spring Harbor Laboratory, New York: Cold Spring Harbor.

79. Feron, V. J., Speek, A. J., Williams, M. I., van Battum, D., and deGroot, A. P. 1975. Observations on the oral administration and toxicity of vinyl chloride in rats. *Food Cosmet. Toxicol. 13:*633–638.

80. Bartsch, H., Malaveille, G., Barbin, A., and Planche, G. 1979. Mutagenic and alkylating metabolites of halo-ethylenes, chlorobutadienes and dichlorobutenes produced by rodent or human liver tissues. Evidence for oxirane formation by P450 microsomal monooxygenases. *Arch. Toxicol. 41:*249–277.

81. Eckardt, F., Muliawan, H., de Ruiter, N., and Kappus, H. 1981. Rat hepatic vinyl chloride metabolites induce gene conversion in the yeast strain, D7RAD in vitro and in vivo. *Mutat. Res. 91:*381–390.

82. Heath, C. W., Dumont, C. R., and Waxweiller, R. J. 1977. Chromosomal damage in men occupationally exposed to vinyl chloride monomer and other chemicals. *Environ. Res. 14:*68–72.

83. O'Berg, M. T. 1980. Epidemiologic study of workers exposed to acrylonitrile. *J. Occup. Med. 22:*245–252.

84. Norris, J. M. 1977. Status report on the 2 year study incorporating acryonitrile in the drinking water of rats. Health and environmental research. pp. 1–14. Midland, Michigan: The Dow Chemical Company.

85. Milvey, P. 1978. (Letter to the Editor.) *Mutat. Res. 57:*110–112.

86. Venitt, S., Bushell, C. T., and Osborne, M. 1977. Mutogenicity of acrylonitrile (cyanoethylene) in *Escherichia coli*. *Mutat. Res. 45:*283–288.

87. Thiess, A. M., and Fleig, I. 1978. Analysis of chromosomes of workers exposed to acrylonitrile. *Arch. Toxicol. 41:*149–152.

88. Jukes, T. H. 1974. Diethylstilbesterol in beef production: What is the risk to consumers? *Prev. Med. 5:*438–453.

89. Herbst, A. L., and Cole, P. 1978. Epidemiologic and clinical aspects of clear cell adenocarcinoma in young women. in A. L. Herbst (Ed.) *Intrauterine exposure to diethylstilbesterol in the human*. pp. 2–7. Chicago: American College of Obstetricians and Gynecologists.

90. Bulow, H., Wullstein, H. K., Bottger, G., and Schroder, F. H. 1973. Carcinomas of the breast under estrogen-treatment for prostatic carcinoma. *Urologe A 12:*249–253.

91. Cutler, B. S., Forbes, A. P., Ingersoll, F. M., and Scully, R. E. 1972. Endometrial carcinoma after stilbesterol therapy in gonadol dysgenesis. *N. Engl. J. Med. 287:*628–631.

92. Gass, G. H., Coats, D., and Graham, N. 1964. Carcinogenic dose–response curve to oral diethylstilbesterol. *J. Natl. Cancer Inst. 33:*971–977.

93. Gass, G. H., Brown, J., and Okey, A. B. 1974. Carcinogenic effects of oral diethylstilbesterol on C3H mice with and without the mammary tumor virus. *J. Natl. Cancer Inst. 53:*1369–1370.

94. Gibson, J. P., Newberne, J. W., Kuhn, W. L., and Elsen, J. R. 1967. Comparative chronic toxicity of three oral estrogens in rats. *Toxicol. Appl. Pharmacol. 11:*489–510.

95. Rustia, M. 1979. Role of hormone imbalance in transplacental carcinogenesis induced in Syrian golden hamsters by sex hormones. *Natl. Cancer Inst. Monogr. 51:*77–87.

96. Glatt, H. R., Metzler, A., and Oesch, F. 1979. Diethylstilbesterol and 11 derivatives. A mutagenicity study with *Salmonella typhimurium*. *Mutat. Res. 67:*113–121.

97. Fluck, E. R., Poirier, L. A., and Ruelius, H. W. 1976. Evaluation of a DNA polymerase-deficient mutant of *E. coli* for the rapid detection of carcinogens. *Chem. Biol. Interact. 15:*219–231.

98. Ishidate, M., and Odashima, S. 1977. Chromosome tests with 134 compounds on Chinese hamster cells in vitro—a screening for chemical carcinogens. *Mutat. Res. 48:*337–353.

99. Ivett, J. L., and Tice, R. R. 1981. Diethylstilbesterol-diphosphate induces chromosomal aber-

rations but not sister chromalid exchanges in murine bone marrow cells in vivo. *Environ. Mutagen. 3:*445–452.

100. Clive, D., Johnson, K. O., Spector, J. F. S., Batson, A. G., and Brown, M. M. M. 1979. Validalion and characterization of the L5178Y/TK $^{+/-}$ mouse lymphoma mutagen assay system. *Mutat. Res. 59:*61–108.

101. Martin, C. N., McDermid, A. C., and Garner, H. C. 1978. Testing of known carcinogens and noncarcinogens for their ability to induce unscheduled DNA synthesis in HeLa cells. *Cancer Res. 38:*2621–2627.

102. Chrisman, C. L. 1974. Aneuploidy in mouse in embryos induced by diethylstilbesterol diphosphate. *Teratology 9:*229–232.

103. National Academy of Science—National Research Council. 1982. Diet, nutrition, and cancer. pp. 14-1 to 14-54. in *Additives and contaminants*. Washington, D.C.: National Academy Press.

104. Dikshith, T. S. S. 1973. *In vivo* effects of parathion on guinea pig chromosomes. *Environ. Physiol. Biochem. 3:*161–168.

105. Huang, C. C. 1973. Effect on growth but not on chromosomes of the mammalian cells after treatment with three organophosphorous insecticides. *Proc. Soc. Exp. Biol. Med. 142:*36–40.

106. Eisenbrand, G., Schmahl, D., and Preussman, N. 1976. Carcinogenicity in rats of high oral doses of N-nitrosocarbaryl, a nitrosated pesticide. *Cancer Lett. 1:*281–284.

107. Schwartz, L. 1943. An outbreak of halowax acne ("table rash") among electricians. *JAMA 122:*158–161.

108. Jelinek, C. 1981. Occurrence and methods of control of chemical contaminants in foods. *Environ. Health Perspect. 39:*143–151.

109. U.S. Food and Drug Administration. 1980. FDA Compliance Program Report of Findings. FY77 Total Diet Studies—Adult (7320.73). Washington, D.C.: Food and Drug Administration, U.S. Department of Health, Education and Welfare.

110. Kutz, F. W., and Strassman, S. C. 1976. Residues of polychlorinated biphenyls in the general population of the United States. in *The national conference on polychlorinated biphenyls, November 1975, Chicago, Illinois*. pp. 139–143. Washington, D.C.: EPA-560/6-75-004. Office of Toxic Substances, Environmental Protection Agency.

111. Makiura, S., Aoe, H., Sugihara, S., Hirao, K., and Ito, N. 1974. Inhibitory effect of polychlorinated biphenyls on liver tumorigenesis in rats treated with 3¹-methyl-4-dimethylaminoazobenzene, N-2-fluorenylacetamide, and diethylnitrosamine. *J. Natl. Cancer Inst. 53:*1253–1257.

112. Preston, B. D., Van Miller, J. P., Moore, R. W., and Allen, J. R. 1981. Promoting effects of polychlorinated biphenyls (Aroclor 1254) and polychlorinated dibenzofuran-free Aroclor 1254 on diethylnitrosamine-induced tumorigenesis in the rat. *J. Nat. Cancer Inst. 66:*509–515.

113. Wertz, G. F., and Fiscor, G. 1978. Cytogenetic and teratogenic test of polybrominated biphenyls in rodents. *Environ. Health Perspect. 23:*129–132.

114. Howard, J. W., and Fazio, T. 1980. Review of polycyclic aromatic hydrocarbons in foods. Analytical methodology and reported findings of polycyclic aromatic hydrocarbons in foods. *J. Assoc. Off. Anal. Chem. 63:*1077–1104.

115. Fritz, W. 1969. Zum Losungrerhalten der Polyaromaten beim Kochen von Kaffee-Ersatzstoffen und Bohnenkaffee. *Dtsch. Lebensm. Rundsch. 65:*83–85.

116. Masuda, Y., Mori, K., Hirohata, T., and Kuratsune, M. 1966. Carcinogenesis in the esophagus. III. Polycyclic aromatic hydrocarbons and phenols in whiskey. *Gann 57:*549–557.

117. Grimmer, G. 1968. Cancerogene kohlenwasserstoffe in der Umgebung des Menschen. *Dtsch. Apoth. Ztg. 108:*529–533.

118. Suess, M. J. 1976. The environmental load and cycle of polycyclic aromatic hydrocarbons. *Sci. Total Environ. 6:*239–250.

119. Fritz, W. 1971. Umfang und Quellen der Kontamination unserer Lebensmittel mit kreb-serzeugenden Kohlenwasserstoffen. *Ernaehrungsforschung 16:*547–557.
120. Soos, K. 1980. The occurrence of carcinogenic polycyclic hydrocarbons in foodstuffs in Hungary. *Arch. Toxicol. Suppl. 4:*446–448.
121. Doll, R., Vessey, M. P., Beasley, R. W. R., Buckley, A. R., Fear, E. C., Fisher, R. E. W., Gammon, E. J., Gunn, W., Hughes, G. O., Lee, K., and Norman-Smith, B. 1972. Mortality of gas-workers—final report of a prospective study. *Br. J. Ind. Med. 29:*394–406.
122. Freudenthal, R., and Jones, P. W. (Eds.) 1976. Carcinogenicity—hydrocarbons: *Chemistry, metabolism and carcinogenesis.* New York: Raven Press.

Chapter 9

Unproven Cancer Diet Claims

LAETRILE

Chemistry

Laetrile (Fig. 9-1) is an amygdalin, a cyanogentic glycoside that is naturally present as a toxicant (poison) in the kernels of apricot pits as well as a number of other stone fruits and nuts (e.g., macadamia nuts). There is a possibility that nature may have put it in the kernels to protect the plant from being eaten.

Cyanogenetic glycosides, which have also been called "laetrile," "nitrilosides," and "vitamin B_{17}," are chemical substances made up of cyanide, aldehyde, ketone, and sugar. Laetrile consists of two parts glucose, one part benzaldehyde, and one part cyanide. Even though some have called laetrile "vitamin B_{17}," laetrile has never been recognized by the scientific community as a vitamin.

The cyanide contained in laetrile is released as hydrogen cyanide (prussic acid) by the hydrolytic action of the enzyme β-glucosidase, or heat, or mineral acids or megadoses of ascorbic acid, especially in the presence of blood.

Toxicology

The released hydrogen cyanide is a colorless weak acid that boils at 25.5°C (well below body temperature of 37°C) to become a gas. The almond oil odor of crushed apricot kernels is associated with the release of the gas. The gas is so toxic a poison that victims have died with 2 min of ingestion of 300 mg hydrocyanic acid in aqueous solution, an amount that one can obtain by mixing saliva with 70 gm (2½ ounces) of some varieties of bitter almond kernels or by mixing saliva with 5 gm (one-sixth of an ounce) of laetrile and vegetables containing β-glucosidase, a plant enzyme.

The claim by laetrile promoters that any dose of cyanide from food or

335

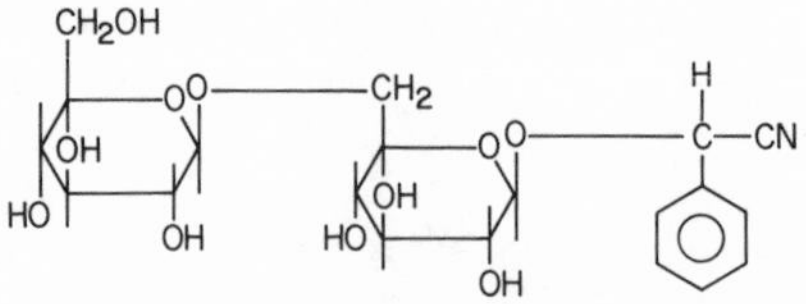

Figure 9-1. Formula of amygdalin (laetrile).

laetrile is immediately detoxified to thiocyanate by rhodanese (mitochondrial sulfer transferase) is probably false. This false claim is proved so by the fact that undetoxified cyanide is measurable in the blood of people poisoned by laetrile or apricot kernels. In addition, thiocyanate is itself toxic, but to a lesser degree. Even though the liver and kidneys contain enough rhodanese to convert several kilograms of cyanide to thiocyanate in 15 min, very little of the enzyme is present in the blood; also, the limiting detoxification factor is not the rhodanese enzyme, but the availability of intracellular cystine, cysteine, and other reducing sulfur as substrate. In addition, thiocyanate can be converted back to cyanide.

While the total daily excretion of thiocyanate in the urine of nonsmoking adults averages 0.65 mg KSCN/24 hr, smokers may urinate a mean of 10 mg potassium thiocyanate (KSCN)/24 hr. Nonsmoking adults may average 0.54 mg/100 ml KSCN in their serum and smokers 1.52 mg/100 ml.

There is a possibility that Leber's hereditary optic atrophy and tobacco amblyopia are both due to defects in the partial detoxification of cyanide to thiocyanate.

Several deaths from laetrile ingestion have been reported. For example, an 11-month-old baby who accidently swallowed 2.5 gm laetrile rapidly went into a coma from cyanide poisoning and died 3 days later. In July 1977 three Los Angeles physicians published a case report in the *Journal of the American Medical Association* about a 17½-year-old Los Angeles girl who drank 3½ ampoules (10.5 gm) laetrile.[1] A coma from cyanide poisoning resulted within 10 min and she died.

Clinical Trial

Historical Background

Amygdalin has been used for medical purposes for many centuries. The use of amygdalin was first documented by Dioscorides of Anazarbos shortly after the birth of Christ. Amygdalin was a common ingredient of herbal prescriptions for a variety of illnesses and is usually administered in the form of bitter almonds. If one were to interpret the ancient pharmacopeias liberally, one might conclude that it was used for cancer treatment. With the advent of the science of medicine, amygdalin, along with most other herbal agents, was abandoned for our modern-day clinical therapy.

Recent Use

However, in 1952 it was revised by Ernest Krebs, Jr., who registered amygdalin with the U.S. Patent Office under the trade name of Laetrile, to be used for the treatment of "disorders from intestinal fermentation," i.e., cancer. In the following years, laetrile completely surpassed any other unorthodox therapy used for any disease in our time.

Laetrile has been used by 27 of our 50 states and is also legal for use nationwide under a federal court order, which, even though it has been reviewed by the U.S. Supreme Court, has not been reserved. It is apparent that these phenomena were not just responses to local minorities, as was shown by a nationwide Harris poll showing that the American public favored legalization by an amazing 30% margin.

Case Reports

In response to the marked public interest, the National Cancer Institute has elected to evaluate amygdalin by requesting that practitioners who use laetrile mail in their test results. Sixty-eight reports were received and cirtically evaluated by several cancer experts, who concluded "The panel judged six laetrile cases to have had a response."[2] Certainly such evidence can be questioned because of a lack of matched control groups. For about a quarter of a century, laetrile has remained a major and unresolved health problem involving many thousands of cancer patients in treatment and causing serious doubts and concerns in many more patients and their families. These humanitarian and scientific issues were the primary considerations.

Chemotherapeutic Use

Moertel et al. studied 178 cancer patients who were treated with amygdalin plus a metabolic therapy regimen consisting of diet, enzymes, and vitamins.[3] All patients selected had histologically proved cancer for which no standard therapy was known to be curative or to extend life expectancy. All patients had no surgery, radiation therapy, or chemotherapy for at least 1 month. One-third of the patients had received no previous chemotherapy. Special emphasis was placed on selecting patients in good general condition, and all patients were ambulatory and able to maintain oral nutrition. Seventy-one percent of patients were capable of working full time or part time. Patients who were totally disabled and bedridden were ineligible for study.

Each patient had either a tumor area that could be measured in two dimensions or malignant hepatomegaly with a clearly defined liver edge extending at least 50 cm below the costal margin. In addition, lesions demonstrable by radioisotopic liver scan or by computered tomographic scan were acceptable if they measured at least 5 cm in diameter. Those patients in whom the tumor size could only be estimated (e.g., those with extrarectal or pelvic masses) and patients with only bone lesions were not eligible for study.

Amygdalin was supplied for intravenous use in vials containing 3 gm lyophilized RS-amygdalin and for oral use in tablets containing 0.5 gm R-amygdalin. The routes, dosage, and schedule of amygdalin administration were chosen to be representative of current Laetrile practice. Amygdalin was administered in 21 daily intravenous injections at a daily dose of 4.5 gm/m² body surface area (BSA). The course of intravenous therapy was administered either on consecutive days (121 eligible patients) or during weekdays only (57 patients). After the initial course, oral maintenance therapy was initiated at a dose of 0.5 gm given three times a day.

In this study, there was some difficulty in obtaining consensus among the major proponents of laetrile on the so-called "metabolic therapy" regimen. Some recommend laetrile only, saying that metabolic therapy was unnecessary and might distort the effects of amygdalin itself. Others recommend megadoses of numerous vitamins as well as an unusual array of unusual ancillary treatments. Moertel et al. elected to compromise between these extremes, using very high but not massive doses of vitamins.[3] The usual pancreatic enzymes were added. The study also anticipated the possible objections of some laetrile practitioners who had not used high enough doses of amygdalin or of vitamins. A smaller group of patients with an extremely high-dose program. One hundred sixty-five patients were treated with the standard-dose treatment and 14 with the high-dose treatment.

One patient was declared ineligible because of an inadequate histological confirmation of malignant disease before therapy. Therapy was administered to a total of 178 eligible patients, who were followed for survival. Three patients could not be evaluated for objective response, two of whom had died suddenly of causes not directly related to cancer within 3 days of the start of therapy, and one because he left the program after only six intravenous injections, claiming that his pain had not been relieved. Four patients whose condition was objectively stable on early evaluations could not be evaluated up to the time of progression. Two patients refused to continue therapy at 5 and 6 weeks because there was no improvement in pretreatment symptoms. One withdrew from the program after 3 weeks due to family problems, and one therapy was discontinued at 5 weeks because blood cyanide levels during the oral regimen had exceeded 3.0 μg/ml. At least partial therapeutic observations could be made in 175 patients, and the clinical courses of 171 patients could be completely followed up to the time of measurable progression of disease.

Tumor types included a preponderance of colorectal, lung, and breast cancers with the standard dose treatments. All patients chosen for the high-dose treatment had colorectal cancer.

Cyanide Levels during the Clinical Trial. After intravenous therapy, cyanide levels were either negligible or not detectable. However, after oral administration, cyanide levels were elevated. These levels tended to increase over the first 48 hr and then stabilized. Eleven patients had levels 2 μg/ml; it was observed that three of these 11 patients had received the high-dose program. The highest level observed was just under 4 μg/ml.

Five patients had evidence of the narrow safety range of this therapy with regard to cyanide intoxication. One patient had typical symptoms of cyanide toxicity associated with rapidly increasing blood cyanide when she took large amounts of raw almonds in association with the amygdalin. Another patient took two amygdalin tablets in the morning to make up for the one she had forgotten the night before. This patient had a peak level of 3.5 μg/ml, but only 0.6 μg/ml when she took amygdalin in the prescribed manner. A third patient had taken two amygdalin tablets half an hour apart, because she had slept late one morning. Symptoms suggestive of cyanide poisoning appeared in this patient, with nausea, vomiting, headache, and mental dullness. These symptoms subsided spontaneously over a period of 2 hr. Two additional patients, in spite of following instructions carefully, still had blood cyanide levels of 3.1 and 3.7 μg/ml without associated symptoms.

Therapeutic Results. Among the 175 patients who were eligible for evaluation of therapeutic response, only one met the criteria for a partial response. This patient had gastric carcinoma with metastases to the cervical lymph nodes. Tumor measurements were unchanged during 5 weeks of treatment and observation of the Mayo Clinic. The patient then moved to the Southwest, where he underwent further treatment. This patient was the only one whose care was transferred to another institution. The first measurements made 5 weeks later at the University of Arizona met the criteria for a partial response, in contrast to those at the Mayo Clinic. This response was maintained for 10 weeks, followed by clear progression while the patient was still receiving treatment. The patient died of cancer 37 weeks after the start of therapy.

Ninety-five patients (54%) had measurable progression of malignant disease at termination of their treatment with intravenous amygdalin. Seventy-nine percent of the 175 evaluable patients had tumor progression by 2 months, and 91%

had tumor progression by 3 months. By 7 months all the patients had tumor progression.

While therapy was in progress, only 6% of patients had gained at least 1 kg of weight, and only 3% maintained this weight gain for 10 weeks. About 7% of the 144 patients with impaired performance status before therapy reported any claims of improvement in performance status. In only 3% of these patients did this improvement continue for 10 weeks. Out of the 153 who had symptoms before therapy, 27% claimed symptomatic benefit at some time during therapy. After 10 weeks, only 5% of patients were still receiving therapy and claimed any degree of symptomatic benefit.

After 15 months 152 of the 178 eligible patients had died (see Fig. 9-2), with the median survival for all patients being 4.8 months from start of therapy. Median survival times among the major tumor groups studied were 5 months for those with lung cancer, 4 months for those with breast cancer, and 3 months for those with melanoma. The survival times in these groups appear to be consistent with the anticipated survivals in similar patient groups, but in patients who had received inactive treatment or no treatment.

Among the 14 patients treated with the high-dose schedule, the results obtained were entirely consistent with those reported above for the study as a whole. In this group, no objective responses were observed and the median time to progression was 24 days. The median survival in this group was five months and only three patients claimed transient symptomatic improvements. Only one patient gained weight, and no patient had improvement in performance status.

Certainly a response rate of less than 1% cannot be regarded as beneficial.

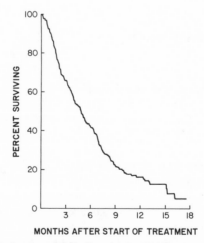

Figure 9-2. Patient survival measured from the start of amygdalin treatment. $N = 178$. (By permission of the *New England Journal of Medicine*, 1982, *306*:201–206.)

The fact that amygdalin therapy neither slowed the advance of malignant disease nor induced "stabilization" is evidenced by the facts that more than one-half of these patients were found to have tumor progression at termination of the intravenous induction therapy. In addition, more than 90% showed progression by 3 months. The very small rates of improvement in symptoms, performance status, and body weight are within a range that can be anticipated with placebo treatment. Patients also died rapidly, with a median survival of only 4.8 months. From the results of Moertel et al.'s experiments, it must be concluded that amygdalin (laetrile) in combination with high vitamin doses, pancreatic enzymes, and a diet commonly used by "metabolic therapists" was of no substantive value in cancer treatment.

PANGAMIC ACID

Pangamic acid, trade named "vitamin B_{15}" has been widely used as a dietary supplement. Pangamic acid has been suggested as a cure for many diseases. However, the Food and Drug Administration regards vitamin B_{15} as "not an identifiable substance—not a vitamin nor a provitamin—in man or animals." B_{15} is a label for any of a number of different formulations sold as pangamate and is not a substance in itself.

Many of the substances sold as B_{15} contain either dimethylglycine hydrochloride or diisopropylamine dichloroacetate. Using the Ames *Salmonella*/mammalian microsome mutagenicity test, dimethylglycine incubated with nitrites proved mutagenic under conditions similar to long-term human ingestion.[4] Dichloroacetate, a component of diisopropylamine dichloroacetate, also demonstrated mutagenicity in the Ames mutagenicity test and has also been shown to be directly toxic to human subjects and animals.[5]

UNPROVEN THERAPIES

Unproven therapies share some common features. These treatment regimens are characterized by a lack of objective, published, verifiable data obtained by careful laboratory and clinical studies according to methods recognized by the scientific community. Procedures to develop new medications in the treatment of cancer require several steps:

Phase I: Testing is performed both *in vitro* and in laboratory animals with tumors to determine the extent of antitumor therapy as well as its potential toxicity. If the new medication is effective in these systems, the new agent is tested in human volunteers.

Phase II: When this pharmacological testing shows relative safety, the agent is tested for antitumor activity on a small scale in relationship to existing drugs.

Phase III: If effective and safe on a smaller scale, the agent is used on a larger scale in therapeutic trials with larger numbers of patients.

In addition, each of the human test phases is done after protocols are developed that are reviewed by experts in the field. The results obtained are openly available so that they may be reviewed by peers, the public, and regulatory agencies. This peer review system screens out drugs or other treatments that are less effective than current treatments. This painstaking and carefully conducted scientific research is in contrast to the untested, often secret, and fanciful claims made on behalf of unorthodox alternative cancer therapies. Some of the unorthodox approaches are the comprehensive approach, combating metabolic abnormalities, pancreatic digestive enzymes, and detoxification.

Comprehensive Approach

One aspect of unorthodox treatment that appeals to a number of patients is the appearance of a logical, comprehensive approach in combination with an effort by the "healer" and his or her staff to bring about a feeling of confidence, rapport, and concern for the patient. In many cases, detailed questionnaires and complex "analysis" may be used in a fairly complicated system of procedures, along with wordy pseudoscientific explanations that sound impressive to those who are not scientifically trained. Even though these systems differ in some ways from one healer to another, there are some similarities in many of the better-known systems. Each approach has its own "theoretical" explanation as to why it is used.

A common claim is a need to combat the "metabolic abnormalities" that develop in cancer patients. Other claims are based on the effectiveness of various extracts that are supposed to transform cancer cells into "normal" cells by unknown or unproved mechanisms. Stress is often blamed on the "anaerobic metabolism" of cancer cells, which is claimed to require some reversal process. Even though it is true that some cancer cells can metabolize anaerobically to a greater extent than normal cells, many cancer cells also have normal metabolic pathways. The idea that the presence of anaerobic metabolism is a major problem in managing cancer patients lacks convincing evidence. There is also no physiological basis for the claims of unorthodox treatment that one improve oxygenation or oxidation of cancer cells by various ways (e.g., oxygen inhalation, infusion of ozone-containing solutions, or large doses of vitamin C or vitamin E).

Pancreatic Enzymes

Another claim made is that cancer cells can be killed by increasing the levels of pancreatic digestive enzymes in the belief that such enzymes are low in cancer patients, hence the advocacy of pancreatic enzymes by mouth or by enema. There is no evidence to support this theory. Pancreatic enzymes are usually present in small amounts in circulating blood, but are in an inactive form, since they are potentially dangerous if they happen to be activated when in contact with living tissues outside the upper intestinal tract. Therefore, oral administration cannot increase blood enzyme levels. In addition, the presence of activated pancreatic enzymes in the colonic mucosa, where they are normally present in very small amounts, may lead to possible erosion of the colonic mucosa.

Detoxification

This concept is based on the belief that increased amounts of toxic materials are derived from tumors and that these tumor products induce illness. It is believed that if one rids the body of such "poisons," the patient will be improved. In addition, detoxification is also supposed to stimulate the liver by ingestion of liver and herb extracts, pancreatic enzymes, and special diets low in animal protein assisted by periodic fasting. The specific nature of the toxins and the chemical changes that occur in detoxification have not been stated. As a clinical factor in the human cancer, no one has been able to demonstrate the presence of specific "toxins." This preoccupation with "detoxification" and "purification" has led to the recommendation that coffee and other enemas be used to cleanse the bowel of toxins. This treatment is not without hazard, as two deaths have been observed after administration of coffee enemas associated with hyponatremia and hypokalemia.[6] In addition, one could also decrease the toxin burden, according to various practitioners of detoxification, by avoiding canned, smoked, and refined foods such as salt, pickles, and meat.

After conventional medically acceptable treatment by oncologists, kidney function may be reduced on occasion by excessive accumulation and deposition of uric acid consequent to massive tumor cell death brought about by radiation or chemotherapy. Hemodialysis will frequently tide the patient over until uric acid can be lowered to relatively normal levels and kidney function returned to normal. This example shows the need for sophisticated support systems, whether they are nutritional or other types, in the rational treatment of cancer. In the writings of practitioners of unorthodox treatments, the need for such support systems is ignored. If such treatments are indeed effective, one should expect to learn of cases in which massive tumor lysis has required hemodialysis. In addition, what happens to patients with advanced cancer who develop infection or organ failure while under the care of those who treat by unorthodox methods? Certainly where these conditions exist, successful treatment by modern medical techniques can prolong life.

Immune Increase

Many of these unorthodox treatment methods also stress the need to maintain a high level of immune status. Many unorthodox treatments claim to increase the immune response. These include injections derived from urine and blood, antitoxins, extracts of herbs, glands, and bacteria, which are often combined with a number of foodstuffs and nutritional supplements in high concentration. Certainly objective data on the effectiveness of such treatments have not been published in reputable medical journals. The field of immunotherapy is still experimental and is only a minor adjuvant in cancer therapy.

Avoidance of Certain Foods

Certain foods should be avoided by reasons which vary with theory. For example, one theory states that cancer is caused by a virus and because all chicken is infected with that virus, chicken should not be eaten. Furthermore, since cattle can be fed chicken-containing products, they might become infected with the virus, hence according to the theory beef must also be avoided.

ANALYSES OF SPECIFIC UNORTHODOX PROGRAMS

Unorthodox Treatment 1

Seven unorthodox treatment programs are listed in Table 9-1.[7] Program 1 is a cancer treatment system directed "toward the restoration of harmony in the metabolism of all internal organs." In the initial treatment stages this program emphasizes intensive detoxification as the most important initial step. Coffee enemas (three tablespoons of ground coffee per quart of water) are given at least every four hours during the first 2 weeks of treatment. Castor oil and 10% caffeine potassium citrate solution are mixed with soapy water to yield the castor oil enema solution which was given to patients every other day to "control pain" and "eliminate the need for sedation." The enema is preceded by the oral intake of castor oil in coffee. In mild cases camomile tea enemas are permitted during the restoration, as opposed to the detoxification period. Colon cancer patients

Table 9-1. Unorthodox Methods of Antitumor Therapy: Dietary, Drug, Other Manipulations[a,b]

Approach	Proponent						
	1	2	3	4	5	6	7
Low-protein diet	+	+	+	+	+		+
High-protein diet						+	
Pancreatic/digestive enzymes	+	+	+	+			+
Metabolic correction[b]	+	+		+			
Detoxification[c]	+	+	+	+			
Laetrile (vitamin "B$_{17}$")		+[d]	+				+
Vitamin supplementation	+	+	+	+		+	+
Spiritual healing		+		+	+		+

[a]From Shils (1982).[7]
[b]Includes electrolyte, mineral supplements.
[c]Includes coffee enemas and vegetable juices.
[d]As raw almonds.

receive green leafy juice enemas to "control pain, odor, discomfort and discharge." Detoxification continues to a lesser extent for up to 1½ years, at which time organ and immune systems should be "restored."

Diet type 1 consists primarily of fruits and vegetables, their juices, potatoes, oatmeal, and special soups and breads. In this diet water intake is discouraged on the grounds that it will reduce the ability to drink the prescribed juices. If the vegetables are not taken raw, they should be cooked slowly without water, supposedly to prevent alternations in vitamin and mineral compositions making them unabsorbable, and to facilitate digestion. After four to six weeks which coincides with the anticipated return of appetite, the diet is expanded to allow unsalted, fermented milk products, and small amounts of meat, fish, eggs, and unfermented dairy products. Meats, eggs, and sweets should total no more than 1 quarter of the diet. Various electrolytes, vitamins, and enzyme prescriptions complete this diet system. The various vitamin recommendations by the seven unorthodox diet therapies are listed in Table 9-2.

Unorthodox Treatment 2

A second unorthodox therapy, named nonspecific metabolic therapy, has been claimed to provide the body with required nutrients to stimulate the glands, to clean out toxins, and to allow maintenance of mental and emotional states. Before treatment, each patient undergoes "metabolic typing" through computerized evaluation of 2500-question questionnaire, blood and urine testing, a "functional metabolic index," and a "malignancy index." The results of this

Table 9-2. Adult Recommended Dietary Allowance versus Vitamin Recommendations in Unproved Antitumor Therapy[7]

	RDA 1980 (adult)	1	2	3	4[c]	5[d]	6[e]	7
Vitamin A (IU)[a]	2,640–3,300	50,000		150,000			25,000	75,000
							300–	300–
Vitamin E (IU)[b]	8–10	400	1,200	1,000			600	2,400
			1,500					2,000
Vitamin C (mg)	60	1,000	4,500				4,000	6,000
		150–						
Niacin (mg NE)	13–19	300						
High-potency B complex					+[d]		+	

[a]1 ug retinol = 3.3 IU vitamin A activity from retinol.
[b]1 IU 1 mg. α tocopherol.
[c]Dosages not available.
[d]Vitamin supplementation not a part of this "system."
[e]Estimate.

questionnaire classify the patient into one of 10 types. The therapy varies with the patient's classification.

The dietary plan also uses detoxification which consists of a 3-day "purge," which begins with the colon cleansing. The patient takes three doses of epsom salt solution, one tablespoon per half cup of water, and drinks diluted citrus juices hourly if hungry. The purge is repeated once every month. The first month of treatment, the patient receives daily coffee enemas, and yogurt enemas are given twice weekly "to restore colon bacteria." The kidneys are also "cleansed" with large volumes of fluids and lemon juice. Nose irrigation and deep breathing "purify" the lungs. In addition, hot showers, apple cider vinegar baths, oil baths, and induced sweating are believed to detoxify the skin. Further antitumor therapy is not allowed without prior initiation of the above treatments to avoid overwhelming the body with "toxins" from tumor destruction.

This treatment type attributes cancer proliferation to pancreatic insufficiency secondary to the ingestion of high protein diets. This theory is based on the idea that the pancreas produces insufficient enzymes for both the digestion of dietary protein and foreign protein (e.g., tumor). This dietary approach discourages the use of meat, dairy products, except yogurt and buttermilk, and peanuts; however a small amount of meat is allowed for patients who have rapid metabolism. At breakfast and lunch regular proteins may be eaten. Raw almonds, raw vegetable juices, and raw whole grain cereal round out the very-low-protein regimen.

This dietary system includes the standardization use of seven nutritional supplements. Almond protein is augmented by liquid predigested protein to "maintain proper amino acid content for cell and tissue health." Vitamin supplements are provided as a therapeutic multivitamin plus 1500–4500 mg vitamin C daily. Blackstrap molasses contributes minerals to "stimulate the liver and general metabolism." This unorthodox dietary approach makes liberal use of pancreatic enzymes, chymotropysin, and pepsin.

Unorthodox Treatment 3

In this diet treatment a diet free of animal protein is also suggested. Proponents of this diet cite pancreatic enzyme deficiency theories in their recommendation to include only fermented milk products in an otherwise all-vegetable diet. This diet emphasizes raw vegetables, fruits, nuts, sprouted seeds, and grains; this diet also promotes incidental ingestion of laetrile and β-glucosidase. Undereating is also recommended with a marked reduction in protein consumption to "avoid liver pancreas and kidney paralysis."

"Autoxemia" is thought to be predecessor to the manifestation of cancer. Therefore, frequent juice fasts are accompanied by daily coffee enemas. Very large doses of vitamins and minerals are promoted in this therapy. Both B_{17} and B_{15} are included in this anticancer plan. Other vitamin, mineral, and enzyme components include brewer's yeast, "vitamin F," essential fatty acids, B-complex vitamins, a digestive enzyme compound and a comprehensive mineral and trace element supplement.

Unorthodox Treatment 4

This treatment categorizes patients on the basis of an in-depth (3000-question), computer-analyzed questionnaire and modifies his approach accordingly. Proponents of this treatment do not state overtly that their system cures cancer, but rather that it enables the restoration of host defenses against disease. After identifying the causes of the health problems, this treatment attempts to heal through toxin elimination, nutritional replenishment, biochemical balance, and revitalization of the life forces.

This treatment advocates enemas, fasts, and dietary supplements. The supplements should be taken during fasting because deficiencies will "lower the body's ability to detoxify." Patient instruction material suggests the following for liver cleansing: cholacol, a "natural" detoxified bile to "correct liver deficiency"; disodium phosphate for those with gallbladder involvement; carbamide to detoxify and help protein action; betacol, a tonic for the liver; and 2 ounces of sesame or sunflower oil in orange juice, twice weekly, in order to lubricate the bile duct. The treatment recommends as many enemas to clean out toxins and promote a feeling of well-being.

This dietary system provides good-quality protein from both animal and vegetable sources. Fermented dairy products, eggs, gelatin, fresh nuts, brewers yeast, and raw and lightly cooked organ meats, fish, and seafood comprise one-quarter of the daily intake. After the first 2 months of treatment, lean meats and poultry are to be taken in moderation. Each patient's specific allotment corresponds to his or her "metabolic type."

This diet has a low-starch content and concentrates on vegetables and fruits and their juices and skins and grains in moderation. Proponents of this diet feel that cooking destroys vital enzymes and minerals and that the described intake impairs liver function. The "C" foods, namely, commercial foods, cakes, cookies, candies, caffeine, canned foods, cheese, and chocolate, should be omitted to protect against liver congestion.

Unorthodox Treatment 5

One macrobiotic center offers lifestyle manipulation enabling a person to "align himself with the flow of the universe." The macrobiotic theory contains both dietary and spiritual components. It suggests that illness develops as a result of the patient's imbalance with universal laws and forces—yin and yang. Yang tumors are thought to arise in compact organs from overconsumption of eggs, dairy products, meats, and fish. Yin tumors in hollow organs arise from soft drinks, sugar, honey, citrus, spices, and chemicals. The tumor type dictates the type of macrobiotic diet recommended to the patient. The yang tumor diet contains 40–50% of the total cooked volume of food as whole cereal grains. In this type of diet a wide variety of dried beans totaling 5–10% of the daily intake, is permitted. Five percent of the diet is contributed by a weak miso, a soup of fermented soy paste and vegetables. Raw salads comprise 10%, the remainder of the diet is allotted as cooked vegetables, weak seaweed, and small amounts of fruit. About 50–70% of the yin tumor diet is made up of grains. On this diet only aduki, a Japanese red bean, garbanzos, and lentils may be eaten. On the yin diet both miso and tea must be of a stronger concentration than on the yang diet. No fruit is permitted. All macrobiotic diets eliminate animal and dairy products, tropical fruits, sweets, processed foods and hot spices. Food preparation and positive throught processes are important aspects of the macrobiotic lifestyle.

Unorthodox Treatment 6

This approach avoids dietary planning for those with malignancies, but applies general principles to protect normal tissues. This dietary approach recommends six small daily high-protein, low-calorie, moderate-fat meals that supply "generous" amounts of antistress factors and all nutrients that appear to inhibit malignant growth. Six times daily, the patient is advised to drink up to two-thirds of a cup of "pep-up," an egg–milk–orange juice-based drink supplemented with vegetable oil, yeast, soy flour, calcium, and magnesium. Digestive enzymes and hydrochloric acid are given to those with digestive disturbances. A general vitamin supplementation meets the patient's requirements during illness; desiccated liver in juice is sometimes added to these vitamin supplements.

Unorthodox Treatment 7

This treatment approach is usually called "laetrile plus" and takes in centers and practitioners who base antitumor therapy upon laetrile in conjunction with medication and such dietary manipulations as nutrition; vitamin C in adequate doses; vitamins, minerals, and enzymes in proper physiological balances; immune system enhancement; appropriate rest and exercise; and importantly, awareness of the mind–body relationship of each patient.

One group believes that processed and cooked foods are the causes of tumor proliferation. Denatured vegetable enzymes by thermal and chemical means "in combination with inadequate "B_{17}" intake is believed to impair the integrity of the antineoplastic surveillance mechanism. Therefore, the laetrile-plus diet relies heavily on raw plant material, with attention to "vitamin B_{17}" sources.

Some of the laetrile-plus systems differ in their allowance of animal protein and some recommend a diet low in protein through the elimination of animal protein.

One group permits fish or poultry prepared without salt or fat. Another comprehensive evaluation and treatment center includes fresh fish, broiled meats and poultry, and limited amounts of eggs and dairy products in their "modified laetrile diet." This strict diet which is used during the early treatment phases, eliminates eggs and dairy products. Even though not exactly quantitated, the laetrile plus diet should be low in protein to conform to its theoretical use.

All of the laetrile plus systems encourage consumption of large amounts of vegetables, fruits, juices, grains, and cereals. Fresh or dried fruits without preservatives are recommended; juices are freshly pressed to preserve enzyme activity; vegetables may be cooked briefly to soften and to prevent "enzyme deactivation." Grain and cereal products also should not contain preservatives. Use of sprouted grains is believed to enhance "B_{17}" intake. Many foods in the laetrile plus diet are believed to contain high concentrations of "B_{17}" thereby augmenting the prescribed daily supplementation. One major proponent recommends fruit seed kernels as excellent sources of the vitamin as well as the enzyme β-glucosidase. However, no analytic methods are given. Roasting is thought to destroy both B_{17} and β-glucosidase and only raw nuts, seeds and kernels are permitted. The chewing, crushing, and grinding processes allow for an interaction between B_{17} and β-glucosidase, producing hydrocyanide.

Accessory therapy utilizes minerals, vitamins, and enzymes. Bone pain is reduced by 1500 mg/day of calcium, as calcium diorotate. One group also supplies thyroid extracts to "raise the basal temperature," 300 mg thiamine hydrochloride to "increase tumor cell respiration and resultant "B_{17} vulnerability," and up to 120 mg. zinc orotate or 150 mg zinc gluconate for "tissue healing." Another group recommends "vitamin B_{15}" 150 mg (claimed without evidence to increase cellular oxygen uptake), 6 gm vitamin C for antioxidation, free radical detoxification, and for liver and kidney stimulation. Up to 2400 IU vitamin E for antioxidation; and 75,000 IU of vitamin A for "epithelia; tissue integrity" are also recommended by this group. In addition, bromelin, an enzyme present in pineapple, is claimed to have a synergistic effect with laetrile. Some of the recommended amounts of vitamins are listed in Table 9-2.

One dietary group suggests that commercial pancreatic enzyme preparations are equally as effective as the more costly Wobe-Mugos enzyme preparation which is available from other groups. The enzymes are taken between meals, during which time no dietary protein is suppose to be present in the gut. This low level of protein is achieved by low protein ingestion. However, there is no evidence to support the intact absorption or the proteolytic theory.

In most laetrile plus systems a positive attitude is also emphasized. One group believes that "the mind, the emotions, and the attitude of a patient play a role in both disease development, including cancer and the response that a patient has to any form of treatment."

The seven systems reviewed here draw on common treatment methodologies. However, there are individual modifications in evaluation, therapy, adjunctive measures, a follow-up widens the spectrum of differences among scientifically unproved systems. Thus, the total cost incurred by the patient varies with the extent of care and the degree of sophistication of metabolic analyses.

REFERENCES

1. Sadoff, L. K., Fuchs, K., and Hollander, J. 1978. Rapid death associated with laetrile ingestion. *JAMA 239*:1532.
2. Ellison, N. M., Byar, D. P., and Newell, G. R. 1978. Special report on Laetrile: the JNCI Laetrile review: Results of the National Cancer Institute's retrospective Laetrile analysis. *N. Engl. J. Med. 299*:549–552.
3. Moertel, C. G., Fleming, T. R., Rubin, J., Kvols, L. K., Sarna, G., Koch, R., Currie, V. E., Young, C. W., Jones, S. E., and Davignon, J. P. 1982. A clinical trial of amygdalin (Laetrile) in the treatment of human cancer. *N. Engl. J. Med. 306*:201–206.

4. Ames, B. N., NcCann, J., and Yamasaki, E. 1975. Methods for detecting carcinogens. *Mutat. Res. 31:*347–364.
5. Herbert, V., Gardner, A., and Colman, N. 1980. Mutagenicity of dichloroacetate, ingredient of some formulations of pangamic acid (Trade-named 'Vitamin B_{15}.'' *Am. J. Clin. Nutr. 33:*1179–1182.
6. Eisele, J. W., and Reay, D. T. 1980. Deaths related to coffee enemas. *JAMA 244:*1608–1609.
7. Shils, M. E., and Hermann, M. G. 1982. Unproven dietary claims in the treatment of patients with cancer. *Bull. N.Y. Acad. Med. 58:*323–340.

Chapter 10

Cancer Cachexia

Cachexia associated with cancer is a frequent occurrence. Although some progress has been made in this area, the basic mechanisms involved have not been fully elucidated in spite of a considerable research effort. The term cachexia is derived from the Greek *kakos,* "bad," and *hexis,* "condition." The patient with cachexia is often considered to embody the classical textbook picture of a cancer patient.

Cancer cachexia has been recognized as a common condition in cancer patients since the first large-scale study was conducted in 1932. The frequency of cancer cachexia varies with tumor type, ranging from 8 to 84%, with gastrointestinal cancers and lung cancer having the greatest incidence.[1] The incidence of cachexia and its relationship to the site of the primary tumor is outlined in Table 10-1.

In addition, anorexia seems to be associated with cancer cachexia. Although weight loss is one component of cachexia, it may have considerable prognostic value. For example, in a large series of cancer patients, progressive weight loss was associated with a poor prognosis and perhaps, just as important, with lower response rates to chemotherapy. The weight loss associated with cancer may have some clinical value because it can be measured easily with noninvasive techniques.

WHAT IS CANCER CACHEXIA?

Cancer cachexia is well characterized by several features: (1) anorexia and nausea, (2) weight loss, (3) anemia of a nonspecific type, (4) altered host metabolism, often associated with an elevated basal metabolism rate, (5) muscle weakness, and (6) malabsorption and diarrhea.

In cancer patients cachexia is not directly correlated with food intake or with the stage' histological type, or site of the tumor. Cachexia may occur with a small primary tumor and may precede the clinical diagnosis. In addition, cancer cachexia is not always associated with patients who have large tumor burdens.

Table 10-1. Incidence of Cachexia in Patients with Cancer[a]

Site of primary tumor	Study group		
	Total N	With cachexia	Incidence (%)
Breast	87	20	33
Cervix	64	10	16
Colon	90	20	22
Kidney	979	338	35
Liver	53	18	34
Lung	221	65	30
Esophagus	60	5	8
Pancreas	449	327	73
Stomach	1112	934	84

[a]Source: From Strain (1979).[1]

Brennan reviewed how cancer cachexia compares with other conditions associated with weight loss such as anorexia, which might occur in uncomplicated starvation or with a major injury or sepsis.[2] The noncancer patient subject to acute starvation develops rapid breakdown of protein from lean body mass, amino acid mobilization, glucoenogenesis, and an increase in urinary nitrogen. These initial responses are later altered by the body to conserve protein and energy. The addition of a major injury or sepsis increases the rate and duration of the response, and the associated high rate of catabolism may persist for some time.

The patient with cancer cachexia shows features of both starvation and injury. Food intake is usually deficient, but the presence of the tumor may decrease the ability to regulate the response to starvation. Cancer cachexia may be more like the condition produced by a major injury or sepsis than that due to simple starvation. Clinically a patient with cachexia looks ill, has weight loss, and has a pale skin, often with edema, anemia, lethargy, and weakness. Some or all of the clinical features noted above may be evident.

PATIENT ASSESSMENT

Biochemical Disorders

A dietary history generally reflects the poor dietary intake associated with the anorexia. The clinical signs of vitamin deficiency may be confirmed by relevant biochemical measurements. A high incidence of subclinical vitamin deficiencies occurs in these patients. Other biochemical measurements often reveal evidence of metabolic disorders including low serum albumin level, electrolyte abnormalities, and trace metal deficiencies. Anthropometric tests confirm the loss of subcutaneous fat and lean body mass. These routine tests help verify the clinical impression; it is not usually necessary to use more complicated investigations and invasive procedures.

Immunological Abnormalities

Immunological abnormalities are often associated with patients with cancer cachexia. At some clinics, routine immunological testing is part of the patient investigation.[3] Delayed hypersensitivity skin testing is widely used and is frequently abnormal in cancer patients. The delayed hypersensitivity response in cancer patients appears to be caused mainly by aging and by malnutrition due to the advanced progression of cancer. The relationship between these abnormalities and the susceptibility of cancer patients to infection has not been proved and requires further definition.

Psychological Problems

The problems of malignant disease and cachectic symptoms may be compounded by the psychological reaction of the patient.[4] The patient may become withdrawn and depressed or increasingly frightened and anxious. Cancer patients with advanced disease associated with cachexia require sympathetic and careful management. Other physical symptoms such as pain, breathlessness, or diarrhea may aggravate the patient's condition and should be alleviated promptly.

PATHOGENESIS OF CACHEXIA

Several factors acting together produce the clinical picture of cachexia. The factors generally considered relevant to the pathogenesis of cachexia are listed in Table 10-2. The significance of these factors depends on the patient, tumor site, and extent of disease.

Decreased Food Intake

Decreased food intake may be related to a mechanical obstruction of the gastrointestinal tract preventing entry of food into the gastrointestinal tract. Malignant disease affecting the head and neck, esophagus, or upper gastrointestinal tract is the most prevalent reason for this problem. Decreased food intake can also be associated with anorexia and early satiety; this decrease in appetite can be observed even when the tumor is very small. This finding suggests that the tumor or an abnormal metabolic response of the body produces substances with an anorectic effect. There are no firm data, however, either to confirm this hypothesis or to refute it.

The regulation of food intake is under central nervous system control in the hypothalamic region of the brain, which either stimulates or suppresses the feeding response. Several receptor sources affect sensory input to the appetite control center, including visceral receptors in the stomach and the intestine sensitive to osmotic, volumetric, and chemical properties of ingested materials, as well as temperature receptors, which monitor the specific dynamic action of food. Other mechanisms rely on monitoring nutrients in the blood giving rise to glucosensitive, liposensitive, and amino acid-sensitive control mechanisms. Whatever the regulatory mechanisms involved, an obvious impairment in function is often associated with the presence of a neoplasm.

In addition to developing anorexia, the cancer patient may find that the taste for food is altered and its palatability affected. The taste aversions accompanying anorexia of cancer may be caused by a zinc deficiency that is known to affect taste. Taste studies have been reported by several investigators, who have observed that the extent of the deficiency seems to be correlated with the disease. It

Table 10-2. Pathogenesis of Cachexia[a]

Feature	Symptom
Decreased food intake	Anorexia
Excessive loss of body protein	Ulceration
	Hemorrhage
	Diarrhea
	Vomiting
Malabsorption	Decreased fat absorption
Increased metabolic rate	Increased T-4, BMR
Abnormal host metabolism	Protein
	Carbohydrate
	Fat
	Hormones
	Water
	Electrolytes
Tumor products	Several
Nitrogen trap by the tumor	
Anemia	Blood hemoglobin

[a]From Calman, *Brit. J. Hosp. Med.* 27:28–29, 33–34, 1982.

is possible that the taste aversions and cravings common in pregnancy are associated with similar experiences of cancer patients. Cancer patients acquire an aversion to certain foodstuffs, and changes in taste sensation could be correlated with a reduction in caloric intake. Reduced levels of glucose or amino acids in the blood have been reported to result in decreased appetite. This mechanism may be important in cancer patients whose amino acid patterns are known to vary. In addition, pain, fever, and anxiety might contribute to the decrease in food consumption.

Anorexigenic substances have been found in the urine from fasted rats and also in a human plasma sample taken from a subject after severe exercise. Some investigators have hypothesized that tumors produce peptides, oligonucleotides, as well as other small metabolites that might have a direct anorexic effect on hypothalamic sensory cells or through peripheral neuroreceptor cells. This latter hypothesis is totally unsupported by experimental data and remains speculative. Thus, the precise reasons for the high incidence of anorexia in cancer patients are poorly understood.

Excessive Loss of Body Protein

Development of cachexia probably does not result from excessive loss of body proteins, but this condition is probably worsened by protein loss. Significant complications of the problem probably result from loss of protein from the gastrointestinal tract through vomiting or diarrhea or the sequestration of protein in pleural or peritoneal cavities. Cancer patients may also have repeated minor bleeds, thereby increasing the risk of developing anemia, which may be associated with the loss of plasma proteins. In addition, there may be increased proteolysis of tissue protein to supply glucose precursors by hepatic conversion through gluconeogenesis.

Experimental models of cachexia have almost invariably used rapidly growing transplantable rodent tumors where symptoms of cachexia only start to appear at the later stages of tumor growth, when the tumor may contain 30–40% of total body weight. These models are unlike the situation in man in whom tumor growth is much slower and in whom the tumor burden rarely exceeds 5% of total body weight.

Malabsorption

Malabsorption also seems to be a component of the pathogenesis of cachexia. The incidence of malabsorption varies widely and seems to be dependent on the tumor type. The malabsorption observed thus far has been related to the histopathology of the gut and to functional biochemical tests of absorption. The mechanism behind the formation of malabsorption is unclear, but it has been suggested that it represents a systemic effect of the tumor. Certainly defects in the functional integrity of the gastrointestinal tract will result in malabsorption, diarrhea, and other disorders that may contribute to the overall weight loss. Patients with carcinoma of the small bowel may also have structural abnormalities of the jejunal mucosa, which reduce the total absorptive surface area. In many cases of lymphoma, there is further involvement of the intestinal tract, which can lead to malabsorption syndromes with flattening of the intestinal villi and steatorrhea or diarrhea.

There are also many instances in which abnormalities of mucosal architecture and disorders of absorption occur with neoplasms arising at sites distant to and not directly involving the gastrointestinal tract. The small bowel mucosa and absorptive function of six such patients was studied; mucosal abnormalities were found to be associated with steatorrhea and weight loss in all but two cases. Other investigators have observed structural abnormalities associated with malabsorption of lipid and carbohydrate. Another study reported malabsorption of xylose and fat in a series of 20 patients with cancer, although villous atrophy was detected in only one patient. Furthermore, other workers have found abnormalities in absorptive function of the gut in the absence of mucosal changes.

Even though the reason for this derangement in absorptive function of the gut can be understood where the primary tumor involves the gastrointestinal tract itself or where there is metastatic involvement, it is not as clear why extra-gastrointestinal tumors give rise to this syndrome. These changes clearly represent distant systemic tumor effects, but no possible humoral agents have been identified. The overall significance of malabsorption in cancer patients is not fully understood, but it is obviously important if essential dietary components are not absorbed.

Increased Metabolic Rate

Another important feature associated with the development of cancer cachexia is an increased basal metabolic rate, as demonstrated in many patients. The increase in metabolic rate should also increase the need for dietary component. This increased metabolic rate is in contrast with the mechanism of starvation, in which the metabolic rate usually decreases. The mechanism is probably complex and has not been observed in all patients.

The mechanism of the increased metabolic rate in cancer cachexia has been studied in both humans and animals. One of the usual explanations proposed is that the tumor has produced low-molecular-weight components such as peptides and nucleotides, which may interfere with intermediary metabolism. In addition, there may be activation of metabolic pathways and energy expenditure because of loss of control or regulation. These claims, however, cannot be fully substantiated.

Energy metabolism is important to almost all metabolic processes. It is therefore not surprising that if the energy supply is not regulated, abnormalities in protein, carbohydrate, and fat metabolism may result. It is also likely that the growing tumor has a requirement for energy. The process of tumor requires energy for cell division and for the synthesis of protein, carbohydrate, and fat.

Abnormal Host Metabolism

Increase in Glycolysis

The early work of Warburg indicated that the tumor metabolism was predominantly glycolytic.[5] Since that work almost three decades ago, numerous investigations have been made to study the metabolism of animals and humans with cancer. Several workers have suggested that the host metabolism is changed because either the tumor produces excess lactic acid (due to an increase in glycolysis), or the body itself develops an abnormal metabolism in the presence of the tumor. A lactic acidosis is produced, and the excess lactate is recycled to glycose by gluconeogensis in the liver and kidneys. This pathway is known as the Cori cycle.

Cori Cycle

The Cori cycle is inefficient in the use of energy, since only 2 mol adenosine triphosphate (ATP) is produced by an aerobic glycolysis in the breakdown of glucose to lactate. However, gluconeogenesis that converts lactate to glucose requires 6 mol ATP. Therefore, the tumor derives little energy from glucose, and the host must expand considerable energy in its resynthesis. As a possible method of controlling tumor growth, Gold tested the effect of compounds that inhibit such pathways.[6] These studies do not completely explain the progressive weight loss associated with cancer, but do suggest that pathways are likely to be contributing factors.

Insulin

In addition to altered metabolic pathways, a variety of other factors have been identified. In relationship to carboydrate metabolism, the secretion of insulin may be modified. A higher proportion of cancer patients have a diabetic glucose tolerance curve than do normal people. The abnormal glucose tolerance curve in malignant cachexia appears to be related to abnormal insulin production and to insulin resistance, which may be due to a decreased receptor affinity of insulin. In cancer patients administered glucose has a disappearance rate significantly lower than in the controls, even though the fasting blood sugar in the cancer group does not significantly differ from that in the controls.

Body Fat

As the patient develops cachexia, body fat is rapidly mobilized, along with associated changes in plasma lipids. In one group of cancer patients a significant increase in the level of unesterified fatty acids in plasma was observed, as well as an increased rate of removal of infused lipids. The caloric expenditure was increased, the calorie deficit was not corrected by hyperalimentation, and the hypermetabolism was associated with an increased utilization of fat per unit time.

The lipid lost from the body during tumor growth must be burned completely, for no significant ketosis has been observed in tumor-bearing animals. In addition, in the cancer patient, the rate of removal of infused lipids from the blood appears to be increased. There is an important question in this regard: How does the tumor induce the host to mobilize fat for energy metabolism?

Peptides exhibiting fat-mobilizing activity have been isolated from the urine of fasted animals and humans. These substances are able to (1) mobilize fat from fat depots, (2) increase the total metabolic turnover of fat in the animals, and (3) increase the total amount of fat in the liver. It was thought at first that these peptides only had anorexigenic properties, but since then peptides with both anorexigenic properties and peptides with lipolytic properties have been separated and partially purified. Peptides displaying fat-mobilizing activity have been detected in the urine of patients with widespread malignant disease, even in those with normal food intake.

Initially it was thought that such peptides were of pituitary origin, but later work demonstrated that the peptides were produced even when the pituitary gland was absent. The lipid mobilizing peptide activity has not only been detected in pituitary extracts, but also in hypothalamic extracts of mammalian species, including humans. In addition, lipolytic activity has been reported in extracts from other parts of the brain.

Protein

Catabolism. Protein metabolism is clearly abnormal in the cancer patient. Protein breakdown sometimes results in the depletion of 30% of the muscle mass within as short a period as 3 weeks; this rapid breakdown of protein can lead very rapidly to death. The clinical picture is one of obvious loss of lean body mass, and hypoalbuminemia is common. The low serum albumin is due not only to the decreased albumin synthesis, but to an increased catabolic rate as well. The primary function of albumin, besides maintaining the proper osmotic balance throughout the body, is as a medium for finding various and diverse substances (fatty acids, calcium, and numerous drugs). In addition to its effect on body mass and albumin, cancer cachexia is frequently associated with a negative nitrogen balance.

Survival is dependent on minimizing protein catabolism and, in chronic starvation, this is done through an adaptive mechanism. Glucose is replaced by the ketone bodies, acetoacetate and β-hydroxybutyrate, as the most important oxidative fuel utilized by the brain, and there is a concomitant decrease in hepatic gluconeogenesis. The resultant fall in oxidative metabolism, metabolic rate, as well as CO_2 output leads to a lowering of the respiratory quotient. These changes, often described as a conversion to "fat fuel economy," will permit a person to survive for prolonged periods under conditions of near starvation. It is difficult to undertake controlled studies with cancer patients in the absence of standardized conditions. Apparently the same metabolic adaptation does not occur in the patient who may or may not be in a semistarved condition, with the additional complication of tumor burden.

Synthesis. Synthesis of muscle proteins is generally depressed in cancer patients. There is some alteration of plasma amino acids in cancer patients with decreases in some amino acids. However, decreased muscle protein synthesis is not simply due to alterations in the precursor pool. Depressed protein synthesis measured in cultures of tissues taken from cancer patients may be only partly corrected by an addition of an excess of amino acids or insulin.

Although the synthesis of muscle proteins is depressed in cancer patients, synthesis of other host proteins may be enhanced. For example, synthesis of liver structural proteins is normal, whereas synthesis of secretory proteins such as acute-phase reactants is increased. Enzyme activities in muscle tissues of tumor-bearing animals and humans show a decrease in the key enzymes of anabolism and increased activity of catabolic enzymes, such as cathepsin. The enhanced activity of catabolic enzymes in muscle tissue from cancer patients can be correlated with a decreased protein degradation, as compared with normal controls. Amino acids released from skeletal muscle are used for tumor protein synthesis and for gluconeogenesis in order to provide glucose for tumor metabolism. This phenomenon results in progressive muscle wasting in the cancer patient.

Electrolyte Balance

Water and electrolyte balance and mineral metabolism may all be abnormal in cancer patients. These abnormalities may be related to the effects of the tumor or to the synthesis of ectopic hormones. The presence of such hormones has been well documented.

Waterhouse and Craig evaluated body composition changes in patients with advanced cancer. Their study involved a more direct calculation of changes in total body water employing the dilution of deuterium oxide (D_2O). These workers observed that cancer patients lost body fat but gained in total body water, which was shared by the intracellular and extracellular compartments of the body. It was also shown that even after hyperalimentation, the weight gained was mainly due to an accumulation of large quantities of intracellular fluid. In this regard, patients with advanced cancer are different from patients who have an insufficient caloric intake attributable to other causes. In the latter situation, only extracellular fluid is increased.

Hyponatremia is the most common clinical electrolyte abnormality in advanced cancer patients. This deficiency is difficult to correct; even if it is corrected, it is difficult to maintain a normal serum sodium level for long periods during advancing cachexia.

In animals inoculated with a tumor, the total weight of the animal, i.e., animal plus tumor, begins to increase and continues to increase up to a few days before death, at which point the total weight begins to decrease. The initial increase in the weight of the animal is probably attributable to an increase in the total body water content of tumor-bearing animals, as the animal carcass is shown to contain less nitrogen and less fat.

In animals with tumors the alimentary canal weight has a normal ratio to total body weight. Most of these animals have a hypertrophied heart and all have a hypertrophied liver. The dry liver:total animal weight ratio is greater than the normal values even when the estimated loss in carcass weight is added to the total body weight. It remains unexplained why the liver gains weight in cancer when all other tissues lose weight. In starvation the liver also loses weight.

The alterations of host metabolism may be extensive, possibly affecting nearly every metabolic process. The mechanisms that produce such effects are diverse, and several different mechanisms may operate simultaneously. The particular abnormalities can only be ascertained by metabolic balance studies in individual patients.

Tumor Products

It has been postulated that for almost every metabolic abnormal change a tumor-derived product is involved in the mechanism. Such products have been reported to affect anorexia, protein, carbohydrate, fat metabolism, the immune response, as well as the psychological state. These products are produced in addition to the well-recognized hormones, which also have been designated toxohormones. Such diffusible factors have been isolated and purified from a variety of animal tumors. These toxohormones have been shown to affect a large variety of processes. However, in humans the isolation and identification of these toxohormone-like substances have been more difficult and still need to be elucidated. Perhaps the recent results with plasmapheresis may help clarify their action. Because these substances have not as yet been identified, one might be skeptical about the presence and function of such tumor-derived products; theoretically, their origin is feasible, and these toxohormones would explain many of the metabolic abnormalities observed in the cancer patient. In addition, other hormones such as glucagon, oncofetal proteins, carcinoembryonic antigen, and α-fetoprotein have been detected in the serum of cancer patients. In rats, plasma-free tryptophan, brain tryptophan, and brain 5-hydroxylindoleacetic acid (5 = HIAA) are also significantly greater in tumor-bearing rats than in controls. This suggests an association between altered brain tryptophan metabolism and feeding behavior in tumor-related anorexia.

Nitrogen Trap by the Tumor

On the basis of animal work, it was suggested that the tumor itself could selectively take up proteins and amino acids for its growth at the expense of the body.[8] Other studies have attempted to confirm this theory. Wiseman and Ghadially concluded that cancer cells could concentrate amino acids more efficiently from the plasma than could normal cells.[9] In addition, albumin could be directly extracted from plasma and used by the tumor.[10]

Norton et al. perfused the limbs of patients bearing sarcomas, and the uptake of glucose, free fatty acids, and amino acids was compared with that in the control non-tumor-bearing limb.[11] These investigators found that the tumor-bearing limb ignores normal control mechanisms in the postabsorption state and continues to use substrate at the expense of the body. The parasitic effect of the tumor on the body's nutritional state is apparently important; however, the overall contribution of this effect requires further study in the individual patient.

Anemia

Anemia in the advanced cancer patient has many causes. Decreased hemoglobin and red cell production, increased red blood cell destruction, and increased red blood cell loss may contribute to the genesis of anemia. Anemia in cancer may contribute to tissue hypoxia, the role of which is unknown. Cardiac cachexia has been attributed entirely to cellular hypoxia.

MANAGEMENT

The best way of dealing with cancer cachexia is to eradicate the malignant disease. If this attempt is successful, the patient's condition improves, appetite returns, and weight gain results. There is a question about the value of nutritional support in those patients who fail to respond to anticancer therapy.

Cancer patients with weight loss could be roughly divided into two groups: The weight loss in one group is mainly due to protein-energy malnutrition, while the weight loss in the other group may be due to a metabolic component and true cancer cachexia. In the former group, nutritional support given orally or intravenously will usually reverse the problem. However, in the latter group reversal may not be easily achieved in spite of aggressive hyperalimentation.

It has been suggested that measurement of the acute-phase response and the catabolic rate of albumin might predict which patients will respond to nutritional support. However, confirmation in a prospective study is needed.

There are two potential disadvantages of feeding cancer cachexia patients: An increase in tumor growth might occur when nutrients are supplied to the patient. There is little firm evidence, but this is theoretically possible. One small group of patients was found to have an increase in the tumor growth rate. In contrast, no increase in tumor growth rate was observed in a group of force-fed patients. Mullen *et al.* studied protein synthesis in patients with gastrointestinal tumors who were given intravenous hyperalimentation before surgery. Comparisons were made in the rates of protein synthesis in the tumor and in the normal gut. No increases were observed in the growth of the tumor. Because of the possible significance of such an effect, further studies would be desirable.

Another management problem arises because of the potentially harmful effects of hyperalimentation in patients with cancer cachexia. In addition, there are technical complications of intravenous hyperalimentation, and the physiological effects of rapid refeeding may be dangerous.

Anorexia

When anorexia is associated with cancer, it can be extremely difficult to control. Dietary advice and the use of appetite stimulants may not be sufficient. In addition, the psychological component may require correction.

Dietary Supplementation

An increasing range of nutritional products can be added to the diet of cancer patients. However, since the sensation of taste may be altered in cancer patients the unpalatability of some of these products may inhibit their use. Adequate vitamin supplementation could also be supplied.

Nasogastric Tube Feeding

An enormous contribution to our ability to feed cancer patients was made when the fine-bore nasogastric tube was introduced. This route is preferable, unless there is an anatomical reason not to use it. This method has been successfully employed in the management of cancer. However, in one series of 52 patients experiencing weight loss, less than one-half showed weight gain after 2 weeks of nasogastric tube feeding.[13]

Intravenous Hyperalimentation

Intravenous hyperalimentation has been extensively used in the management of cancer both to correct weight loss and to enhance the effect of anticancer therapy. The hyperalimentation can reverse cachexia in some patients, but not all cancer patients, and can prevent the weight loss associated with treatment by chemotherapy.[4] Hyperalimentation does not reverse cachexia in all patients. This implies that either insufficient nutrients are being supplied or that the metabolic defect in cachexia cannot be reversed simply by feeding. This also may be an area in which the ability to predict the response to feeding may have important clinical implications. Whether hyperalimentation improves the response to chemotherapy and radiotherapy is yet to be determined. If any form of nutritional support is used in cases of cancer cachexia, it should be undertaken only after the patient has been fully assessed, with accurate staging and tumor measurement, and with a clear goal in mind.

Plasmapheresis

Removal of plasma from the cancer patient is a method that has been used for many years. Interest in this procedure has increased because of the possibility of extracting from the plasma a variety of substances that may include some of the tumor-derived products (pp. 362–363). Plasmapheresis may become an experimental technique in the investigation of the cachexia patient. Changes in appetite, in pruritus, and in the immunological responses have been observed in cancer patients who have undergone plasmapheresis.

Nutritional Effects of Cancer Treatment

It is likely that almost all forms of cancer treatment can affect the nutritional status of the patient and may therefore complicate the problems of cachexia. In addition, patients with cachexia may be less able to withstand the effects of cancer treatment, and there is appreciable evidence that drug metabolism may be abnormal in cancer patients.[15] Methods of nutritional support for the cancer patient will most probably continue to be developed, even though there may be a greater selectivity in the choice of patients for hyperalimentation. Further investigations are needed on the effect of treatment on nutritional status. With more knowledge of the nutritional effects on the cancer process, more effective treatments will likely be found that, in combination with chemotherapy, will further extend life or even reverse the cancer process. At this time, however, chemoprevention offers the most immediate reward in the nutrition and cancer area.

REFERENCES

1. Strain, A. J. 1979. Cancer cachexia in man: A review. *Invest. Cell Pathol. 2:*181–193.
2. Brennan, M. 1977. Uncomplicated starvation versus cancer cachexia. *Cancer Res. 37:*2359–2364.
3. Dudrick, S. J., MacFadyen, B. V., Souchon, E. A., Englert, D. M., and Copland, E. M. 1977. Parenteral nutrition techniques in cancer patients. *Cancer Res. 37:*2440–2450.
4. Schmale, A. H. 1977. Psychological aspects of anorexia. *Cancer 43:*2087–2092.
5. Warburg, O. 1956. On the origin of cancer cells. *Science 123:*309–314.
6. Gold, J. 1974. Cancer cachexia and gluconeogenesis. *Ann. N.Y. Acad. Sci. 230:*103–110.
7. Craig, A. B., and Waterhouse, C. 1957. Body-composition changes in patients with advanced cancer. *Cancer 10:*1106–1109.
8. Mider, G. B., Fenninger, L. D., Haven, F. L., and Morton, J. J. 1951. Energy expenditure of rats bearing Walker carcinoma 256. *Cancer Res. 11:*731–736.
9. Wiseman, G., and Ghadially, F. N. 1955. Studies in amino acid uptake by RD3 sarcoma cell suspensions *in vitro. Br. J Cancer 9:*480–485.
10. Busch, H., Fujiwara, E., and Firszt, D. C. 1961. Studies on the metabolism of radioactive albumin in tumour-bearing rats. *Cancer Res. 21:*371–377.
11. Norton, J. A., Burt, M. E., and Brennan, M. F. 1980. In vivo utilization of substrate by human sarcoma-bearing limbs. *Cancer 45:*2934–2939.
12. Mullen, S. L., Buzby, G. P., Gertner, M. H., Stein, T. P., Hargrove, W. C., Oram-Smith, J., and Rosata, E. F. 1980. Protein synthesis dynamics in human gastrointestinal malignancies. *Surgery 87:*331–338.
13. Trotter, J. M., Scott, R., MacBeth, F. R., Merie, J. G., and Calman, K. C. 1981. Problems of the oncology outpatient: Role of the liaison health visitor. *Br. Med. J. 282:*122–124.
14. Samuels, M. L., Lanzotti, V. J., Holuge, P. Y., Boyle, L. E., Smith, T. L., and Johnstone, D. E. 1976. Combination chemotherapy in germinal cell tumors. *Cancer Treatm. Rev. 3:*185–204.
15. Higuchi, T., Nakamura, T., and Uchino, H. 1980. Antipyrine metabolism in cancer patients. *Cancer 45:*541–544.

Index